Manual of Dermatology in Chinese Medicine

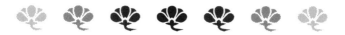

Shen De-Hui

Wu Xiu-Fen

Nissi Wang

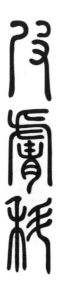

EASTLAND PRESS ◆ SEATTLE

© 1995 by Eastland Press, Inc.
P.O. Box 99749
Seattle, WA 98139, USA
www.eastlandpress.com

All rights reserved.

No part of this book may be reproduced or transmitted in any form or by any means, electronic or mechanical, including photocopying, recording, or by any information storage and retrieval system, without the prior written permission of the publisher, except where permitted by law.

Library of Congress Catalog Card Number: 94-61962
ISBN: 978-0-939616-60-2

2   4   6   8   10   9   7   5   3

Cover design by Patricia O'Connor and Lilian Bensky
Book design by Gary Niemeier

Table of Contents

Preface vii

PART I

CHAPTER 1   History of Traditional Chinese Dermatology 1
CHAPTER 2   Etiology 7
CHAPTER 3   Diagnostics 13
CHAPTER 4   Differentiation 19
CHAPTER 5   Treatment 29

PART II

CHAPTER 6   Pruritus 43
CHAPTER 7   Bacterial Infections 51
    Impetigo 51
    Folliculitis 56
    Furuncles 60
    Carbuncles 65
    Erysipelas 72
    Lupus Vulgaris 80
    Leprosy 84

CHAPTER 8 Viral Infections ... 93
- Herpes Simplex ... 93
- Herpes Zoster ... 98
- Common Warts ... 106
- Venereal Warts ... 112
- Measles ... 115
- Chickenpox ... 121

CHAPTER 9 Fungal Infections ... 127
- Tinea Corporis ... 127

CHAPTER 10 Spirochete Infections ... 135
- Syphilis ... 135

CHAPTER 11 Dermatoses Caused by Arthropods ... 141
- Scabies ... 141
- Pediculosis ... 144
- Insect Stings and Bites ... 148

CHAPTER 12 Dermatoses Due to Environmental Influences ... 151
- Chilblain ... 151
- Sunburn ... 156

CHAPTER 13 Dermatitis ... 161
- Contact Dermatitis ... 161
- Atopic Dermatitis ... 165
- Lichen Simplex Chronicus ... 173
- Seborrheic Dermatitis ... 179
- Diaper Dermatitis ... 186

CHAPTER 14 Inflammatory Reactions ... 191
- Drug Eruptions ... 191
- Erythema Multiforme ... 198
- Urticaria ... 204

CHAPTER 15 Scaling Disorders ... 215
- Psoriasis ... 215
- Pityriasis Rosea ... 225

CHAPTER 16 Autoimmune Rheumatologic Skin Diseases ... 229
- Lupus Erythematosus ... 229
- Scleroderma ... 234
- Dermatomyositis ... 238

TABLE OF CONTENTS

CHAPTER 17 Disorders of the Sweat Glands..........245
    Miliaria..........245
    Bromhidrosis..........248

CHAPTER 18 Acne and Rosacea..........253
    Acne..........253
    Rosacea..........259

CHAPTER 19 Disorders of Hair..........263
    Alopecia..........263

CHAPTER 20 Circulatory Disorders..........273
    Purpura..........273
    Leg Ulcers..........279

CHAPTER 21 Disorders of Pigmentation..........289
    Vitiligo..........289

CHAPTER 22 Disorders of Keratinization..........297
    Ichthyosis..........297
    Corns..........302

APPENDIX A Supplemental Materia Medica..........305
APPENDIX B General References..........327
APPENDIX C Historical References..........329
APPENDIX D *Pinyin*-English Cross Reference of Formula Names..........333

Formula Index..........343
Point Index..........353
Materia Medica Index..........357
General Index..........371

Preface

As traditional Chinese medicine becomes a more widely accepted form of healing in the West, the variety of diseases that practitioners are encountering is also expanding. Skin diseases are a new challenge to many practitioners. For them we are pleased to present this manual of traditional Chinese dermatology. Students of Chinese medicine will also find this book of value, especially in gaining further insight into the process of instituting treatment based on pattern differentiation.

While a number of skin diseases, such as psoriasis and the dermatites, are universally prevalent, others, such as those due to tropical parasites, have a low incidence in the West. Since our readers are mainly practitioners in the developed countries of the West, we have focused on skin conditions commonly seen in these countries.

This book is organized according to biomedical categories since we felt this to be the most practical and cogent way of presenting such material to modern-day readers. Based on the work of Chinese medical historians, the biomedical names of the skin diseases represented in this book are for the most part the equivalent terms of the ancient Chinese names. Because in ancient times many diseases had more than one name, the only way to determine what their modern-day equivalents are is to study their symptoms and patterns as described in the classical Chinese medical literature. Thus, for example, when we state that herpes zoster was first described in *Discussion of the Origins of Symptoms of Diseases* (610), we are not saying that herpes zoster, the present-day biomedical term, first appeared in that text. Instead, we are referring to the description of the set of symptoms that largely corresponds to herpes zoster that first appeared in that work.

There are many methods of treatment in Chinese medicine. We have attempted to include all suitable forms of therapy for the skin diseases discussed in this text. In addition to the more familiar herbs and acupuncture, lesser known external remedies such as plasters, washes and steaming (among others) are presented as well. We also include empirical remedies where appropriate, since treatment in Chinese medicine continues to be based on clinical experience. For many patterns, more than one formula and/or remedy is presented. It is assumed that readers who use this book are at a level where they can discern which remedy is appropriate for the given pattern. For skin diseases in particular, it is often more effective to administer internal and external remedies simultaneously, rather than relying on just one or the other.

The treatment section for each disease is followed by a comparison of traditional and biomedical therapies. We hope that this section will serve as a guide to practitioners who may be uncertain as to which type of treatment is more effective. There are some diseases, such as early syphilis, where traditional treatment is in fact not superior to biomedical therapy, which in this case consists of a single, one-injection dose of penicillin that effects a cure within one week. Nevertheless, the traditional remedies are also presented, since there are some patients who, as in the case of syphilis, are allergic to penicillin and may thus benefit from alternative treatment. For many other skin conditions, however, particularly chronic ones like the dermatites, traditional therapy proves to be superior since it is able to resolve the root of the problem.

The purpose of this book is to serve as a framework for practitioners to refine their own skills. It is not intended to be *the* authoritative work on Chinese dermatology. For it would be impossible and pointless to list every existing remedy for every skin disease. Therefore, in selecting which remedies to include—since for some diseases there are countless ones—we chose those that are effective and that can be prepared with relative ease, and for which the ingredients can be readily obtained in the West.

It is expected that practitioners who use this book are familiar with the cautions, contraindications and toxicities of the various materia medica that are mentioned. Some of the remedies (especially external ones) can be toxic if used long-term or in large doses. When warranted, such toxicities are mentioned in a clinical note following the remedy.

For each condition, the traditional etiology is presented. These are the *common* patterns encountered in the clinic. But they may not be the *only* cause(s) of the given condition. Thus, when applying the information in this book, practitioners should not be confounded when in the clinic they encounter a variation or an altogether different pattern of a particular disease. A diagnosis can still be reached and a treatment strategy instituted by following the principles of traditional pattern differentiation—the heart of Chinese medicine.

Readers will find that we have eliminated the capitalization of all traditional Chinese terms, with the exception of the organs when used in their traditional sense, since we feel that practitioners are now sophisticated enough to understand such terminology within the traditional context.

Dermatology is a visual specialty. We therefore suggest that color atlases be consulted when readers use this book, especially to aid in diagnosis. A list of such volumes is provided among the references in the back. Although we have described the biomedical causes and symptomatologies for each of the diseases, readers are again urged to consult biomedical dermatology textbooks for further information about laboratory diagnoses, biomedical treatments and the like.

We are grateful to many people for their support and encouragement throughout this project. We are particularly indebted to our colleagues and professors at the Beijing College of Traditional Chinese Medicine and affiliated hospitals for their help and insight as we compiled our information. We thank Professor Zou Mingxi for reviewing the initial draft of the manuscript. To our many patients who so willingly gave of their time as we studied their conditions, we cannot thank them enough.

Rendering a manuscript about Chinese medicine from Chinese into English is never an easy task, and we would like to thank Richard Feit for helping with the editing of the English. Eastland Press has been enormously patient and supportive of this project, and for this we are deeply grateful.

We would like to thank our families—their acceptance and sacrifice are what made this book possible. Nissi thanks Bruce and Colin, and especially her parents, for their love and encouragement.

CHAPTER 1

Historical Perspective of Traditional Chinese Dermatology

Not until the mid-twentieth century, with the appearance of several texts devoted solely to skin diseases, was dermatology recognized as a separate specialty in traditional Chinese medicine. Before then skin diseases were studied within the general category of external diseases, which, in addition to dermatological conditions, included sores and abscesses, rectal diseases, trauma, lacerations, and maladies of the eye, ear, nose and mouth. Although there are numerous references to skin diseases in classical medical textbooks, they are scattered among several works, and do not comprise an independent body of medical literature.

Shang (Yin) Dynasty (c. 1700–1100 B.C.)

Inscriptions on bones excavated from Shang dynasty ruins show that Chinese characters describing skin conditions were used as early as the fourteenth century B.C. It is certain that these characters (e.g., *jiè* (疥), meaning scabies) represent descriptions of unusual physiologic occurrences. There is no indication, however, that such observations of the human physical condition coincided with an understanding of the cause, pathogenesis or treatment of these phenomena.

Zhou Dynasty (c. 1100–221 B.C.)

In the Zhou dynasty it was recognized that the occurrence and transmission of certain skin disorders was seasonal in nature. The ancient Chinese classic *Zhou Annals* (attributed to the Duke of Zhou during the Warring States period, 475–221 B.C.) contains the following description of infectious skin diseases whose appearance coincided with specific seasons:

> Skin disorders are present in all four seasons: in the spring, pain of the head is common; in the summer, scabies; and as midwinter turns to spring, people often contract pestilent sores.

Such observations eventually led to attempts to discover the causes of these diseases.

Methods of treatment were also first described during this era. Externally-applied medicines, as well as the techniques of scraping and surgical debridement, appear in the *Zhou Annals*. The use of lard as a vehicle for topical medication is discussed in Chapter 81 of the *Divine Pivot,* while a form of lancing is described in Chapter 7 of this book: "Repeated needling [means] the needle is inserted superficially straight in and out numerous times until blood is drawn. This is for treating carbuncles and swellings."

The *Yellow Emperor's Inner Classic* is the representative medical work of this era, the culmination of medical knowledge in China during the Spring-Autumn and Warring States periods (770–221 B.C.). It is during this time that the "contention of a hundred schools of thought" occurred, when scholarly factions vied for dominance, and great strides were made in Chinese culture and medicine. The *Inner Classic* is acknowledged as the cornerstone of traditional Chinese medicine. Through the centuries and dynasties that followed its publication, the development of Chinese medicine and its specialties—including dermatology—has been dependent upon this book.

The *Inner Classic* records more varieties of skin disorders than any previous work, often in terms that are still used today. Examples include *féi* (疿) for miliaria; *yǎng jiè* (痒疥) or *qí yǎng* (奇痒) for itching disorders; *tū* (秃) for eczema or tinea of the head; *làn* (烂) for ulcer; *yóu zhuì* (疣赘) for warts; and *lì fēng* (疠风) for leprosy.

Not only does the *Inner Classic* describe the signs and symptoms of various skin diseases, it also elaborates on their etiology and pathology. Consider, e.g., the following passages from Chapter 74: "Painful and itching sores are all due to the Heart . . . Sweating, and then exposure to wind, results in miliaria." A central principle of Chinese medicine is thus brought to light: although a disease may appear on the exterior, its cause is often found in the interior, as a function of the disharmony of the Organs.

Qin, Han and Jin Dynasties (221 B.C.–420 A.D.)

The period comprising the Qin, Han and Jin dynasties was one of great advancement in Chinese culture and science, with perhaps the greatest contributions made in the field of medicine. This period is best exemplified by the work of the eminent physician Zhang Zhong-Jing (150–219) of the Han dynasty. Zhang carried forward the principles of the *Yellow Emperor's Inner Classic* and, combining his own experience and knowledge with that of other medical scholars and texts, wrote *Discussion of Cold-induced Disorders* (c. 196), a work that was later revised into two volumes: *Discussion of Cold-induced Disorders* and *Concise Prescriptions from the Golden Casket*. In these works, Zhang Zhong-Jing discussed cold-induced disorders in relation to the six channels, and miscellaneous disorders in relation to the Organs. He also proposed that the underlying pattern of a disease must be differentiated before effective treatment could be instituted.

Thus the principle of diagnosing according to patterns was incorporated into Chinese dermatology. It was recognized, e.g., that urticaria was caused by the "conflict between wind and heat" which have lodged in the skin, an insight that led to the treatment strategy of "clearing wind and heat."

The etiology, pathogenesis, diagnosis and treatment of skin diseases were well documented at this time. *Concise Prescriptions from the Golden Casket* mentions skin disorders not previously described, such as *yǐn zhěn* (瘾疹) for urticaria, and *jìn yín chuāng* (浸淫疮), which closely corresponds to exfoliative dermatitis. *Hú huò bìng* (狐惑病), an ailment characterized by eye problems and lesions of the skin and genitalia (among other symptoms), is believed by Chinese medical historians to correspond to Behcet's syndrome—an entity not recognized in the West until the twentieth century. The treatment for *hú huò bìng* described in *Concise Prescriptions from the Golden Casket* itself represents a significant advance in Chinese medicine, namely the combination of internal and external remedies within a single treatment strategy. For example, Radix Glycyrrhizae Uralensis *(gan cao)* is taken orally, while the external lesions are steamed and washed with Sophora Decoction *(ku shen tang)*.

Sui and Tang Dynasties (581–907)

In 610, during the Sui dynasty, Chao Yuan-Fang completed his *Discussion of the Origins of Symptoms of Diseases,* a work important for its discussion of almost one hundred skin disorders, and its detailed descriptions of disease etiology. The level of understanding that had been reached at this time about the causes of disease is exemplified by Chao's discussion of pigmented contact dermatitis and scabies. About pigmented contact dermatitis he wrote:

> Man has an innate aversion to paint, and upon contact will be poisoned by its toxin. There are also those who are resistant, and can [participate in producing] paint by boiling it and are never harmed.

Clearly, this shows a recognition of the cause of this disease as early as the seventh century, as well as an understanding that resistance varied from individual to individual. Today it is known that pigmented contact dermatitis is due to chemically-induced photosensitivity.

Chao demonstrated a similar level of insight into the method of transmission of scabies:

> Scabies often manifests between the fingers and toes, and slowly infests the body . . . Its lesions have minute insects that are most difficult to see. Infants often contract the disease through contact while being breast fed.

In other words, Chao not only knew that scabies is transmittable, but also that it is caused by a parasite—predating Linne's observation by 1100 years.

The study of skin diseases was further developed during the Tang dynasty when Sun Si-Miao (581–682) published his *Thousand Ducat Formulas* and *Supplement to Thousand Ducat Formulas.* Sun recorded 197 medicinal substances that were used in the treatment of skin disorders, including minerals such as

Cinnabaris *(zhu sha)* and Alumen *(ming fan),* botanicals such as Radix Angelicae Sinensis *(dang gui),* Radix Ginseng *(ren shen)* and Herba Ephedrae *(ma huang),* as well as substances derived from animal sources like Gelatinum Corii Asini *(e jiao)* and Mylabris *(ban mao).*

Sun Si-Miao also described in great detail his observations of leprosy, gleaned from the more than six hundred cases that he treated. Perhaps Sun Si-Miao can justly be considered the earliest medical expert on leprosy in China.

Song through Yuan Dynasties (960–1368)

The Song dynasty saw the introduction of several new methods for treating skin diseases. Bloodletting, also known as the "stone needle method" or "flying needle method," utilized a pyramidal needle, knife point or the sharp edge of a porcelain shard to prick the skin lesion or its surroundings to induce bleeding. This method was used for draining stagnant-heat toxins from the body via the blood to relieve swelling and pain. It was developed from the method known as "repeated needling," first identified in the *Divine Pivot* as one of the Nine Needling Methods. The *Complete Records of Sage-like Benefits* (completed between 1111 and 1117) mentions the "sickle-cutting method" to treat erysipelas. Later, in the Yuan dynasty, Qi De in *Essence of External Diseases* (1335) introduced the term "stone needle-sickle method," which was used thereafter in medical texts.

Another method introduced in the Song dynasty was "drainage," also known as "medicinal thread method," or "medicinal spill method." This technique involves the insertion of a small roll or twist of medicine-soaked paper into a pustulant skin lesion or fistula in order to drain the pus and dead tissue. This technique is described in the *Complete Book of Ulcer Experience* (1695) by Dou Han-Qing:

> [A]fter incising [the lesion], make a cotton paper spill, soak it in medicinal oil so that the pus will gather [be absorbed by the spill]. Remove after half a day and the pus will dry easily.

The medicinal spill was also utilized as a probe. The *Book of Health Benefit Treasures* (anonymous, completed c. 1170) describes it thusly:

> Existing lesions can be probed. . . . It is necessary to use good paper to make a large spill so that it can be inserted [into the lesion] and looked through.

In the Yuan dynasty, Qi De-Zhi in his *Essence of External Diseases* (1335) introduced the method of wet compress, which is still used today.

Ming and Qing Dynasties to the Opium War (1368–1840)

Dermatology during the Ming and Qing dynasties matured with the publication of several volumes that presented external diseases in a systematic manner. In *Precise Treatment of Patterns* (1602) the Ming dynasty physician Wang Ken-Tang (1549–1613) categorized skin diseases according to anatomical regions and described them in such detail that the book became a convenient bedside manual. The physician Shen Dou-Yuan, also of the Ming, wrote *Profound Insights on External Diseases* (1604), one of the first Chinese medical texts to include diagrams, and considered to be China's first atlas of skin diseases. This work describes over one hundred skin disorders.

Two of the earliest Chinese texts on leprosy were published during the Ming dynasty: *Fundamental Gatherings of Disclosure of Diseases* (1550) by Shen Zhi-Xiang, and *Secrets on Pestilent Sores* (1554) by Xue Ji. Both works detail the etiology, symptoms, treatment and prevention of leprosy.

In the fifteenth century syphilis was brought to China by traders. First known as "Guangdong sores" *(guǎng chuāng)* because the lesions were originally found among people of Guangdong province in southern China, syphilis was most commonly known as "mold or mildew sores" *(méi chuāng)* because of the moldy and necrotic appearance of the surface of the lesions. The premier text on the subject, Chen Si-Cheng's *Secret Records on Bayberry Flower Sores* (1632), describes the disease as being transmitted through direct contact by "unclean sexual intercourse," inheritance (passed from mother to fetus) or indirect exposure. Chen also described the different stages of syphilis, and introduced the use of cinnabar and arsenic in its treatment. (This is the earliest known record of the use of arsenic in the treatment of syphilis). Also mentioned are methods of syphilis prevention.

Qing Dynasty through the Republican Period (1840–1949)

Following the Opium War, China underwent great economic and social changes that profoundly influenced the field of medicine. During this time biomedicine began to take root in China, and new methods and medicines, such as ether anesthesia and antibiotics, were gradually introduced. Although traditional medicine was still widely practiced among the great majority of the population at the beginning of the twentieth century, it began to be eclipsed by biomedicine in more cultured circles. One by one, traditional schools of medicine were closed by the Nationalist government, which intended to shut down all such institutions by 1929. Fortunately, through the efforts of a few traditional medical scholars who established societies and schools of traditional Chinese medicine in the 1920s and 30s, this form of medicine was preserved.

Yet even during this period when biomedicine was moving toward a position of prominence in China, traditional Chinese medicine continued to evolve. Several works published during this time had a significant impact on external medicine and skin diseases. Noteworthy among these were *Sores and Ulcers* (1840) by Zou Han-Huang, *Essentials of Ulcers* (1876) by Zhang Shan-Lei and *Collection of Cases on External Diseases* (1894) by Yu Jing-He.

People's Republic of China (1949–Present)

After the victory of the communists, traditional medicine was acknowledged as having played an important role in saving lives during the previous war-torn era, and, above all, as being a medicine of the people. Official recognition was thus restored to traditional medicine in 1949, and schools, hospitals and research institutes specializing in traditional medicine were established thereafter.

Formal dermatological textbooks were published in the 1960s, and classics on external diseases were reprinted. With the arrival of modern medical technology, methods of diagnosis and treatment were improved through the integration of traditional medicine and modern biomedicine. Several dermatological disorders, such as scleroderma and lupus erythematosus, are now successfully treated by using this combined approach. Yet, partly because of the number of Chinese publications and journals that focus on the use of traditional remedies for skin diseases, it would appear that traditional methods still predominate as the treatment of choice in modern Chinese dermatology.

CHAPTER 2

Etiology

Traditional Chinese medicine views all disease according to the same fundamental premise: the body as a whole—indeed, all aspects of the patient—must be assessed in order to fully understand a disorder. Skin diseases are viewed from the same perspective. Although their manifestations are external, their root causes are often complex, and involve internal imbalances between yin and yang, deficiency or excess of qi and blood, or dysfunction of the Organs.

Modern principles of Chinese dermatology categorize the causes of disease as either internal or external. (A third category—"neither internal nor external"—that originally referred to burns, cuts or improper diet, has now been subsumed into these two categories, and is no longer used.) However, even externally-caused disease is often seen as having an internal relationship: "When normal qi is harbored internally, harmful factors cannot affect [the body]" *(Basic Questions,* Chapter 33). This process is exemplified in a passage from *Discussion of the Origins of Symptoms of Diseases,* in which the causes of ulcers on the face are traced from the external factors of wind and dampness to an internal dysfunction of the Lung:

> Ulcers of the head and face are specifically due to internal heat and external deficiency, and wind and dampness taking advantage [of the weakness]. The Lung governs the qi and controls the skin; qi deficiency results in opening of the skin [pores], thus wind and dampness take advantage.

Internal Causes

INJURY OF THE SEVEN EMOTIONS

The seven emotions—elation, anger, worry, pensiveness, sadness, fear and terror—are psychological and physiological reactions to one's surroundings. Each emotion has an Organ with which it is related. Under ordinary circumstances, emotional reactions will not cause disease. However, when any emotion is provoked beyond the body's capacity to regulate it, the corresponding Organ will be affected. Chapter 5 of *Basic Questions* identifies these correspndences: "Anger injures the Liver, elation injures the Heart, pensiveness injures the Spleen, worry injures the Lung, terror injures the Kidney." The effects of traumatic emotions on the qi are described in Chapter 39: "Anger causes qi to ascend, elation causes qi to slow, sadness causes qi to weaken, fear causes qi to sink, pensiveness causes qi to gather." Thus, e.g., individuals who experience an instance of deep anger may develop red spots or swellings on the skin because the Liver qi has stagnated, causing the blood to stagnate and accumulate. Pensiveness may cause acne by disturbing the Spleen's transformative function, resulting in accumulation of fluids and dampness, which, if allowed to progress, will give rise to phlegm and heat. Damp-heat with phlegm then stagnate in the skin and produce acne.

IMPROPER DIET

That an improper diet can lead to disease was recognized by the ancient Chinese. Consider the following passage from Chapter 10 of *Basic Questions:*

> Too much bitter food causes dryness of the skin and the falling out of body hair; too much spicy food causes spasm of the tendons and dryness of the nails; too much sweet food causes pain of the bones and the falling out of head hair.

Many skin disorders are caused by damp-heat toxin. A diet of rich and/or spicy foods can cause dysfunction of the Spleen, resulting in the internal production of damp-heat toxin. Coupled with harmful external factors, conditions such as carbuncles, phlegmon and furuncles may arise. This was described in Chapter 3 of *Basic Questions:* "Injury from fatty meat and refined rice may result in nail-like boils of the foot."

It should be noted that skin disorders caused solely by external factors are usually less severe than those resulting from a combination of external factors and internal dysfunction.

IMBALANCE OF ACTIVITY AND LEISURE

Normal work and exercise facilitate the flow of qi and blood and the harmonious functioning of the Organs. Overwork and excessive exercise may consume qi and injure blood; lack of exercise can cause qi and blood to stagnate. For example, overindulgence in sexual activity harms the Kidney essence, causing accumulation of Kidney fire; upon exposure to external wind, skin disorders such as erysipelas of the leg may occur.

NATURAL INTOLERANCE

Certain individuals are constitutionally sensitive to exposure to various factors. The resulting skin disorders that may develop fall into two categories: contact dermatitis and urticaria.
- Contact dermatitis—allergic skin disorder caused by substances coming in contact with the skin.
- Urticaria—allergic skin disorder due to an allergy to drugs, foods or beverages.

External Causes

THE SIX EXCESSES

Whenever any of the six climatic factors (wind, cold, summerheat, dampness, dryness, fire) becomes excessive at a time when the body's protective qi is deficient, it can contribute to disease. They are therefore called the six excesses or harmful factors. The symptoms associated with external excesses are often quite similar to those associated with internal dysfunction; thus differentiation is critical to effective treatment. The discussion of each of the six excesses that follows will therefore include consideration of the related internal manifestations of excess for comparison.

Wind. This is a significant factor in the etiology of skin disease. It is usually prevalent in the spring, although diseases caused by wind may arise during any season. Dryness, cold, dampness and heat will often "ride" with wind into the body, giving rise to symptoms of wind-dryness, wind-cold, wind-dampness and wind-heat. Chapter 42 of *Basic Questions* notes that "[w]ind is the chief of many diseases."

The etiology and symptomatology of wind-related disorders reflect the characteristics of wind as a force of nature. Wind is a yang excess characterized by an "opening up," and by an upward and outward nature. Wind diseases usually affect the upper body first, producing sores and ulcers of the head and face. Wind has the propensity to move and change, thus there is usually no predictable location for diseases caused by wind. Urticaria, known in Chinese as "wind-type concealed rash," is such a skin condition.

Diseases caused by wind are characterized by rapid onset and resolution, and a short course; a propensity to move about, without a fixed location in the body; itching (in skin disorders); a tendency to attack the surface of the body and the head; an aversion to wind; and, like the spreading and dispersing nature of wind itself, by the opening of the pores, with sweating.

Internal wind is related to the Liver. The Liver stores blood; if blood is deficient and unable to nourish the Liver, wind can arise. Internal wind can also occur due to the presence of heat toxin, which injures yin. Although the internal movement of wind is different from the external excess wind, there are similarities in their clinical symptoms. Such is the case with pruritus and seborrhea, which are caused by protracted wind transforming into dryness.

Cold. This is a yin excess that injures yang. Cold causes blood stasis and the stagnation of qi, as in frostbite or chilblain. It can also cause coldness, pain and masses in the extremities, as well as chronic open sores.

Skin diseases caused by cold are characterized by purple, darkened skin and the absence of redness and warmth in the affected area; slow resolution of swelling; slow formation of pus; and confined localization of the pain.

Internal cold generally results from yang failure and qi deficiency, and is thus also known as deficiency cold. Yang deficiency results in yin flourishing and the loss of internal warmth, hence the build-up of internal cold.

Summerheat. This is a yang excess, a transformation of fire-heat, which occurs during the summer months. Summerheat is upward-moving and spreading in nature; thus when it attacks, it causes the pores to open and sweating to increase. Increased sweating injures the fluids and allows qi to be lost (through the sweating), causing qi deficiency.

Summer rains often cause summerheat to combine with dampness. This type of weather increases the sweating even more and can lead to such skin disorders as heat rash or even inflammation of the sweat glands.

Skin disorders caused by summerheat are characterized by redness, swelling and a burning sensation in the affected area; pus-forming lesions which, if protracted, may necrose; and pain that generally diminishes upon exposure to cold.

Dampness. This factor is more dominant during the summer, although it can occur throughout the year. It can also occur when individuals are exposed to a damp or wet environment, or to rain. Dampness has a heavy, sinking nature. Diseases caused by dampness are often accompanied by heaviness and fatigue of the limbs.

Skin disorders caused by dampness are characterized by open sores with pus or necrosis of the affected area; by a protracted course (because they are refractory to treatment); and by swelling of the affected area.

Internal dampness is often caused by dysfunction of the Spleen's transportive and transformative mechanisms. This leads to a build-up of fluid, and eventually to dampness. If the fluids accumulate in the skin, intense itching, blistering, swelling or necrosis may occur.

Dryness. This factor predominates during the autumn, and is thus known as "autumn dryness." It often enters through the nose and mouth, with the disorder starting in the Lung. Dryness is of two kinds: warm-dryness and cool-dryness. If there is a long spell of clear skies without rain, and with wind and heat dominating, individuals succumbing to these conditions will often suffer from the warm-dryness variety. On the other hand, the breezes of autumn tend to be cool, especially those out of the west, and individuals succumbing to this climatic condition will often develop the cool-dryness variety.

Skin diseases due to dryness are generally of the warm-dryness variety. Dryness consumes body fluids, causing the skin to crack easily. Other harmful factors take advantage of the cracked skin and enter the body, giving rise to conditions such as carbuncles, or furuncles of the hands and feet.

Skin diseases caused by dryness are characterized by dryness, cracking and scaling of the affected area. The hands, feet and mucous membranes are most susceptible.

Internal dryness is related to the Lung. The Lung governs the skin. Insufficiency of Lung yin causes dryness of the skin. Other causes of dryness of the skin include internal heat which consumes fluids; yin deficiency with internal heat; and long-term use of bitter, cold and dry medicines, or those that promote diuresis, which results in injury to yin and consumption of blood. The latter can transform into blood heat/wind-dryness or blood deficiency/wind-dryness. The skin loses its nourishment and becomes dry and scaly, as happens in psoriasis.

Fire. Fire and heat arise from an excess of yang. Although their natures are similar, and they are often spoken of together as fire-heat, there are subtle differences between them. Heat is more intense than warmth, and fire is an extreme form of heat. Heat often occurs in combination with other excesses to produce wind-heat, summerheat or damp-heat. Fire, on the other hand, is often produced internally, as the result of Organ dysfunction (e.g., Heart fire rising, exuberant Liver fire, excess Stomach fire), or from overstimulation of the emotions, which, under certain conditions, can transform into fire.

Two distinctive characteristics of fire-heat are that it readily transforms into fire and/or toxin, and that the conditions it causes are extremely serious. Such is the case, e.g., with wind-heat that transforms into fire toxin in erysipelas of the head; damp-heat sinking that transforms into fire toxin in erysipelas of the shins; and summerheat that transforms into fire toxin in hidradenitis (inflammation of the sweat gland). Fire also has an ascending nature, and diseases due to fire often occur on the face and head, e.g., erysipelas of the head.

Skin diseases caused by fire are characterized by sudden or rapid onset; redness and a burning sensation in the affected area; by the sheen of the skin in the area of swelling; intense pain; purulence and necrosis; and development of red or purple macules, often because fire is carried by the blood and burns the channels and collaterals, thus causing intradermal bleeding (petechiae).

Internal fire is primarily caused by dysfunction of the Organs or provocation of the emotions, resulting in an imbalance of yin and yang. Internal fire can be further categorized as excessive or deficient. Heart/Small Intestine fire, Liver/Gallbladder fire, Spleen/Stomach fire and Lung/Large Intestine fire are regarded as excessive in nature because these Organs are most affected by overabundant yang. Kidney fire (fire of the gate of vitality) is deficient in nature since this Organ is most affected by yin deficiency. Examples of skin disorders caused by internal fire include Heart fire blazing upward causing sores in the mouth; flourishing Heart/Liver fire causing shingles; accumulating Spleen/Stomach fire causing heat sores; flourishing Lung fire causing acne rosacea; and flourishing Kidney fire resulting in melasma.

EPIDEMICS (PESTILENCES)

Epidemic diseases differ from external excesses in that the former are considered highly contagious while the latter are not. Epidemic pestilences *(yì lì)* are very serious and are thought to have a highly toxic nature. Early Chinese medical records refer to pestilences by such names as "pestilent factor" *(lì qì)*, "perverse factor" *(yàn qì)*, "abnormal factor" *(yì qì)* and "poisonous factor" *(dú qì)*.

The characteristics of an epidemic disease are rapid onset, severe and intense symptoms, similar or identical signs and symptoms among individuals afflicted with the same disease, and extreme contagiousness. The route of transmission of contagions "through the mouth and nose" was described as early as the Ming dynasty by Wu You-Xing in his *Treatise on Febrile Pestilences* (1642). Contagious skin diseases include smallpox, leprosy, chickenpox and rubella.

INSECTS AND PARASITES

Insects and parasites are common causes of skin diseases. They can be divided into three categories: insect bites and stings, visible parasites and microscopic parasites.

Insect bites and stings. These include bites from mosquitos, fleas, bedbugs and chiggers, which cause local itching and wheals. Insects that sting include wasps, bees and centipedes, whose stings result in pain and swelling. Skin disorders from bites and stings usually subside in a matter of days.

Visible parasites. These usually come about because of unsanitary conditions or lack of personal hygiene. Mites, which cause scabies, and lice, which cause pediculosis of the head, body or pubic area, are examples of such parasites. The skin of the affected area generally itches, and presents with papules, hives, pyoderma, oozing and scaling.

Microscopic parasites. Examples of skin conditions caused by microscopic organisms are leishmaniasis and leprosy. Leishmaniasis is caused by a protozoan, and is characterized by cutaneous papules that develop into nodules, break down to form ulcers, and finally heal, leaving depressed scars. Leprosy is caused by a bacteria that gives rise to nodules, leading to nerve pain and eventually numbness and ulceration, and even disfiguration.

MISCELLANEOUS

Other external causes of skin disorders include animal bites, cuts, abrasions, trauma and burns. These will not be discussed in this book since they are mechanical causes and are readily treated with modern biomedicine.

CHAPTER 3

Diagnostics

In order to fully understand a disease and its effect on the body, the Chinese through the ages have developed four methods of diagnosis: looking, listening/smelling, asking and palpation. All four methods rely on the practitioner's own senses to assess a patient's condition. Used together they provide a thorough description of the body and its functions, and form the basis for effective treatment strategies.

Looking

Three observations are significant in diagnosing dermatological disorders: the appearance of the skin itself, the overall appearance of the patient, and the appearance of the patient's tongue.

Appearance of the skin. Skin diseases may be differentiated according to the area of skin surface on which they occur, their coloration and their physical form. Furuncles, e.g., usually appear on the head, face, breasts and buttocks; shingles occurs in the hypochondriac region; psoriasis generally involves the scalp and the extensor surfaces of the extremities, particularly the elbows and knees. Red lesions are a sign of heat; pale lesions a sign of cold; purple or dark lesions indicate stagnation; and brown or black lesions (when not variations in pigmentation) indicate tissue necrosis. A detailed description of skin lesion types is set forth in Chapter 4.

Overall appearance of the patient. Spirit (*shén*) is derived from essence (*jīng*) and qi, and is the external reflection of the condition of the internal Organs' qi and blood. The condition of the spirit is thus reflected in an individual's general appearance—in the posture, facial expression and manner of speech: When a patient is spirited and responsive, with clear eyes and normal breathing, the condition is usually not a serious one. When a patient shows a lack of spirit, has a dull complexion and eyes and shallow breathing—all signs of decline of normal qi—the condition is probably more serious. People with serious skin diseases (e.g., bacterial infections like erysipelas) will show confusion, restlessness and rapid and uneven breathing—indications that the excess has entered the nutritive (*yíng*) level, and that the toxin has been transmitted to the Pericardium.

An individual's physical type can reveal predispositions to certain conditions. Overweight people usually harbor dampness and/or phlegm, while thin people are prone to conditions of fire or heat. Awareness of such predispositions can be useful in diagnosing such diseases as eczema, which may be caused by dampness, heat or wind.

Appearance of the tongue. Inspection of the tongue is an important aspect of diagnosis in Chinese medicine. The tongue is connected to the Organs via the channels and collaterals, and thus reflects the condition of the blood and qi. Changes in the tongue's shape, color and coating during the course of a disease are indicative of the nature of the pathology; the specific area of the tongue on which such changes occur indicates the specific Organ that is involved.

A dry tongue indicates yin deficiency, and is seen in diseases such as severe systemic lupus erythematosus. A wet tongue indicates yang deficiency, and is present in conditions such as the early stages of scleroderma.

A normal tongue body with a thin white coating indicates an exterior disorder such as the onset of hives. A red or scarlet tongue with a yellow coating that turns black indicates an interior disorder such as late-stage pemphigus vulgaris. A pale tongue without coating is found in deficiency disorders such as late-stage scleroderma. A purple tongue with a thick sticky coating indicates an excessive disorder such as poisoning.

A fat wet tongue with a pale or white coating is present in disorders associated with cold, such as Raynaud's syndrome. A dry and red or purple tongue with a grayish coating signifies a heat pattern, as is seen in skin disorders caused by drug overdose.

Listening/Smelling

The quality of a person's breathing, speech and cough may also be indicative of the nature of his or her condition. Loud, excessive talking accompanied by restlessness is often a sign of heat. A weak, low voice is usually an indication of deficiency. Heavy breathing is generally associated with excess, while shallow and soft breathing are signs of deficiency.

The odor of the exudates of a skin lesion can be significant. Odorless lesions are usually less serious, heal more rapidly and are generally easier to treat than are malodorous lesions.

Asking

Questioning the patient about his or her condition yields essential information about the etiology, progression and present state of the illness. In dermatology, specific information should be sought about the patient's fever and chills, perspiration, stools and urine, appetite and diet, occupation and medical history.

Fever and chills. Fever and chills are signs of the conflict between normal qi and the factor of excess. Skin disorders accompanied by fever and/or chills, e.g., bacterial infections of the skin such as those caused by staphylococci, are generally more serious, and indicate that the excess is flourishing.

Fevers are divided into three phases: rising, plateau, and reduction. During the rising phase, if the fever rises gradually to between 37.5°C and 38°C, the condition has been caused by flourishing fire toxin and attack by external wind. In cases in which chills accompany fever, if the chills are stronger than the fever, the condition is one of wind-cold; if the fever predominates, then the condition is one of wind-heat. During the plateau phase the fever ranges between 38°C and 39°C, and the skin lesions become red, edematous and tender—often signs of pus formation. During the reduction phase the fever subsides and the pus is discharged. If the fever persists after the reduction phase, the toxin has not been overcome by normal qi. If chills and high fever persist after the discharge of pus, then the toxin has "sunk in," and treatment will be more difficult.

Perspiration. In skin disorders like carbuncles, if sweating occurs while a fever is subsiding, then the factor of excess is successfully being expelled with the sweat. If there is sweating without a break in the fever, then the excess is still flourishing and pus is forming.

Stools and urine. In general, hard stools, and yellow, cloudy and scanty urine, are signs of flourishing damp-heat. If the stools are loose and the urine is clear and copious, then the condition is generally due to cold-dampness.

Appetite and diet. An individual's desire for food is indicative of the condition of Spleen/Stomach qi. When there is a desire for food, the Spleen/Stomach qi is still sufficient, and the condition is not serious. When there is no desire for food, however, the Spleen/Stomach qi is deficient, and the condition is deeper and more serious.

Some skin disorders are caused by improper diet. For example, hives are often due to a diet too rich in meat, shellfish, alcohol or spicy foods, all of which result in a build-up of dampness that becomes lodged in the skin.

Occupation. The etiology of certain skin diseases can be traced to an individual's occupation. People who work with chemicals (e.g., house painters) and those who are regularly exposed to wet and damp environments (e.g., fishermen) are especially vulnerable to skin problems.

Medical history. The practitioner should encourage the patient to reveal as much as possible about his or her medical history, particularly if the condition has appeared previously. A detailed account should be sought of the present condition, the circumstances of its onset, its progression and any prior diagnoses and treatment. A family history should also be considered in cases in which the condition is contagious (e.g., impetigo or scabies) or hereditary (e.g., inherited ichthyosis). (See Table 3-1.)

Palpation

Two categories of palpation are utilized in the diagnosis of skin disorders: palpation of the radial pulses, and palpation of the affected dermal area. By palpating the radial pulses the practitioner can ascertain the level of the disease, the dynamics of the factor of excess, and the strength of the normal qi. Palpation of the locally-affected area serves to confirm and focus the diagnosis, and helps differentiate between excess and deficiency, heat and cold.

Pulses. Since other textbooks of Chinese diagnostics offer detailed descriptions of the various pulse types, we will confine our discussion here to the pulses associated with common dermatological disorders.

- A floating pulse indicates an exterior disorder caused by wind-cold or wind-heat. It may also mean that the wind-heat toxin is located in the upper part of the body.
- A submerged pulse indicates that the condition is situated at a deep level.
- A slow pulse signifies a cold disorder and/or that qi and blood are deficient. When there is a skin infection, a slow pulse may indicate that the toxin has lost its virulence, and that the normal qi is weak.
- A rapid pulse reflects disorders of heat. When there is a skin infection, a rapid pulse means that the heat toxin has not yet cleared, and that the normal qi is weak.
- A slippery and rapid pulse indicates the presence of phlegm and flourishing heat, or the presence of pus.
- A choppy pulse signifies stagnation of qi and blood.
- A large pulse indicates that the excess and the normal qi are locked in great conflict.
- A thin pulse means that the normal qi is unable to overcome the excess. It may also indicate deficiency of both qi and blood.

Changes in the pace of the pulse (in beats per minute) during the different phases in the progression of a disease should also be noted. Conditions that are yang in nature usually present with a slightly rapid pulse (80-84 beats/minute) at the outset of the disease, an accelerated pace (84-100 beats/minute) during the suppurative (pus formation) phase, and a return to normal after the lesions have broken. If the condition worsens as a result of the excess traveling to a deeper level, the pulse will race (100-120 beats/minute).

Yin conditions will generally start with a moderate pulse (less than 72 beats/minute), increase as the condition progresses (to 80-100 beats/minute), and then return to normal during the recovery phase.

Palpation of local areas. Areas that are red, swollen and clearly demarcated, that are warm or hot to the touch, and that are painful upon light pressure usually indicate a condition of excess. If the affected area is neither swollen nor unusually warm, and only slightly painful upon strong pressure, the condition is generally one of deficiency. Skin presentations that are only slightly elevated and not easily palpable have usually not yet suppurated; lesions that are raised and that can be distinctly palpated usually contain pus. (Chapter 4 contains descriptions and illustrations of skin lesion types.)

Table 3-1 Principles of Dermatologic Diagnosis

Present Complaint	Nature, site, duration
History of Present Condition	• Details of onset • Signs, symptoms, distribution • Course (rapidity of spread, interval of recurrence, severity) • Accompanying generalized symptoms • Previous laboratory studies and diagnosis • Previous treatment, if any (prescriptive, over-the-counter, home remedies, and alternative, including name of remedy, dosage, results) • Factors, i.e., diet, menstrual, occupational, seasonal • Patient's opinion about cause or nature of problem
Medical History	Present and previous medical conditions, operations, allergies, medications, drug intolerances
Patient's Personal History	Race, occupation, hobbies, diet, emotional status; women should be asked about their menstrual history; family members with same condition presently or previously, members with allergies, asthma, hay fever, etc.
Examination of Skin Lesions	• Location and distribution (use good lighting and vary the angle and intensity to pick up less conspicuous skin changes; use magnification to see markings otherwise invisible to the naked eye) • Primary or secondary lesion, size, number, appearance, color (ascertain fading upon pressure), texture and hardness, superficial appearance, appearance of borders (see Chapter 4 for description and illustrations of lesions); inspection should be both visual and tactile • Examine other areas (e.g., in mouth, behind ears, on scalp, between fingers and toes) to ascertain spread or initial site of condition. • If disorder is not identifiable, consult a color atlas or more experienced practitioner or dermatologist.
Pathologic and Laboratory Analyses	When a diagnosis cannot be reached using the gross methods above, then a biopsy and/or laboratory test may be required.

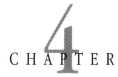

CHAPTER 4

Differentiation of Patterns

In Chinese medicine, diagnostic information can be organized into patterns according to various systems. Three such systems are significant in dermatology: patterns based on the eight guiding parameters, patterns based on yin and yang Organ *(zàng fǔ)* functions and relationships, and four-level patterns for heat-induced disorders. In addition, the subjective skin sensation (as reported by the patient) and the type of skin lesion itself offer two further categories by which raw diagnostic data can be organized into clinically significant patterns—a process known in Chinese medicine as differentiation.

Eight Guiding Parameters of Differentiation

All diseases can be generally described using four ranges of disease characteristics, each range defined by two parameters of an opposite nature: yin/yang, interior/exterior, cold/hot, deficient/excessive. The yin/yang range characterizes the general form of the condition, and is defined in part by the disease attributes described by the remaining parameters (diseases that are interior, cold and of a deficient nature are considered yin; diseases that are exterior, hot and of an excessive nature are considered yang). The interior/exterior range describes the level or depth of the disease. The cold/hot range defines the thermal nature of the disease. And the range between deficiency and excess shows the conflict between the normal qi and the factors of excess. Through careful assessment of all the signs and symptoms of a disease in relation to each of these eight parameters, the overall nature of the disease can be understood, and a comprehensive treatment strategy developed.

Disease is a dynamic and complex process. During the course of a disease any attribute may transform toward its polar opposite—an exterior condition may become interior, a cold condition may transform into one of heat. Opposite disease attributes may also exist simultaneously, e.g., signs of heat as well as cold, or excess as well as deficiency. Certain conditions may present one attribute disguised as another, as in cases of true heat and false cold, or true deficiency and false excess. Thus, in applying the eight guiding parameters to differentiate patterns, it is important to grasp the most prominent aspects, as well as the relationship among the different stages of a given condition.

Dermatological diseases that are yang, exterior, hot and excessive are usually acute, intensely itchy, rapidly changing and produce local redness, swelling and pain. The patient may have a dry mouth, thirst, constipation, yellow urine, restlessness, fever and a flushed face, with a pulse that may be floating, slippery, rapid or strong, and a tongue that may be red (or have a red tip) and with a greasy yellow coating.

Skin diseases that are yin, interior, cold and deficient are generally chronic, moist and present with locally darkened skin. These symptoms may be accompanied by a bland taste in the mouth, loss of appetite, normal or loose stools, or bloating. The pulse may be submerged and moderate, or submerged and thin, or slow. The tongue may be slightly pale, fat or tooth-marked, with a white and slippery, or white and sticky coating.

Differentiation of Skin Diseases According to the Organs

Differentiation according to the Organs is based on observation of the manifestations of the physiology and pathology of the Organs in order to understand a disease—its nature, etiology and location, and the balance between the normal qi and the factor of excess. Wang Bing, the famous Tang dynasty physician, once noted that while the Organs are located internally, they manifest externally. Although the following descriptions are limited to the coupled yin and yang Organ systems, it should be remembered that the comprehensive system of channels and collaterals links all the Organs together as a unified whole, and that pathological disorders in one Organ may affect one or more other Organs in a variety of ways under a diverse range of conditions.

Heart and Small Intestine. Symptoms of Heart/Small Intestine dysfunction presenting on the skin may include red macular eruptions, papules, burning and redness, crusting, pus formation and necrosis. All conditions induced by fire toxin associate and resonate with the Heart. If the heat is intense, there will be pain; if the heat is slight, there will be itching. Accompanying symptoms may include ulcers of the tongue, restlessness, palpitations, dry mouth, yellow tongue coating and a rapid pulse.

Common skin disorders associated with Heart/Small Intestine dysfunction are boils, furuncles, carbuncles and pemphigus.

Liver and Gallbladder. Symptoms of Liver/Gallbladder dysfunction presenting on the skin may include papules, burning red macular eruptions, necrosis and vesicles. Whenever an emotional upset precipitates the skin disorder, or if the condition appears in the hypochondria, genitalia or near the eyes, then the Liver/Gallbladder system is most likely involved. Accompanying symptoms may include redness of the eyes, anger, depression, bitter taste in the mouth, dry throat and a wiry pulse.

Common skin disorders associated with Liver/Gallbladder dysfunction are shingles, tinea cruris and vulvitis.

Spleen and Stomach. Symptoms of Spleen/Stomach dysfunction presenting on the skin may include papules, vesicles, ulcers and lichenification. Disorders related to dampness usually arise because of weak Spleen yang that results in dysfunction of the Spleen's transformative function, and a corresponding build-up of dampness. Accompanying symptoms may include ulcers of the mouth and/or tongue, poor appetite, loose stools, diarrhea, greasy tongue coating and a moderate pulse.

Common skin disorders associated with Spleen/Stomach dysfunction include eczema and various forms of dermatitis.

Lung and Large Intestine. Symptoms of Lung/Large Intestine dysfunction presenting on the skin may include red macules, papules, pustules and excoriation. The Lung governs the skin, and is also the Organ most affected by wind. Thus, a skin condition accompanied by such symptoms as dry nose and throat, dry cough, dry white tongue coating, and a thin, floating and rapid pulse is associated with the Lung. Common skin disorders associated with Lung/Large Intestine dysfunction include acne, acne rosacea and hives.

Kidney and Bladder. Symptoms of Kidney/Bladder dysfunction presenting on the skin may include dark brown patches on the face, and loss of head hair. Accompanying symptoms may include forgetfulness, low back pain, tinnitus, chills and fever, spontaneous sweating, or pale complexion, bloating, edema, loose stools, cold extremities, deep red tongue and a thin, rapid pulse.

Common skin disorders associated with Kidney/Bladder dysfunction include systemic lupus erythematosus and melasma.

Differentiation According to the Four Levels

Four-level differentiation is applied primarily to acute febrile diseases, and to serious skin diseases that involve the entire body. Developed by the Qing dynasty physician Ye Tian-Shi (1667-1746), the four levels refer to the individual patterns associated with the protective *(wèi)*, qi *(qì)*, nutritive *(yíng)* and blood *(xuě)* aspects of energetic physiology, and describe the depth to which a disease has penetrated, as well as its origin and severity. For skin diseases that involve systemic symptomatology, differentiation according to the four levels can be used in conjunction with other methods of differentiation.

Protective-level patterns and qi-level patterns are closely related in terms of their clinical manifestations, and together in many ways form a continuum of symptomatology that ranges from less severe (protective level) to more severe (qi level). Nutritive-level patterns and blood-level patterns have a similar clinical relationship. Thus, in clinical practice, these four patterns are often considered as two pairs of related groups of patterns —protective/qi and nutritive/blood— and patterns are differentiated between them.

Protective level. Protective qi defends the body against harmful external influences, and is the organism's first line of defense. Thus patterns involving the protective level are those that are seen when a harmful factor has just entered the body. Such patterns are usually associated with the Lung. Skin symptoms related to protective-level patterns include intense itching and hives, accompanied by fever, headache, sore throat, joint pain and other bodily discomfort.

Common skin disorders at the protective level of penetration include acute hives.

Qi level. If a disease is not stopped at the protective level it will continue inward to the qi level, where the excess and the normal qi become locked in conflict, generating a significant accumulation of heat. At this level the excess can invade the Organs; the resulting patterns will thus vary. The affected skin may be flushed, red and painful, accompanied by high fever, restlessness, thirst with desire to drink, dry stools, rapid and forceful pulse and a yellow and dry tongue coating.

Common skin disorders at the qi level of penetration include pemphigus, shingles, inflammatory reactions of the skin (such as drug eruptions and photosensitivity eruptions) and acute dermatitis.

Nutritive level. A disorder of heat that persists in the qi level will consume fluids and cause the excess to sink into the nutritive level. Skin lesions such as purple patches will often be diffuse or indiscernible. The skin may be moist and flushed, or edematous. Blisters and/or pustules may be present. These symptoms may be accompanied by restlessness, sleeplessness, high fever, raving, thirst, fever that is more pronounced at night, scarlet tongue and a thin, rapid pulse.

Common skin disorders at the nutritive level include purpura and exfoliative dermatitis.

Blood level. If the heat penetrates to the blood level, the presenting patterns will relate primarily to the Heart, Liver and Kidney. Symptoms appearing on the skin are associated with bleeding, and may include petechiae and telangiectasia, which can be accompanied by vomiting of blood, bleeding from the nose or passing of bloody stools. The tongue is scarlet and the pulse rapid.

Common skin disorders at the blood level include systemic lupus erythematosus, exfoliative dermatitis and purpura.

Differentiation According to Subjective Skin Sensation

Itching, pain and numbness are the most common symptoms in dermatology. The correct differentiation of these symptoms is vital to understanding a skin disease and instituting the proper treatment.

ITCHING

Wind. The nature of wind excess is one of motion and changeability, and a propensity to affect the upper part of the body. Itching due to wind therefore often occurs on the head, face and ears, though other parts of the body may be affected as well.

If the condition is more hot in nature, the itching usually arises suddenly, and is frequently accompanied by small papules which, if persistently scratched, may produce redness, fissures and elongated crusts along the scratch lines.

Signs of pus or necrosis are generally absent. Heat often exacerbates the itching, and exposure to cool breezes tends to ameliorate it.

If the condition is more cold in nature, the itching usually occurs on the exposed areas of the head, face, ears and hands. This type of wind itching is more pronounced during the cooler parts of the day than during the midday hours. There is also a seasonal recurrence, with the condition becoming worse in winter than in summer. Scratch marks and pale papules or wheals may be present.

Dampness. The nature of dampness is heavy and sticky, with a tendency to sink. Diseases associated with dampness usually affect the lower portion and/or yin aspects of the body. Skin lesions include blisters, crusting and necrosis. Itching generally leads to scratching. If the skin is broken, oozing occurs, which may remain on the skin and cause erosion and further itching, thus developing into a chronic cycle.

If heat accompanies this disorder, the affected skin is flushed and slightly edematous, and the erosion and itching are equally intense. If the condition is accompanied by cold, the affected area is thickened and dark red or purple in color, with the itching worse than the erosion.

Dryness. Dryness readily injures the fluids. Skin symptoms associated with dryness include dry skin and episodic itching. Scratching often results in long scaling marks. Dry itching can result from either excess or deficiency. Patterns of excess are caused by blood heat or wind-dryness, with intense burning, dryness and scaling, and a yellow tongue coating, such as in the early stages of psoriasis. Patterns of deficiency are the result of blood deficiency leading to wind-dryness, and to malnourishment of the skin. This causes the skin to become dry and to itch, with pronounced scaling, as in the chronic stages of psoriasis (see discussion of itching due to deficiency below).

Heat. Heat is an intense excess that readily injures the fluids, qi and blood. Because of its rising nature, itching associated with heat characteristically occurs on the head and face. However, as the heat rises its intensity may cause itching to break out in other areas. Lesions are primarily red papules or macules that may be diffuse or coalesced. Subjective sensations, which range from burning to prickling, are exacerbated by exposure to heat. If the skin is broken when scratched, bleeding and possibly the formation of pus may occur.

Insect bites and stings. Common bites and stings are those from bees, wasps, ants, ticks, fleas and mosquitos. Itching may be transient or, in hypersensitive individuals, intense. Differentiation should be based on past reactions to insect bites or stings, and on the presence of wheals, blisters, localized swelling or edema.

Poisons. Itching associated with poisons refers to an intolerable dose of drugs, and is similar to drug eruptions in modern biomedicine. A passage in *Discussion of the Origins of Symptoms of Diseases* observes that "[a]ny medicine that is strongly toxic should not enter the mouth, nose, ears or eyes." The result is severe and persistent itching. If the dose is too great, the toxin will affect the Organs. Skin lesions vary from mild rashes to edematous wheals to the more life-threatening toxic epidermal necrolysis (peeling of the epidermis).

Food sensitivities. These are similar to food allergies in modern biomedicine. Seafood, including fish, crab and shellfish, can cause itching in hypersensitive individuals because of the tendency of these foods to generate internal wind. The itching is accompanied by generalized wheals and edematous rashes. Restlessness and disorientation may occur in severe cases. If this disorder is not resolved at the outset, the toxin may attack the interior leading to nausea, vomiting, diarrhea and other generalized symptoms.

Stagnation. This type of itching is so intense that no amount of scratching can relieve it. The skin lesions may be dark red papules or small nodules that may be generalized or localized into patches, and that penetrate into the skin.

Alcohol. Some individuals may experience itching following intake of alcohol. In some of these cases, a maculopapular rash that resembles measles may also appear. Usually, once the alcohol leaves the body through the sweat or urine, the itching and rash disappear.

Deficiency. With blood deficiency the skin loses its nourishment and becomes dry. Itching is intense and generalized, and may feel like crawling insects; the itching is more severe at night. If there is also qi deficiency, resistance to the six excesses is low, and changes in the weather may aggravate the itching. If there is yang deficiency, the itching will be more pronounced around the end of autumn or beginning of winter; middle-age to elderly males are often affected. If there is yin deficiency, the skin will be extremely dry and lackluster, and after scratching will become scaly. (This type of itching is often seen in persons who have a history of yin deficiency.)

PAIN

Heat. Skin pain associated with heat is generally caused by Heart or Liver fire. The skin is scarlet red and burns, and the pain is relieved by cold.

Blood stasis. At the outset of this type of skin disorder the pain is vague, and accompanied by slight swelling and heat, and dark red skin. As the condition progresses, the skin becomes purple and the pain and swelling more pronounced. In some instances nodules may develop. The pain is localized.

Cold. The skin color is unchanged and is not hot. The pain is usually that of soreness.

Deficiency. Skin pain associated with deficiency is relieved with pressure and warm applications.

Excess. This kind of pain rejects pressure and is relieved by cold applications.

NUMBNESS

Numbness indicates that the blood and qi are flowing poorly or not at all. When the skin lacks nourishment from qi and blood, numbness may result.

Differentiation According to Skin Lesion

Almost all skin diseases are distinguished by their lesions. Recognizing these lesions is important both for diagnosis and for discovering any latent conditions.

Primary lesions. In any skin disorder, primary lesions refer to the earliest dermal changes to appear.

Macule *(bān).* A flat spot on the skin that is discernible only by difference in color or texture.
- Red macules that fade upon pressure are regarded as a manifestation of heat in the qi level. Those that do not fade are caused by heat in the blood level, or by blood stasis.
- Purple macules are generally caused by heat stagnation in the yang-brightness channels.
- Black macules are due to Kidney deficiency.
- White macules are a sign of qi stagnation, or disharmony between the blood and qi.

Plaque *(bān).* A flat (not elevated) and palpable discolored spot. Traditionally, these were not distinguished from macules.

Papule *(qiū zhěn).* A small, circumscribed, solid elevation of the skin.
- Red papules usually present with a burning sensation and intense itching. They are generally associated with Heart fire or external wind excess.
- Chronic lichen planus papules are generally attributable to deficiency dampness of the Spleen.

Vesicle *(shuǐ pào).* A circumscribed lesion less than 5mm in diameter that contains serous fluid. (A lesion greater than 5mm is termed a bulla, or blister.) A collection of liquid or semisolid material that is enclosed by a capsule is called a cyst. These are usually caused by dampness or damp-heat. Deep-seated lesions are associated with Spleen deficiency leading to unresolved and extreme dampness, or with an attack by cold or dampness.

Pustule *(nóng pào).* A small, visible blister that contains pus, usually caused by heat toxin or fire toxin.

Wheal *(fēng tuán).* A smooth, raised lesion resulting from local edema, which after receding does not leave any mark.
- Pale wheals are caused by wind-cold or weakness of yang.
- Red wheals are due to wind-heat or yin deficiency leading to fire rising.

Nodule *(jié jié).* A small lump of tissue that may or may not protrude from the skin surface.
- Red nodules are associated with blood stasis.
- Nodules without specific color may be caused by qi stagnation leading to blood stasis, or by accumulation of phlegm-dampness.

Secondary lesions. Secondary lesions result either from the natural progression of a primary lesion, or from the patient's manipulation of the primary lesion.

Scales *(lín xiāo).* Dried, horny epidermis that is layered on the skin.
- Dry scales are attributable to wind-dryness caused by blood deficiency leading to lack of nourishment of the skin.
- Oily scales are caused by damp-heat accumulation in the skin.

Crack *(jūn liè)*. A split or fissure in the skin, often resulting from cold-dryness.

Excoriation *(zhuā hén)*. A scratch or abrasion of the skin. If the skin is broken, crusting may occur.

Erosion *(mí làn)*. A gradual breakdown of part or all of the epidermis that heals without scarring. This may be seen with vesicles or pustules, and is generally attributable to damp-heat.

Ulcer *(chuāng)*. A breakdown of the epidermis and at least part of the dermis. Usually associated with an invasion of toxin such that heat sears the blood and causes blockage to the flow of qi and blood, thus giving rise to an ulcer. In most cases, a scar remains after healing.

Crust scab *(jiā)*. Solid material formed on the skin by drying of blood, exudate, or pus.
- Yellowish serum that dries into a crust is associated with damp-heat.
- Crust formed from dried blood is associated with blood heat.
- Crust formed from dried pus is associated with heat toxin.

Pigmentation *(sè sù chén zhuó)*. Discoloration of the skin attributable to disharmony between blood and qi; generally arises in the wake of chronic skin disorders.
- Light pigmentation is caused by blood deficiency leading to malnourishment of the skin.
- Dark discoloration is associated with Kidney deficiency.

Scar *(bān hén)*. A mark remaining after the healing of destroyed dermis.

DIFFERENTIATION OF PATTERNS

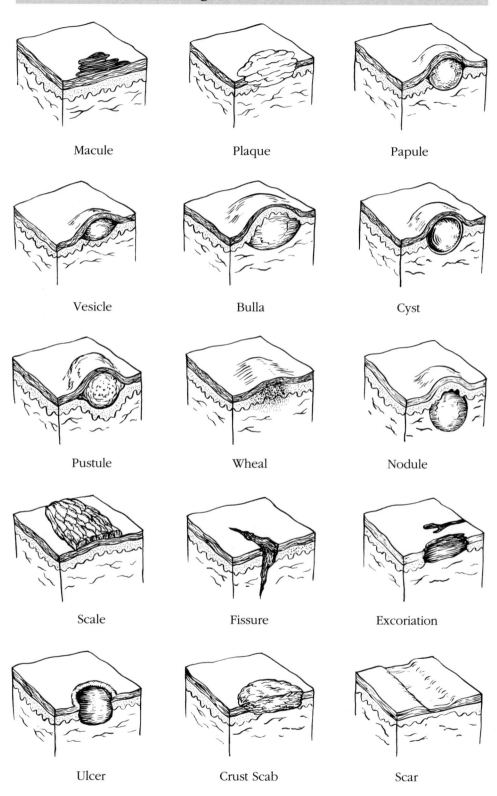

Figure 4-1 Skin Lesions

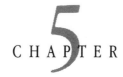

CHAPTER 5

Treatment

Although skin diseases manifest on the exterior surfaces of the body, their occurrence usually reflects the health of deeper physiologic functions—the Organs, channels and collaterals, and bodily substances (qi, blood and fluids). Thus, in traditional Chinese medicine, skin diseases are treated both internally, to affect the whole system (through oral medication), as well as externally, to treat the local manifestation of the disorder (through topical application of the medication).

TREATMENT STRATEGIES

Whether treatment is internal or external, to develop an appropriate strategy the practitioner must differentiate the pattern of the disorder, and then identify the current stage in the progression of the disease. Many skin diseases progress through three stages: prodromal, pustular, and ulcerated. Each stage requires its own general treatment strategy: *elimination* for the prodromal stage, *expulsion* for the pustular stage, and *tonification* for the ulcerated stage. Once the general strategy is developed, a more specific treatment regimen can be determined.

General Strategies

ELIMINATION

Elimination is used in the early or prodromal stage of skin diseases, and is applied to skin lesions that have not yet formed pus. It is aimed at resolving the condition (if caught early enough) or reducing its severity. The number of strategies that can be used during the prodromal stage is as varied as the causes of skin disease, including releasing the exterior, clearing heat, resolving dampness, promoting the qi, etc.

If pus has already formed, elimination should not be used. If it is, this will lead to dispersal instead of elimination of the harmful factor, resulting in injury

EXPULSION

Expulsion is used when the skin lesions have developed pus. The goal of treatment is to tonify and benefit the qi and blood, and to support the normal qi, so that pus will be expelled and the toxin will not sink to a deeper level. This is appropriate for conditions that present with deficiency of normal qi and flourishing of toxin. For conditions that present with flourishing of toxin but no signs of qi deficiency, medications that encourage discharge of pus may be used in order to prevent the pus from penetrating to a deeper level.

TONIFICATION

Tonification is used when lesions have ulcerated, the toxin has been relieved, source qi is deficient and weak, and the pus has turned clear and less viscous. Through tonification, normal qi is restored so that new tissue growth is nourished and the healing of the ulcerated lesion is accelerated. Tonification strategies include regulating and harmonizing the Spleen and Stomach, tonifying and nourishing the Liver and Kidney, and tonifying and nourishing the qi and blood.

If the toxin is not yet relieved (i.e., the lesions have yet to ulcerate), tonification should not be used. To do so could lead to a harboring of the toxin and its subsequent spread.

Specific Strategies

DISPELLING WIND

Wind is the result of either external attack or internal imbalance. For external wind the treatment principle is to expel and disperse wind; for internal wind, the principle is to anchor yang and extinguish wind.

Dispersing wind and clearing heat. Used for conditions of wind-heat. When wind-heat is lodged in the skin, the nutritive and protective levels are out of harmony, giving rise to red papules (such as those of urticaria).

Expelling wind and clearing heat. Used for wind-heat that has stagnated in the tissues, giving rise to such skin conditions as impetigo, erythema multiforme and eczema. The treatment principle is to expel wind and clear heat, and invigorate blood and relieve toxicity.

Expelling wind and scattering cold. Used when the protective level is weak and yang is insufficient, allowing wind and cold to readily enter the body and give rise to such conditions as urticaria.

Dispelling wind and clearing dampness. Used for conditions of wind and dampness in which itching is prominent. When wind excess is mild, so is the itching; when wind is severe, the itching is also severe. If accompanied by damp-heat, blisters may result; if the damp-heat is severe, vesicles will arise, accompanied by redness of the skin.

Dispelling wind and overcoming dampness. Used when damp-heat has stagnated internally and is accompanied by exposure to wind, resulting in papular urticaria consisting of papules, small wheals or small blisters.

Nourishing blood and extinguishing wind. Used when the blood is injured and/or becomes deficient, thus giving rise to wind. Injury to the blood may result from the Liver losing its ability to nourish blood, which causes the blood to become deficient; and from pre-existing wind and dryness. Aging also results in insufficient qi and blood, which leads to a lack of nourishment of the skin and tissues. Conditions such as intense itching of the vagina or scrotum may result.

DISPELLING DAMPNESS

Dampness is a sticky, heavy type of excess that tends to accumulate and is difficult to remove. Dampness often combines with heat, wind, cold or summerheat to cause a variety of disorders; it may also transform into dryness or cold. Therefore, a strategy of dispelling dampness is often combined with heat-clearing, wind-dispelling, cold-scattering or summerheat-clearing strategies.

Dampness is dispelled using one of four methods, each of which is described in more detail below: resolving dampness, transforming dampness, drying dampness, and leaching out dampness. Heavy dampness requires drying or transforming; mild dampness requires resolving or leaching out. Because dampness-resolving herbs can harm the yin, their use must be carefully monitored in skin disorders involving yin deficiency, and completely avoided in treating yin-deficient individuals.

Clearing heat and resolving dampness. Used in treating serious damp-heat disorders such as recurrent eczema, especially when it affects the entire body.

Strengthening the Spleen and transforming dampness. Used in treating dampness of the Spleen that causes blisters accompanied by itching. Such cases present with no outright symptoms of heat, and the skin will generally not appear flushed. Other symptoms include stomach pain, fullness in the upper abdomen, lack of appetite, and watery stools.

Clearing heat and drying dampness. Used for damp-heat that is lodged in the Spleen/Stomach and that rises to the head and face, causing skin disorders such as folliculitis or impetigo.

Neutral leaching and resolving dampness. Used for damp-heat in the lower extremities that causes such skin disorders as chronic ulcers of the leg.

CLEARING HEAT

Treatment strategies for dealing with heat disorders should be based on the principle of "that which belongs to heat should be treated with cold medicines" *(Basic Questions,* Chapter 74). To properly utilize this method, one must differentiate between waxing heat and waning heat, and distinguish fire excess from that due to deficiency.

The bitter and cold herbs that are commonly used in clearing heat must be prescribed with prudence. Their continued use, especially after ulcers have begun to heal, can hinder complete healing. Overuse may lead to such gastric disturbances as acid regurgitation, unformed stools and loss of appetite. Formulas that clear heat should include herbs to support Stomach qi.

Cooling blood and clearing heat. Used in treating blood heat. Flourishing heat in the blood may result in diseases such as erysipelas, which is accompanied by flushed and burning sensations of the skin.

Clearing heat and relieving toxicity. Used in treating heat toxin that presents with such symptoms as redness, swelling, burning and pain (as in impetigo).

Clearing the nutritive level and relieving toxicity. Used in treating heat toxin in the nutritive level. Symptoms include high fever, red skin eruptions and blisters (as in pemphigus).

Enriching yin and relieving toxicity. Used in treating heat toxin injuring yin. When heat toxin enters the nutritive level, yin is injured and fluids are consumed. Skin symptoms include burning, redness and pain (as in exfoliative dermatitis).

MOISTENING DRYNESS

The strategy of moistening dryness is used in treating blood dryness, a pattern of wind-dryness that is caused by either blood heat or blood deficiency.

Cooling blood and moistening dryness. Used in treating blood heat/wind-dryness (a pattern of excess). Protracted blood heat gives rise to wind, which, if untreated, intensifies and transforms into dryness. Symptoms include dry skin or scalp, scaling and itching (as in seborrhea).

Nourishing blood and moistening dryness. Used in treating blood deficiency/wind-dryness. Long-standing wind harms the nutritive level and consumes blood. Symptoms include pale skin, dryness and scaling (as in pruritis).

WARMING AND CLEARING

Warming and clearing is used in treating patterns of cold. This strategy should not be used in treating disorders of yin deficiency accompanied by heat, because warm and drying herbs can exacerbate fire and seize yin.

Warming yang and clearing the channels. Used when wind-cold blocks the channels, preventing yang from reaching the extremities (as in chilblain or even frostbite).

Clearing channels and dispelling obstruction. Used when wind, cold or dampness blocks the channels, resulting in obstruction of blood and qi (as in scleroderma).

INVIGORATING BLOOD

The strategy of invigorating the blood is applied to conditions of blood stasis. The treatment method involves regulating qi and invigorating blood, or invigorating blood and dissolving stasis.

Herbs that invigorate blood are usually warm and hot, and should not be used in treating disorders caused by fire toxin. Also, because these herbs invigorate the blood and open the channels, they should be used with caution when treating pregnant women, or women who have excessive menstrual flow, and in cases of blood deficiency without signs of stasis.

Regulating qi and invigorating blood. Used in treating blood stasis caused by qi stagnation. When qi stagnates, blood stasis soon follows, and the channels become blocked (as in erythema nodosum).

Invigorating blood and transforming stasis. Used in treating long-standing blood stasis that obstructs the channels and prevents the generation of new blood. Conditions such as hair loss and advanced acne rosacea may result.

SOFTENING MASSES

The strategy of softening masses is used for treating masses caused by the accumulation of phlegm or the stagnation of qi.

Eliminating phlegm and softening masses. Phlegm that accumulates may become lodged between the skin and the tissues (as in lipoma).

Invigorating blood and softening masses. When qi stagnates, blood stasis ensues. The channels become blocked, phlegm accumulates, and nodules may form (as with keloids).

TONIFYING THE KIDNEY

This strategy is applied to patterns of Kidney yin deficiency and Kidney yang deficiency.

Enriching yin and directing fire downward. Used when insufficient Kidney yin leads to deficiency fire blazing upward. Symptoms include tidal fever, low back pain, night sweats and loss of hair (as in yin-deficiency type systemic lupus erythematosus).

Warming the Kidney and strengthening yang. Used when yang deficiency causes a preponderance of cold. Symptoms include spontaneous sweating, facial pallor, and pain and coldness of the low back and knees (as in yang-deficiency type systemic lupus erythematosus).

INTERNAL TREATMENT

The following types of herbal formulations are commonly used for oral administration in the treatment of skin diseases in Chinese medicine.

Decoctions

Almost all skin diseases can be treated with decoctions. In preparing a decoction, the medicinal ingredients are placed in water or other liquid (e.g., a mixture of wine and water) and boiled for a specified length of time. The dregs are strained and the liquid is ingested. Decoctions are absorbed quickly by the body, and their effects are almost immediate.

Cooking vessels used in preparing decoctions should be earthenware, ceramic, glass or stainless steel. If herbs are cooked in metal pots other than stainless steel, especially those made of aluminum and iron, there may be chemical reactions between the herbs and the metal in the containers. All pots should have tight-fitting lids.

The decocting liquid should cover the herbs by about one inch. Most Chinese sources recommend that for every 30 grams of herbs, 200-300 milliliters of water should be used. Allow the herbs to soak for awhile so that the active ingredients are effectively extracted during decoction. The decoction should be brought to a boil with high heat, and then cooked over low to medium heat for 20-30 minutes, or until about 200 milliliters (about one cup) of liquid remain.

While there are several methods of preparing decoctions, the most common is to decoct the herbs twice. After the first boiling the liquid is poured off and saved; fresh liquid (about four-fifths the amount used for the first boiling) is added to the left-over herbs, and again cooked until about one cup remains. The liquid from the two boilings is combined and the herbs discarded.

Decoctions should be taken warm, and administered in either two or three equal doses evenly spaced during the day. Patients with high fevers and/or bleeding may take decoctions cold. For disorders of the upper burner, decoctions should be taken *after* meals so as to prolong the formula's effects in the upper burner. For disorders affecting the middle and lower burners, decoctions should be taken *before* meals so that the medicine's effects reach their targets rapidly. Formulas that contain cloying and/or tonifying ingredients should be taken on an empty stomach. Formulas that have powerful effects, or that irritate the stomach, should be administered after meals.

CLINICAL NOTE: When taking decoctions, patients should avoid foods and beverages that are not easily digested, or that are stimulating. Those taking decoctions that are warming in nature should either avoid or moderate their intake of foods that are cold in nature, such as tofu, bean sprouts or cold beverages. Those on formulas that are cooling should avoid or moderate their intake of foods that are warm or hot in nature, such as garlic or chili peppers. After taking formulas that relieve the exterior, patients should rest in bed covered with heavy bed clothes in order to promote sweating.

Powders

Powders are prepared by grinding together dried medicinal substances into a coarse or fine consistency. Powders are mixed with approximately one to one-and-a-half cups of water, steeped or decocted, and then strained. Fine powders require only a few minutes of steeping time before the liquid can be ingested; coarse powders should be decocted for 5-10 minutes before straining the liquid and ingesting (this is known as a "draft"). Powders are almost as readily assimilated as decoctions.

Although many skin disorders are treatable with infusions of herbal powders, powders are more commonly prepared for external application (described below).

CLINICAL NOTE: Powders should always be stored in a cool, dry environment and in an airtight container to preserve their effectiveness.

Pills

Pills are traditionally prepared by combining finely powdered herbs with honey, vinegar, wine, fresh herb juice, rice paste or flour paste, and forming the product into round pills. Depending on the formula, pills range in size from that of a mung bean to a small chestnut.

Pills are commonly used in treating chronic disorders associated with deficiency (due to their slow rate of absorption), and as a delivery system for formulas that contain ingredients that should not or cannot be decocted, such as aromatic or toxic substances. Formulas are often produced in pill form and saved for later use in treating acute disorders in which the time required to prepare a decoction or powder would unduly delay immediate care. Chronic skin diseases, especially those in the pustular or ulcerated stages, can be effectively treated with pills.

CLINICAL NOTE: In general, the dosage for pills is small, and patients should be instructed to follow carefully the required dosage to avoid injury of the

Spleen/Stomach system. Proper storage is essential to maintain the efficacy of pills. As noted above, they should always be stored in a dark, cool and dry environment. In particular, pills that contain aromatic ingredients should be stored away from any source of heat. All pills should be checked regularly for infestation, and should always be used within one year of their preparation.

Special Pills

Pills are considered "special" when they contain any particularly expensive and/or specially processed ingredients. Classically, "special pills" referred to elixirs that contained such ingredients as mercury or sulfur and were taken to promote longevity.

Medicinal Wines

Medicinal wines are prepared by soaking medicinal substances in rice wine, sorghum wine or other spirits (such as vodka), in which the alcohol acts as a solvent. After the dregs are discarded, the liquid is taken orally. Since the wine itself nourishes and invigorates the blood and unblocks the channels, medicinal wines are commonly used to treat deficiency, or pain caused by wind-dampness or trauma. Thus skin disorders like scleroderma, which is often caused by deficiency of Kidney yang and the invasion of wind-cold into the skin, can be treated with medicinal wine formulas.

CLINICAL NOTE: Medicinal wines are typically hot in nature. Individuals who show signs of damp-heat, yin deficiency/yang exuberance, or those with high blood pressure or other abnormalities of the (biomedical) heart, lungs and liver, should not use medicinal wines. Patients with a history of alcohol abuse should also avoid them. Because medicinal wines can readily give rise to heat and dampness, prolonged use should be avoided. Individuals with damp-heat skin disorders should likewise avoid this type of remedy.

EXTERNAL TREATMENT

External treatment methods are an important component of traditional Chinese dermatology; even the ancient Chinese physicians understood the effectiveness of externally-applied medicines. As the prominent eighteenth-century physician Xu Da-Chun observed in *Discussion of the Origin and Development of Medicine,* "External diseases emphasize external [treatment] methods the most."

External methods are effective alone (as in the treatment of sores), or in combination with internal treatment (for more complex pathologies). As with internal medicines, the proper use of topical treatment depends on accurate pattern differentiation according to traditional methodology.

Because external medicines are applied directly to the skin, they are absorbed quickly and react rapidly. Following application, the skin, as well as the patient, should be observed closely for signs of adverse reaction.

External medicines are composed of two parts: the active ingredient and the vehicle (base or carrier). The active ingredient treats the condition itself; the concentration of the active ingredient determines the medicine's pharmacological effectiveness. The vehicle, on the other hand, determines the medicine's physical form— liquid, powder, ointment, etc. The efficacy of the medicine ultimately depends on selection of the proper vehicle. The common formats for traditional external medications, and their applications in dermatology, are described below.

Powders

Powders are prepared by grinding together dried medicinal substances into a powder of either coarse or fine consistency. They are then either sprinkled directly on the affected area, combined with juice from fresh vegetables or medicinal herbs to make a poultice, or mixed with a liquid (such as water, honey, vegetable oil, egg white, rice vinegar or an herbal decoction) to make a lotion or liniment.

Powders can function to protect, absorb and/or dry, depending on the desired therapeutic outcome. Their traditional functions include clearing heat, clearing toxin, transforming necrosis and promoting tissue growth, relieving itching and pain, and stopping bleeding. Suitable disorders for the use of powders include acute inflammation, superficial ulcerations and bleeding.

CLINICAL NOTE: Powders should not be applied directly to weeping lesions (use a wash instead), nor should they be applied to areas where hair re-growth is expected, such as the scalp. Herbal powders should be stored in airtight glass or porcelain containers in order to keep them fresh, and, more importantly, to maintain dryness.

Washes

Washes are prepared by first decocting herbs, and then applying the liquid (after suitable cooling) as a local swab, compress or bath. Washes biomedically function to cleanse, disinfect, soothe, cool and promote tissue healing. Their traditional functions include clearing and regulating the blood vessels, stopping oozing and relieving toxin to stop pain and itching. Washes are appropriate for treating skin disorders that present with oozing, and for itching of the skin, external genitalia and rectal area.

CLINICAL NOTE: Whenever possible, decoctions should be prepared on a daily basis, rather than in batches for use over several days; the fresher the decoction, the more effective it will be.

Ointments

Ointments are prepared by thoroughly combining powdered herbs with an oleaginous base such as a vegetable oil (safflower, soybean, corn, almond, or sesame oil are commonly used), animal grease (like pig or goose lard), lanolin or petroleum jelly. Ointments are either rubbed directly onto the affected area (an application especially appropriate for chronic or lichenified areas) or spread onto gauze and then bandaged over the skin.

Ointments are used to lubricate; to protect lesions with thick crusts, lichenification, or heaped-up scales; to prevent bacterial entry; and to promote healing.

CLINICAL NOTE: Ointments should not be applied to skin lesions that show erosion or constant oozing.

Plasters

Plasters are oil- or wax-based medications affixed onto a backing material, such as rice paper or cloth, and applied topically when long-term effects are required. The thickness of the plaster varies depending on whether the etiology of the disorder is external or internal. Thin plasters are used for treating exterior disorders, and function to relieve swelling, promote suppuration, clear necrosis, alleviate pain, promote healing and protect the skin. Thick plasters are used to treat interior disorders, and function to dispel wind-cold, harmonize the qi and blood, transform phlegm, strengthen the sinews and bones, and scatter masses. Thick plasters can be retained for longer periods of time (from a week to as long as a month) than thin plasters, which must be changed daily or every few days.

Skin disorders appropriate for treatment with plasters include chronic, localized and uniformly elevated lesions; ulcers that are superficial and flat; and other localized lesions, such as tinea and warts.

CLINICAL NOTE: Careful preparation of plasters is important in order to achieve maximum therapeutic effect. Plasters should be thin and applied evenly for superficial flat lesions, and thick and moist when applied to treat nodules. Careful removal of plasters is essential to avoid injury to the skin below. If the plaster is stuck to the skin, vegetable oil applied with a cotton swab to the points of adhesion will help loosen it. Patients exhibiting signs of allergy to plasters should discontinue treatment immediately. Allergic reactions (known in Chinese medicine as "plaster wind") include intense itching, redness, hives, blisters, or even oozing or ulceration, and should be treated like contact dermatitis.

Fumigation

Fumigation is a treatment method used in Chinese medicine since ancient times for both external and internal diseases. There are two methods of fumigation: medicinal steam and medicinal smoke. Medicinal steam is prepared by decocting an herbal preparation and then exposing the area to be treated to the vapors of the hot decoction. Medicinal smoke fumigation involves exposing the affected area to smoldering herbs or smoldering pieces of dried herbal syrup (a decoction that has been boiled to a concentrated liquid and then allowed to dry).

The function of fumigation is to kill parasites in order to relieve itching, warm the channels and promote the flow of qi and blood. Lesions treatable with fumigation include those that have undergone lichenification, chronic cold-type pustules, and chronic ulcers in general.

CLINICAL NOTE: Fumigation should not be used for acute skin inflammation. Individuals who suffer from hypertension or who are extremely deficient should also avoid this treatment.

Infusions

Infusions are prepared by soaking either single herbs or an entire herbal formula in water, vinegar or alcoholic spirits (e.g., rice or sorghum wine). Herbs are generally soaked for three to ten days, during which time the mixture is occasionally shaken. The liquid is then decanted and used for treatment, usually as a wash. Depending on the herbs used, infusions act to kill parasites in order to relieve itching, scatter stasis and reduce swelling, and to stimulate pigment regeneration. Indicated skin disorders include itching, hypopigmentation, some types of tinea, and hair loss.

Tinctures

Tinctures are made by soaking chopped or powdered herbs in ethyl or methyl alcohol; spirits such as vodka or brandy are commonly used as well. The mixture is stored in an amber glass or porcelain container with an airtight lid at a constant temperature for three to five days, during which time it is shaken once or twice a day. When ready, the tincture is strained through cheesecloth, and the dregs pressed to express the residual liquid. Depending on the herbs used, tinctures function to activate blood, reduce swelling, alleviate pain, or kill parasites in order to relieve itching.

Among the conditions suitable for treatment with tinctures are lesions that have not ulcerated.

CLINICAL NOTE: Because most tinctures have a stimulatory nature, lesions that are on the verge of ulcerating or that have already ulcerated should not be treated with tinctures.

Medicinal Spills

Medicinal spills are helical twists of absorbent paper inserted into deep ulcers, abscesses and fistulas in order to drain pus and necrotic debris. The traditional paper used for spills is made from mulberry bark. In the West, imported rice paper used for Asian watercolor painting may be substituted. The size of the paper used can range from six to eighteen centimeters in length, and from one to four centimeters in width (the length of the strip corresponds to the depth of the lesion).

Two methods are used to render a medicinal spill. In the first, a medicinal formula (in any format) is spread onto the paper strip, which is then twisted into the spill. In the second method, which is more commonly used today, the paper is twisted into a spill first, steam sterilized, and desiccated in a sterile environment. It is then moistened with sterile water and then dipped into herbal powder.

The medicinal spill should be gently inserted as far as possible into the lesion, leaving a 1–1.5 centimeter piece of the spill projecting outside the lesion and directed downward. The combination of the spiral form of the twist and the force of gravity causes the lesion to drain.

CLINICAL NOTE: As the lesion begins to heal from the inside, the depth of insertion of the medicinal spill should be reduced accordingly. Continued prodding of the new tissue will prevent effective healing. Also, if there is no longer any drainage, use of the spill should then be discontinued, and medicines to promote healing and tissue growth should be applied.

> **Table 5-1** General Principles of External Application
>
> - For the acute stage of skin inflammations presenting with redness, wheals or vesicles, and absent any signs of oozing, washes and powders are preferred, although compresses may sometimes be appropriate.
> - When lesions are oozing, or extreme redness is present, only compresses should be applied.
> - When oozing or erosion is minimal, and redness is diminished, ointments may then be used.
> - For chronic skin disorders with lichenification of the skin, ointments are preferred.
> - When inflammation is present, the initial treatment strategy should be to clear heat and relieve toxin. Once the inflammation is controlled, the underlying cause of the skin condition may then be addressed.
> - A low dosage and/or low concentration preparation should be prescribed at the outset of treatment; higher doses and/or higher concentration preparations may be introduced as treatment progresses and as the condition warrants.
> - Patients should be monitored constantly for signs of allergic reaction or negative side effects to the external preparation. If a reaction appears, medication should be discontinued, and the reaction treated immediately.

ACUPUNCTURE AND MOXIBUSTION TREATMENT

Acupuncture and moxibustion can be used to great effect, either alone or in conjunction with other therapies, in the treatment of dermatological diseases. Acupuncture is especially effective for treating ulcers, eczema and hives; moxibustion is usually indicated for chronic disorders, such as recalcitrant weeping ulcers.

Acupuncture

FILIFORM NEEDLING

When using acupuncture the principles of draining excess and tonifying deficiency should be followed. Conditions of excess require point prescriptions and needle manipulation techniques that drain to relieve the excess. Conditions of deficiency require points and manipulation techniques that tonify to relieve the deficiency.

> **Table 5-2** Common Points Used in Treating Skin Diseases

LI-11 *(qu chi)*	Urticaria, dryness of the skin, scrofula, skin allergies
LI-4 *(he gu)*	Urticaria, scabies, edema of the face, various types of pain
ST-36 *(zu san li)*	Skin allergies, skin disorders of the external genitalia
SP-6 *(san yin jiao)*	Eczema, urticaria, neurodermatitis, skin disorders of the external genitalia

SP-10 *(xue hai)*	Urticaria, neurodermatitis, itching
BL-40 *(wei zhong)*	Furuncles, leprosy, impetigo
GV-14 *(da zhui)*	Eczema, acute urticaria, herpes zoster
GB-20 *(feng chi)*, GB-31 *(feng shi)*	Acute urticaria, itching
BL-20 *(pi shu)*, BL-23 *(shen shu)*	Acute urticaria, alopecia, rashes during menstruation
CV-6 *(qi hai)*	Acute urticaria, eczema, neurodermatitis

Table 5-3 Point Prescriptions Used in Treating Common Skin Diseases

Acute urticaria	LI-11 *(qu chi)*, SP-10 *(xue hai)*, ST-36 *(zu san li)*, SP-6 *(san yin jiao)*
Alopecia areata	ST-36 *(zu san li)*, SP-6 *(san yin jiao)*, SP-10 *(xue hai)*, GB-20 *(feng chi)*
Eczema	GB-20 *(feng chi)*, GV-14 *(da zhui)*, ST-36 *(zu san li)*, BL-40 *(wei zhong)*, CV-6 *(qi hai)*
Neurodermatitis	LI-11 *(qu chi)*, LI-4 *(he gu)*, SP-10 *(xue hai)*, BL-40 *(wei zhong)*
Pruritis	LI-11 *(qu chi)*, SP-10 *(xue hai)*, BL-40 *(wei zhong)*, GV-14 *(da zhui)*
Psoriasis	LI-11 *(qu chi)*, LI-4 *(he gu)*, ST-36 *(zu san li)*, BL-15 *(xin shu)*, BL-18 *(gan shu)*
Seborrheic Dermatitis	LI-11 *(qu chi)*, LI-4 *(he gu)*, GB-20 *(feng chi)*, GV-16 *(feng fu)*, BL-20 *(pi shu)*
Herpes zoster	LI-11 *(qu chi)*, LI-4 *(he gu)*, ST-36 *(zu san li)*, SP-6 *(san yin jiao)*, SP-10 *(xue hai)*

TRI-ENSIFORM NEEDLING

Also known as bloodletting, this method is used primarily to clear heat and relieve toxicity, and to invigorate the blood and dissipate clumps. A tri-ensiform or pyramid needle is usually employed, although disposable lancets are becoming popular for this procedure. Suitable indications for bloodletting include psoriasis, acne, erysipelas and swelling due to furuncles. Three methods of bloodletting are used: pricking, clumping, and circumscribed.

Pricking. The needle is inserted rapidly into the point to a depth of about 0.1 *cun* (unit) and then quickly removed. A drop of blood will form spontaneously, or upon slight squeezing. Indications include swelling due to furuncles, and erysipelas.

Clumping. With this method the needle is lightly tapped over an area of the skin until it becomes flushed, or until a few drops of blood appear. Indications include acne and eczema.

Circumscribed. The needle is lightly applied around the lesion or swollen area until a few drops of blood appear. Indications include skin obstruction and shingles.

PLUM-BLOSSOM NEEDLING

This method is also known as dermal needling or seven-star needling. The plum-blossom needle is tapped over the skin until it becomes flushed. This method may be applied to the affected skin, to selected acupoints or to the skin along the course of a channel. Indications include eczema, neurodermatitis and pruritus. This method should not be used on swollen or necrotic skin.

Moxibustion

Moxibustion is an important and perhaps underutilized therapeutic method in traditional Chinese medicine. It may be used alone or in combination with other modalities such as acupuncture. In *Introduction to Medicine* (1575) Li Chan observed that "[w]henever a disease is not in time to be treated by herbs, or the effects of acupuncture are ineffective, then moxibustion must be used."

This method involves the burning of moxa (*Artemisia vulgaris,* or common mugwort) on or above the skin at the location of specific acupoints, or on or near the lesion itself. The heat of the cauterization, as well as the properties of the moxa itself, serve to warm the qi and blood in the channels, expel cold and dampness, restore yang, and in general help to regulate the Organs and restore health.

Moxibustion therapy consists of two types: direct and indirect.

DIRECT MOXIBUSTION

Direct moxibustion, which involves the burning of cone-shaped quantities of moxa directly on the skin, is of two kinds: non-scarring and scarring.

Non-scarring. A small moxa cone is burned on the skin. As the patient experiences pain, the cone is moved slightly to the side, or removed from the skin altogether, until the pain subsides; it is then replaced on the point. This process is repeated until the cone is consumed. Several cones may be burned successively over the same point in this manner until the skin is flushed (usually after the third to fifth cone). Suitable conditions for non-scarring moxibustion include eczema, psoriasis and neurodermatitis.

Scarring. With this method the skin is purposely scorched so that a blister forms, followed by a scar. The scar is a constant stimulation to the acupoint, thus achieving a therapeutic effect. Usually seven to nine moxa cones are burned successively on the skin. When pain is experienced, the practitioner may tap the skin nearby to lessen the pain. A local anesthetic may be administered if the pain is too severe. Generally, a blister will form within a few days, and then a scar within a month. This method is applied mainly to chronic and recalcitrant disorders such as warts, eczema and psoriasis.

INDIRECT MOXIBUSTION

This type of moxibustion is performed using an herbal medium between the moxa cone and the skin. The medium is selected for its specific therapeutic effect. For skin disorders the common mediums are garlic and ginger root.

Garlic. A garlic wafer about one-third of an inch in thickness is perforated with tiny holes, placed on the acupoint, and a medium-size moxa cone is set on the garlic and ignited. As the cone smolders, heat penetrates into the acupoint. If the patient experiences pain, the entire wafer may be lifted off the skin and then replaced after a moment. This procedure is repeated until the skin is flushed. Because garlic is a local irritant, after treatment a dry cotton ball should be used to wipe the excess garlic juice from the skin to prevent blistering. Garlic has acrid and warm properties, and is used to kill parasites, relieve and extract toxins, and reduce swelling and masses. Indirect moxibustion on garlic can be used in treating carbuncles, furuncles and other skin infections, and for insect bites and stings, such as those from mosquitos, wasps and scorpions.

Ginger. A ginger wafer is prepared and applied to the skin in the same manner as garlic. Ginger, whose properties are acrid and hot, functions to regulate the nutritive and protective levels, dispel cold and release the exterior, clear the channels and invigorate the collaterals, and treat wind, cold and dampness. Skin conditions suitable for treatment with indirect moxibustion on ginger include chilblain (non-ulcerative) and phlegmon due to skin obstruction.

CLINICAL NOTE: Moxibustion should not be used for patients with fevers or profuse sweating, or on the lower back or abdomen of pregnant women, which might induce miscarriage. Direct moxibustion should not be applied on the face.

CUPPING

Cupping is a method for treating disease by causing local congestion. Jars are heated to create a partial vacuum and then applied to the skin. The underlying tissues are drawn up, and local blood stasis is induced. The ancients first used cupping to drain pustulated sores. Through the centuries other disorders and indications have been found to respond well to cupping. This method may be used alone or in conjunction with other therapies, especially acupuncture. Skin disorders suitable for treatment by cupping include swelling due to insect bites or stings, snake bites, carbuncles and furuncles (especially those that do not readily come to a point).

CLINICAL NOTE: Cupping is contraindicated for patients with high fevers, convulsions, cramps or allergic skin disorders. Cupping should be avoided on areas of the skin that have little muscle or that have bony protuberances. Cupping is also contraindicated on the lower back or abdomen of pregnant women.

CHAPTER 6

Pruritus

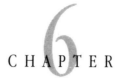

yăng fēng, "itching wind"

Pruritus, or itching, is a sensation that provokes the desire to rub or scratch the skin to obtain relief. It is described in many Chinese medical texts, including the *Divine Pivot,* Chapter 75:

> Harmful factors that traverse into and accumulate in the skin and tissues will be expelled outwardly, so that the interstices are opened . . . and the harmful factors move to and fro, thus causing itching.

Later works, such as the following passage from *Compendium of External Medicine* (1665), explained the causes of and treatment for itching: "Whenever wind-heat lodges in the skin, itching and small bumps arise. Treatment should be to disperse wind."

Itching is a characteristic of many skin diseases, and can be either localized or generalized. Diseases in which itching is most severe include scabies, pediculosis, insect bites, urticaria, dermatitis, contact dermatitis, lichen simplex chronicus and miliaria. Dry skin, especially in the elderly, often causes severe generalized itching. Systemic diseases associated with Liver or Kidney disorders, as well as polycythemia, lymphoma, leukemias and other cancers, are also known to cause itching. During the latter months of pregnancy, itching may occur without any sign of primary lesions. A psychogenic etiology may be considered when no other cause is found.

Signs & Symptoms

Redness, excoriation, fissures, and crusting can result from continuous scratching. Chronic rubbing and scratching can lead to thickening of the skin and discoloration. However, some individuals who complain of intense systemic pruritus will often show no signs of rubbing or scratching.

Traditional Chinese Etiology

Blood deficiency. This pattern is typically seen in the elderly, and in individuals with long-term illnesses, such that there is pre-existing deficiency of qi and blood resulting in deficiency of Liver blood. The Liver's function of dispersing blood is thus disturbed so that the skin lacks nourishment and becomes dry. Also, Liver blood deficiency gives rise to internal wind, which, because of its yang nature, spreads outward and lodges in the skin, thus producing pruritus.

Blood heat. Individuals prone to emotional disturbance, stress or anger often suffer from this pattern. Emotional disturbance causes stagnation of blood, which then transforms into heat and combines with the blood to form blood heat. Others who may present with this pattern include those who overindulge in foods that produce heat, such that this excess enters and contends with the blood. Protracted blood heat sears the Liver channel and provokes wind, which spreads outward and lodges in the skin, causing itching.

Wind. This type of pruritus occurs when the pores and interstices are not compact, which allows wind to enter the body. Protracted wind gives rise to heat, which causes pruritus.

Wind-dampness. This pattern is seen in individuals with pre-existing dampness who are then attacked by external wind. Pruritus is due to the contention between dampness and wind.

Wind-cold. Individuals with pre-existing yang deficiency are often affected by this type of pruritus after being attacked by wind-cold, which lodges in the skin.

Treatment

While most itching involves wind, one should be mindful that wind has various sources and that successful treatment of pruritus first requires careful pattern differentiation.

INTERNAL

Blood deficiency. Itching is more pronounced during autumn and winter, and less so during the spring and summer. The skin is usually dry, and chronic scratching results in lichenification; scaling may be extensive. Some patients may present with blood crusts due to scratching. Generalized symptoms may include lackluster complexion, palpitations, insomnia, light-headedness, a pale tongue with no coating and a wiry, thin pulse. Treatment strategy is to nourish the blood and moisten dryness, and dispel wind and stop the itching.

Formulas recommended for this pattern include Nourish the Blood and Moisten the Skin Decoction, or Tangkuei and Cooked Rehmannia Decoction to Nourish the Blood.

❦ Nourish the Blood and Moisten the Skin Decoction
养血润肤饮
yǎng xuè rùn fū yǐn

Radix Angelicae Sinensis (dang gui)	9g
Radix Rehmanniae Glutinosae Conquitae (shu di huang)	12g
Radix Rehmanniae Glutinosae (sheng di huang)	12g
Radix Astragali Membranacei (huang qi)	12g
Tuber Asparagi Cochinchinensis (tian men dong)	6g
Tuber Ophiopogonis Japonici (mai men dong)	6g
Rhizoma Cimicifugae (sheng ma)	3g
Radix Scutellariae Baicalensis (huang qin)	3g
Semen Persicae (tao ren)	2g
Flos Carthami Tinctorii (hong hua)	2g
Radix Trichosanthis Kirilowii (tian hua fen)	4.5g

PREPARATION & DOSAGE: Decoct and administer while still warm. One dose daily.

MODIFICATIONS: For dry stools, add 9-15g each of Semen Cannabis Sativae (huo ma ren) and Semen Pruni (yu li ren). For wind-dominant patterns that present with severe itching, add 4.5g of Rhizoma Gastrodiae Elatae (tian ma).

❧ Tangkuei and Cooked Rehmannia Decoction to Nourish the Blood

当熟养血汤

dāng shú yǎng xuè tāng

Radix Angelicae Sinensis (dang gui)	9g
Radix Rehmanniae Glutinosae Conquitae (shu di huang)	9g
Radix et Caulis Jixueteng (ji xue teng)	9g
Semen Zizyphi Spinosae (suan zao ren)	9g
Semen Biotae Orientalis (bai zi ren)	9g
Fructus Schisandrae Chinensis (wu wei zi)	9g
Herba seu Flos Schizonepetae Tenuifoliae (jing jie)	9g
Radix Ledebouriellae Divaricatae (fang feng)	9g
Radix Ligustici Chuanxiong (chuan xiong)	6g
Radix Polygoni Multiflori (he shou wu)	6g
Radix Glycyrrhizae Uralensis (gan cao)	6g

PREPARATION & DOSAGE: Decoct and administer while still warm. Three doses daily.

Blood heat. With this type of pruritus, scratching often produces red scratch marks that may ooze forth small amounts of blood. Generally, warmth or warm weather aggravates the itching, while coolness relieves it. Generalized symptoms may include thirst, restlessness, a red tongue or tongue tip with a thin yellow coating, and a wiry and rapid or slippery and rapid pulse. The strategy is to cool the blood and clear heat, and eliminate wind and stop the itching. The formula recommended for this pattern is Cool the Blood and Eliminate Wind Powder.

Cool the Blood and Eliminate Wind Powder
凉血消风散
liáng xuè xiāo fēng sǎn

Radix Rehmanniae Glutinosae (*sheng di huang*)	30g
Radix Angelicae Sinensis (*dang gui*)	9g
Herba seu Flos Schizonepetae Tenuifoliae (*jing jie*)	9g
Periostracum Cicadae (*chan tui*)	6g
Radix Sophorae Flavescentis (*ku shen*)	9g
Fructus Tribuli Terrestris (*bai ji li*)	9g
Rhizoma Anemarrhenae Asphodeloidis (*zhi mu*)	9g
Gypsum (*shi gao*)	30g
Radix Glycyrrhizae Uralensis (*gan cao*)	6g

PREPARATION & DOSAGE: Decoct and administer in one dose daily.

Wind. This pattern is often seen during the spring. Typically, the entire body is affected and the itching is not fixed. Chronic scratching may lead to thickening and even lichenification of the skin. The tongue is often red with a thin yellow coating, and the pulse is usually wiry and thin. The strategy is to collect wind and clear heat, and stop the itching. The formula recommended for this pattern is Zaocys Dispel Wind Decoction.

Zaocys Dispel Wind Decoction
乌蛇驱风汤
wū shé qū fēng tāng

Zaocys Dhumnades (*wu shao she*)	9g
Periostracum Cicadae (*chan tui*)	6g
Herba seu Flos Schizonepetae Tenuifoliae (*jing jie*)	9g
Radix Ledebouriellae Divaricatae (*fang feng*)	9g
Radix et Rhizoma Notopterygii (*qiang huo*)	9g
Radix Angelicae Dahuricae (*bai zhi*)	6g
Rhizoma Coptidis (*huang lian*)	6g
Radix Scutellariae Baicalensis (*huang qin*)	9g
Flos Lonicerae Japonicae (*jin yin hua*)	9g
Fructus Forsythiae Suspensae (*lian qiao*)	9g
Radix Glycyrrhizae Uralensis (*gan cao*)	6g

PREPARATION & DOSAGE: Decoct and administer in one dose daily.

Wind-dampness. Pruritus of this type is usually worse during the summer and autumn. Scratching often leaves wheals or blisters that may eventually erode. The tongue often has a yellow and sticky coating, and the pulse is slippery and rapid. The strategy is to scatter wind, eliminate dampness and stop the itching. The formula recommended for this pattern is Scorpion Formula.

PRURITIS

❧ Scorpion Formula
全虫方
quán chóng fāng

Buthus Martensi *(quan xie)*	6g
Spina Gleditsiae Sinensis *(zao jiao ci)*	12g
Fructus Gleditsiae Sinensis *(zao jiao)*	15-30g
Dry-fried Fructus Sophorae Japonicae Immaturus *(chao huai hua mi)*	15-30g
Radix Clematidis *(wei ling xian)*	12-30g
Radix Sophorae Flavescentis *(ku shen)*	6g
Cortex Dictamni Dasycarpi Radicis *(bai xian pi)*	15g
Cortex Phellodendri *(huang bai)*	15g

PREPARATION & DOSAGE: Decoct and administer in 1-2 doses daily.

CLINICAL NOTE: While taking this formula, the patient should abstain from foods that are spicy, and should also avoid lamb, capon and shrimp. Do not use this formula to treat itching caused by blood deficiency. Because of the toxicity of Buthus Martensi *(quan xie)*, this formula should not be used long-term. The recommended dosage is daily for 7-10 days, followed by three days' rest, then resume at a reduced dosage, e.g., once every other day.

Wind-cold. Pruritus of this pattern often occurs during the winter, and affects the head and face, neck, chest, hands and other exposed areas. Cold often exacerbates the itching, and warmth or sweating relieves it. The skin is dry and scaly. The tongue is often pale with a white coating, and the pulse is usually floating and moderate. The strategy is to dispel wind and scatter cold. The formula recommended for this pattern is Combined Cinnamon Twig and Ephedra Decoction.

❧ Combined Cinnamon Twig and Ephedra Decoction
桂枝麻黄各半汤
guì zhī má huáng gè bàn tāng

Ramulus Cinnamomi Cassiae *(gui zhi)*	5g
Radix Paeoniae Lactiflorae *(bai shao)*	3g
Herba Ephedrae *(ma huang)*	3g
Semen Pruni Armeniacae *(xing ren)*	3-6g
Honey-toasted Radix Glycyrrhizae Uralensis *(zhi gan cao)*	3g
Rhizoma Zingiberis Officinalis Recens *(sheng jiang)*	3g
Fructus Zizyphi Jujubae *(da zao)*	4 pieces

PREPARATION & DOSAGE: Decoct and administer in three daily doses. Note that some sources specify that the proper manner to decoct this formula is first to add Herba Ephedrae *(ma huang)* to the water, and when it boils, remove the froth and add the other ingredients.

EXTERNAL

For acute itching of any pattern, decoct together 30-60g of any two or three of the following herbs in equal amounts, and apply the decoction as a warm wash:

Fructus Kochiae Scopariae *(di fu zi)*
Fructus Xanthii Sibirici *(cang er zi)*
Herba Lemnae seu Spirodelae *(fu ping)*
Herba Leonuri Heterophylli *(yi mu cao)*
Fasciculus Vascularis Luffae *(si gua luo)*
Herba Equiseti Hiemalis *(mu zei)*
Rhizoma Cyperi Rotundi *(xiang fu)*
Excrementum Bombycis Mori *(can sha)*
Herba Lysimachiae *(jin qian cao)*
Fructus Evodiae Rutaecarpae *(wu zhu yu)*
Flos Lonicerae Japonicae *(jin yin hua)*

Afterward, apply Clearing and Cooling Powder (see sunburn in Chapter 12) or Stemona Tincture (see pediculosis in Chapter 11) to the affected sites. Internal remedies should be continued in order to resolve the root cause of the disorder.

ACUPUNCTURE

Filiform needling. For all patterns, the recommended acupoints include LI-11 *(qu chi)*, ST-36 *(zu san li)*, LI-4 *(he gu)*, SP-6 *(san yin jiao)* and SP-10 *(xue hai)*. Draining manipulation is applied, with or without needle retention. Treat once daily during acute outbreaks, and at least twice weekly thereafter to consolidate the effect.

Ear acupuncture. Recommended points include Occiput, Shenmen, Lung and Adrenal. During acute outbreaks, treat once daily, retaining needles for 30 minutes, and once or twice weekly thereafter.

CUPPING

Cupping may be used at two sets of points: [A] GV-14 *(da zhui)*, BL-12 *(feng men)*, BL-18 *(gan shu)*; [B] GV-12 *(shen zhu)*, BL-13 *(fei shu)*, BL-15 *(xin shu)*, BL-20 *(pi shu)*. Treat once daily or every other day, alternating the sets of points. Acupuncture may be applied to the points prior to cupping.

Traditional vs. Biomedical Treatment

In many cases, traditional treatment of pruritus is more effective than biomedical intervention, provided the pattern is correctly differentiated and appropriate treatment instituted, in order to resolve the root of the problem. Unless a physical cause is found and properly addressed, biomedical treatment is aimed solely at relieving the itch with antipruritics. Once such medications are discontinued, however, recurrence is common.

Prevention

Practitioners may be tempted to attribute all itching to the general category of wind. However, in treating pruritus, the root cause of wind must first be identified through careful pattern differentiation.

Additionally, biomedical causes such as systemic disorders should be sought and corrected. If possible, all medications should be stopped. Irritating clothing such as woolens should be avoided. Bathing should be minimized, as it may aggravate generalized itching.

Foods and beverages that provoke wind, particularly shellfish and alcohol, should likewise be avoided.

CHAPTER 7

Bacterial Infections

Impetigo
脓疱疮
nóng pào chuāng

Impetigo is a contagious superficial infection of the skin characterized by vesicles and pustules. The disease was first described during the Song dynasty in a work entitled *Complete Book of Ulcer Experience.* Through the ages impetigo has also been known as "yellow fluid sores" *(huáng shuǐ chuāng)*, "pus-dripping sores" *(dī nóng chuāng)* and "heavenly blister sores" *(tiān pào chuāng)*.

Biomedically, impetigo is caused by group A ß-hemolytic streptococci or *Staphylococcus aureus*.

Signs & Symptoms

Impetigo can affect any region of the body, but is usually confined to the arms and legs, and especially the area around the nose and mouth in children. The condition may occur after a skin abrasion, or it may be secondary to other lesions caused by insect bites, skin infections, or dermatitis. The skin first reddens and becomes itchy. Small vesicles and pustules develop. When these break, a thick yellow crust forms from the exudate.

Differential Diagnosis

Impetigo should be differentiated from other skin conditions that weep. These include insect bites, bullous diseases and the dermatites.

Chickenpox usually occurs in winter and spring. The lesions are the characteristic "teardrop" vesicles that contain clear fluid and stand out from their red areolas. Eruption may be generalized, with the upper trunk the most frequent site. Unlike impetigo lesions, those of chickenpox may even occur on the mucous membranes, such as in the mouth and upper respiratory tract.

Some forms of dermatitis may present vesicular lesions. However, the dermatites will have either distinct etiologies, such as contact dermatitis which is caused by substances in contact with the skin, or distinct locations, such as stasis dermatitis which usually affects the skin of the lower legs.

Traditional Chinese Etiology

Impetigo is caused by damp-heat attacking the protective level and then accumulating in the skin. The condition appears more frequently during the late summer when summerheat and dampness (humidity) are both present, which causes the skin pores to open and thereby become susceptible to attack by toxins and other pathogenic factors. Generally, a greater abundance of lesions on the upper half of the body indicates a preponderance of wind-heat, while a larger number on the lower half suggests a preponderance of damp-heat. If the condition progresses, fluids are consumed and source qi is injured, resulting in deficiency of qi and yin.

Treatment

INTERNAL

The pattern of damp-heat transforming into toxin is characterized by acute onset of symptoms, with large vesicles and large areas of erosion. Generalized symptoms may include ulcers of the mouth and tongue, fever, thirst, restlessness, dry stools, yellow urine, a red tongue with a thin yellow or dry yellow coating, and a thin, rapid pulse. The strategy is to clear heat and transform dampness, and to cool the blood and relieve toxicity. The formula recommended for this pattern is Clear the Spleen and Remove Dampness Decoction.

❦ Clear the Spleen and Remove Dampness Decoction
清脾除湿饮
qīng pí chú shī yǐn

Sclerotium Poriae Cocos *(fu ling)*	15g
Radix Rehmanniae Glutinosae *(sheng di huang)*	15g
Fructus Forsythiae Suspensae *(lian qiao)*	15g
Herba Artemisiae Yinchenhao *(yin chen hao)*	15g
Rhizoma Atractylodis Macrocephalae *(bai zhu)* (fried)	10g
Rhizoma Atractylodis *(cang zhu)* (fried)	10g
Tuber Ophiopogonis Japonici *(mai men dong)*	10g
Rhizome Alismatis Orientalis *(ze xie)*	10g
Dry-fried Fructus Gardeniae Jasminoidis *(chao zhi zi)*	10g
Rhizoma Cyperi Rotundi *(xiang fu)* (fried)	10g
Radix Astragali Membranacei *(huang qi)*	6g

PREPARATION & DOSAGE: Decoct and administer in three daily doses.

Chronic conditions show lesions that have sticky exudates and scaling over large areas that do not easily resolve. Generalized symptoms may include thirst without the desire to drink, fatigue, shortness of breath, incoherent speech, restlessness, disturbed sleep, a pink tongue with thin pale or little coating, and a thin, submerged pulse. The strategy is to benefit qi and nourish yin, and to clear and relieve toxicity. The formula recommended for this pattern is Codonopsis, Astragalus, and Anemarrhena Decoction.

❧ Codonopsis, Astragalus, and Anemarrhena Decoction
参芪知母汤
shēn qí zhī mǔ tāng

Tuber Asparagi Cochinchinensis *(tian men dong)*	12g
Tuber Ophiopogonis Japonici *(mai men dong)*	12g
Radix Dioscoreae Oppositae *(shan yao)*	12g
Radix Astragali Membranacei *(huang qi)*	12g
Radix Codonopsitis Pilosulae *(dang shen)*	12g
Herba Artemisiae Annuae *(qing hao)*	12g
Radix Ampelopsis Japonicae *(bai lian)*	12g
Rhizoma Atractylodis *(cang zhu)*	9g
Rhizoma Atractylodis Macrocephalae *(bai zhu)*	9g
Radix Rehmanniae Glutinosae *(sheng di huang)*	9g
Radix Rehmanniae Glutinosae Conquitae *(shu di huang)*	9g
Radix Paeoniae Rubrae *(chi shao)*	9g
Radix Paeoniae Lactiflorae *(bai shao)*	9g
Cortex Poriae Cocos *(fu ling pi)*	15g
Rhizoma Anemarrhenae Asphodeloidis *(zhi mu)*	15g
Semen Coicis Lachryma-jobi *(yi yi ren)*	30g

PREPARATION & DOSAGE: Decoct and administer in three daily doses.

EXTERNAL

Where the affected skin is more confined in area, Clearing and Cooling Ointment is recommended.

❧ Clearing and Cooling Ointment
清凉膏
qīng liáng gāo

Lime	0.5 liters (dry measure)
Water	2 liters

PREPARATION & DOSAGE: Mix the lime with the water, allow to settle. Gently blow the floating lime powder to one side, and remove the mid-level fluid. Combine one part fluid with one part sesame oil until the mixture is emulsified. Apply once daily.

CLINICAL NOTE: Because of the caustic properties of lime, do not use this formula long-term. Daily application is suggested for 4-5 days. If symptoms do not improve, discontinue and consider other remedies.

For lesions with excessive exudate and erosion, Black Solanum Compress may be applied, followed by Indigo Powder.

❧ Black Solanum Compress
龙葵湿敷剂
lóng kuí shī fū jì

Herba Solani Nigri *(long kui)*	15g
Galla Rhois Chinensis *(wu bei zi)*	15g
Pericarpium Punicae Granati *(shi liu pi)*	30g

PREPARATION & DOSAGE: Decoct and apply as a wet compress for 10-15 minutes, 1-2 times daily. Then apply Indigo Powder.

❧ Indigo Powder
青黛散
qīng dài sǎn

Indigo Pulverata Levis *(qing dai)*	60g
Gypsum *(shi gao)*	120g
Talcum *(hua shi)*	120g
Cortex Phellodendri *(huang bai)*	60g

PREPARATION & DOSAGE: Grind the ingredients together into a fine powder. Mix with sesame oil to form a paste. Spread onto sterile gauze and affix to the affected area.

Other external remedies that may be applied include Evodia Ointment, or Formula to Wash Sores.

❧ Evodia Ointment
吴茱萸膏
wú zhū yú gāo

Fructus Evodiae Rutaecarpae *(wu zhu yu)* (ground)	1g
Petroleum Jelly	9g

PREPARATION & DOSAGE: Thoroughly mix the herbal powder and petroleum jelly. Allow to steep for two days. Apply 1-2 times daily.

❧ Formula to Wash Sores
洗疮方
xǐ chuāng fāng

Cortex Phellodendri *(huang bai)*	30g
Radix et Rhizoma Rhei *(da huang)*	30g
Radix Sophorae Flavescentis *(ku shen)*	30g

Herba Taraxaci Mongolici cum Radice *(pu gong ying)* 20g
Radix Stemonae *(bai bu)*... 20g
Flos Lonicerae Japonicae *(jin yin hua)*........................... 20g

PREPARATION & DOSAGE: Decoct and wash the affected area 3-5 times daily. Lesions that present sticky exudate or crusting should first undergo cleansing with warm, dilute saline before applying the herbal remedy.

EMPIRICAL REMEDIES

[A] For impetigo of the scalp, Fresh Houttuynia Wash[1] may be applied by first decocting 250g of Herba cum Radice Houttuyniae Cordatae *(yu xing cao)* in 3 liters of water until 2 liters of fluid remain. Steam the affected area with the hot decoction. Then, after the decoction has sufficiently cooled, apply the decoction with a washcloth to the affected area as a hot compress. When the decoction cools even further, wash the affected area. The entire process should take about 20 minutes. Apply once daily.

[B] For protracted cases that show deficiency of normal qi along with deficiency of qi and blood, such that the lesions are chronically ulcerated and non-healing, Modified Tonify the Middle and Augment the Qi Decoction[2] is recommended.

❦ Modified Tonify the Middle and Augment the Qi Decoction
补中益气汤加减
bǔ zhōng yì qì tāng jiā jiǎn

Radix Astragali Membranacei *(huang qi)*........................... 50g
Rhizoma Atractylodis Macrocephalae *(bai zhu)*..................... 15g
Radix Codonopsitis Pilosulae *(dang shen)*......................... 15g
Radix Angelicae Sinensis *(dang gui)*.............................. 15g
Honey-toasted Radix Glycyrrhizae Uralensis *(zhi gan cao)*......... 10g
Rhizoma Cimicifugae *(sheng ma)*................................... 10g
Radix Lateralis Aconiti Carmichaeli Praeparata *(fu zi)*........... 10g
Dry-fried Myrrha *(chao mo yao)*................................... 10g
Dry-fried Gummi Olibanum *(chao ru xiang)*......................... 10g
Radix Angelicae Dahuricae *(bai zhi)*.............................. 10g
Cortex Cinnamomi Cassiae *(rou gui)*............................... 5g

PREPARATION & DOSAGE: Decoct and administer in one dose daily.

[C] Bake one cucumber vine with the leaves removed in an oven until crisp. Grind into a fine powder and mix with sesame oil to form a paste. Apply to the affected area 1-2 times daily.[3]

[D] Decoct 60-150g fresh pomegranate skin in water until a concentrated liquid remains. Wash or apply to the affected area three times daily.[4]

[E] Combine together one mashed unripe papaya (about 500g) with 25ml rice vinegar and 30g salt. Extract the liquid by pressing or pouring through a strainer. Apply the liquid to the affected area 1-2 two times daily.[5]

Traditional vs. Biomedical Treatment

Traditional treatment of impetigo may not necessarily be more effective in shortening the course of disease. It may, however, be less harsh than biomedical therapy, which usually consists of administering oral antibiotics that can lead to untoward side effects or bacterial resistance. One advantage of traditional treatment is that herbs which strengthen the immune system can be used to help the body's own defense mechanisms combat the bacterial infection.

Prevention

In children it is important to strengthen the Spleen/Stomach energy so that the protective level is able to ward off attacks of summerheat and dampness.

Patients with impetigo and their families should be advised about personal hygiene and the importance of regular bathing and frequent hand-washing. This is especially important during hot, humid weather during which there is a greater chance for skin trauma and insect bites owing to exposed extremities; the skin is also moist at such times, which favors bacterial growth. Infected individuals should be advised to apply topical antibiotics immediately to cuts, abrasions, insect bites and infected lesions in order to prevent further spread of impetigo.

Impetigo in infants can be highly contagious. It is a serious condition that requires prompt treatment.

Folliculitis
毛囊炎
máo náng yán

Folliculitis is a bacterial infection of the hair follicle that results in a pustule. In Chinese medicine different names are given to this condition depending on the location of the lesions. Those that appear at the hairline, especially at the nape, are called "hairline sores" *(fà jì chuāng)*. Lesions that appear in the bearded areas in men are known as "swallow's nest sores" *(yàn wō chuāng)* or "goat's beard sores" *(yáng hú zǐ chuāng)*.

Biomedically, folliculitis is usually caused by *Staphylococcus aureus* or *Pseudomonas* bacteria.

Signs & Symptoms

Pain, itching, and minor burning occur upon manipulation of the hair. The scalp and extremities are most often affected. Chronic folliculitis can affect areas that have deep follicles and which undergo persistent trauma, such as the bearded areas in men and the axillae in women.

Differential Diagnosis

Folliculitis should be differentiated from carbuncles, furuncles and acne. Folliculitis affects the openings of the hair follicles, whereas furuncles and carbuncles are inflammations of the entire hair follicle. Furuncles and carbuncles are contagious under conditions of poor hygiene and are seen in patients who are immuno-compromised. Carbuncles may be accompanied by fever. While acne is also characterized by inflamed nodules and pus-filled cysts, the presence of either blackheads and/or whiteheads differentiates it from folliculitis.

Traditional Chinese Etiology

Two primary patterns of folliculitis are accumulation of damp-heat combined with attack by external wind, or, if the condition becomes chronic, deficiency of both the qi and blood.

Accumulation of damp-heat combined with attack by external wind. This pattern is commonly seen in overweight individuals who often have an abundance of internal dampness and phlegm. Overindulgence in greasy and sweet foods can also result in accumulation of dampness, which will impair the Spleen's transportive and transformative functions and lead to build-up of damp-heat. The lesions appear when the pre-existing condition of damp-heat is followed by an attack of external wind.

Deficiency of both the qi and blood. If the acute condition remains untreated, or is not treated properly, chronic lesions develop such that the qi and blood are consumed and the normal qi is weakened. The toxin (pus) is not relieved and continues to accumulate, thus giving rise to repeated lesions.

Treatment

INTERNAL

Accumulation of damp-heat combined with attack by external wind. Cases presenting with this pattern are of short duration, and lesions exhibit redness and swelling or moistness and swelling, oozing of pus upon pressure, constant pain and thick scars after healing. The tongue is red with a thin yellow, or yellow and slightly sticky coating, and the pulse is soft and rapid. The strategy is to clear and resolve damp-heat, and invigorate the blood and relieve toxicity.

Formulas recommended for this pattern include Hornet Nest Powder, or Five-Ingredient Decoction to Relieve Toxin.

❧ Hornet Nest Powder
蜂房散
fēng fáng sǎn

Nidus Vespae *(lu feng fang)*	6g
Rhizome Alismatis Orientalis *(ze xie)*	12g
Herba cum Radice Violae Yedoensitis *(zi hua di ding)*	12g
Sclerotium Poriae Cocos Rubrae *(chi fu ling)*	12g
Radix Paeoniae Rubrae *(chi shao)*	12g
Flos Lonicerae Japonicae *(jin yin hua)*	15g
Herba Taraxaci Mongolici cum Radice *(pu gong ying)*	15g
Radix et Rhizoma Notopterygii *(qiang huo)*	4.5g
Bombyx Batryticatus *(jiang can)*	9g

PREPARATION & DOSAGE: Decoct and administer once daily.

CLINICAL NOTE: This formula should not be used long-term as several of the ingredients are cold in nature. Administration once daily for 7-10 days is recommended. If symptoms do not improve, discontinue and consider other remedies.

❧ Five-Ingredient Decoction to Eliminate Toxin
五味消毒饮
wǔ wèi xiāo dú yǐn

Flos Lonicerae Japonicae *(jin yin hua)*	9g
Flos Chrysanthemi Indici *(ye ju hua)*	3g
Herba Taraxaci Mongolici cum Radice *(pu gong ying)*	3g
Herba cum Radice Violae Yedoensitis *(zi hua di ding)*	3g
Herba Begoniae Fimbristipulatae *(zi bei tian kui)*	3g

PREPARATION & DOSAGE: Decoct the herbs. Add half a small rice bowl of rice wine, then bring the decoction to a rolling boil again, and remove immediately from heat. Administer the decoction while hot. Induce sweating by having the patient rest in bed covered by heavy bedclothes.

Deficiency of both the qi and blood. Lesions of this pattern present with mild or undemarcated swelling, clear or opaque exudate, and are painful, especially upon pressure. The tongue is pale with thin or little coating, and the pulse is thin. The strategy is to benefit qi and nourish yin, and support the normal qi in order to expel the pus. The formula recommended for this pattern is Astragalus and Paris Decoction.

❧ Astragalus and Paris Decoction
黄芪蚤休饮
huáng qí zǎo xiū yǐn

Honey-fried Radix Astragali Membranacei *(zhi huang qi)*	12g
Flos Lonicerae Japonicae *(jin yin hua)*	12g
Rhizoma Paris Polyphyllae *(zao xiu)*	10g
Radix Angelicae Sinensis *(dang gui)*	10g
Bulbus Fritillariae Thunbergii *(zhe bei mu)*	10g
Radix Scrophulariae Ningpoensis *(xuan shen)*	10g
Semen Phaseoli Calcarati *(chi xiao dou)*	30g
Radix Dioscoreae Oppositae *(shan yao)*	30g
Radix et Rhizoma Notopterygii *(qiang huo)*	3g
Rhizome Alismatis Orientalis *(ze xie)*	6g

PREPARATION & DOSAGE: Decoct and administer in one daily dose.

EXTERNAL

For acute outbreaks of folliculitis, either Daphne Wash or Xanthium and Kochia Wash may be used.

Daphne Wash
芫花水洗剂
yuán huā shuǐ xǐ jì

Flos Daphnes Genkwa *(yuan hua)*
Fructus Zanthoxyli Bungeani *(chuan jiao)*
Cortex Phellodendri *(huang bai)*

PREPARATION & DOSAGE: Grind equal amounts of the herbs together into a coarse powder, and put into a cloth bag. Boil in 2.5-3.0 liters of water for 30 minutes. Apply the decoction as a warm compress or as a wash for 15 minutes twice daily.

CLINICAL NOTE: Flos Daphnes Genkwa *(yuan hua)* is toxic. Avoid contact with the eyes and mouth.

Xanthium and Kochia Wash
苍肤水洗剂
cāng fū shuǐ xǐ jì

Fructus Xanthii Sibirici *(cang er zi)*	15g
Fructus Kochiae Scopariae *(di fu zi)*	15g
Radix Clematidis *(wei ling xian)*	15g
Folium Artemisiae Argyi *(ai ye)*	15g
Fructus Evodiae Rutaecarpae *(wu zhu yu)*	15g

PREPARATION & DOSAGE: Decoct the ingredients in 1.75 liters of water for 25 minutes. Apply the warm decoction as a wet compress or as a wash for 15 minutes, 3-5 times daily.

For lesions that show swelling but no ulceration, use either Jade Dew Powder (see herpes simplex in Chapter 8) or Golden-Yellow Powder According to One's Wishes.

Golden-Yellow Powder According to One's Wishes
如意金黄散
rú yì jīn huáng sǎn

Radix Trichosanthis Kirilowii *(tian hua fen)*	50g
Radix et Rhizoma Rhei *(da huang)*	25g
Cortex Phellodendri *(huang bai)*	25g
Tuber Curcumae *(yu jin)*	25g
Radix Angelicae Dahuricae *(bai zhi)*	25g
Rhizoma Arisaematis *(tian nan xing)*	10g
Pericarpium Citri Reticulatae *(chen pi)*	10g
Rhizoma Atractylodis *(cang zhu)*	10g
Cortex Magnoliae Officinalis *(hou po)*	10g
Radix Glycyrrhizae Uralensis *(gan cao)*	10g

PREPARATION & DOSAGE: Grind the ingredients together into a fine powder, then add sesame oil to form a paste. Apply 1-2 times daily to the affected area.

ACUPUNCTURE

For individual lesions a 1-unit 32-34 gauge needle may be inserted horizontally into the tissue underlying the eruption. Treat once daily using even manipulation, and retain needle for 15 minutes. In general, symptoms are alleviated after 1-2 treatments.

For multiple eruptions, needle GV-14 *(da zhui)*, BL-13 *(fei shu)*, BL-15 *(xin shu)*, BL-17 *(ge shu)*, BL-18 *(gan shu)* and GV-12 *(shen zhu)*. Treat once daily using even manipulation, and retain needles for 15-20 minutes. Ten treatments are considered one course of therapy. Symptom improvement should be evident after one course.

MOXIBUSTION

Burn moxa cones or moxa roll on GV-14 *(da zhui)*, BL-17 *(ge shu)* and at the lesion site. Treat for 20 minutes, once daily. Ten treatments are considered one course of therapy. Symptom improvement should be evident after one course.

Traditional vs. Biomedical Treatment

Traditional treament is probably more effective than biomedical intervention in addressing folliculitis. In the latter, topical medications are usually prescribed, but the condition may recur once medication is discontinued. According to Chinese medicine, recurrence happens when one has failed to address the root of the problem. Therefore, since traditional treatment is aimed at resolving the root, folliculitis should not recur if the pattern is correctly differentiated and treated accordingly.

Prevention

Folliculitis should be treated immediately to prevent the condition from becoming chronic. The patient should avoid picking and/or squeezing the lesions, especially in bearded areas.

Furuncles
疖
jiē

A furuncle, commonly known as a boil, is an infection of the deepest portion of the hair follicle in which the inflammation spreads to the surrounding skin. One of the earliest records of furuncles in the ancient Chinese medical literature is found in the 5th century compilation, *Liu Juanzi's Formulas Passed Down from a Spirit*. In *Principles and Experiences of External Diseases* (1531) furuncles are described as "arising suddenly, with redness and burning pain, swelling of the skin, size of one to two units, and healing after exudate is released." Because furuncles often break out during the summer, other popular terms for the condition are "summer furuncles" *(shǔ jiē)* and "heat furuncles" *(rè jiē)*.

Bomedically, furuncles are caused primarily by *Staphylococcus aureus* bacteria.

Signs & Symptoms

The lesions most often appear on the face, scalp, thighs, buttocks, perineum, or in the axillae. The primary lesion is a small, round, painful subcutaneous nodule that later becomes raised, tender, shiny, and bright red. As it matures, the furuncle turns fluctuant and is capped with a pustule. Spontaneous rupture of the lesion may result. When the lesions are many and recurrent, with the possibility of an accompanying slight fever, the condition is known as furunculosis.

Differential Diagnosis

Furuncles should be differentiated from carbuncles and folliculitis. Carbuncles are a cluster of furuncles in which the infection has spread subcutaneously, resulting in deep suppuration. Carbuncles develop more slowly than single furuncles, and may be accompanied by fever and prostration. Diabetes mellitus, debilitating diseases and old age are predisposing factors for carbuncles.

Folliculitis is an infection of the *opening* of the hair follicles, while furuncles are inflammations and necroses of *entire* hair follicles.

Traditional Chinese Etiology

Most cases of furuncles arise in patients with a pre-existing condition of accumulated heat. Toxin arises either internally from the accumulated heat, or externally from attack by damp-summerheat, which then gathers in the skin and gives rise to the lesions.

Treatment

INTERNAL

Lesions of damp-heat toxin show pronounced redness, swelling and pain at onset. Generalized symptoms may include fever, aversion to cold, a thin yellow tongue coating and a rapid pulse. The strategy is to clear heat (or summerheat) and resolve dampness, and relieve toxicity. The formula recommended for this pattern is Chrysanthemum Decoction to Defeat Toxin.

❧ Chrysanthemum Decoction to Defeat Toxin
野菊败毒汤
yě jú bài dú tāng

Flos Chrysanthemi Indici *(ye ju hua)*	9g
Radix Scrophulariae Ningpoensis *(xuan shen)*	9g
Fructus Forsythiae Suspensae *(lian qiao)*	9g
Herba cum Radice Violae Yedoensitis *(zi hua di ding)*	9g
Flos Lonicerae Japonicae *(jin yin hua)*	12g
Herba Taraxaci Mongolici cum Radice *(pu gong ying)*	15g

Bulbus Fritillariae Thunbergii *(zhe bei mu)* 6g
Radix Glycyrrhizae Uralensis *(gan cao)* 3g

PREPARATION & DOSAGE: Decoct and administer in three doses daily.

CLINICAL NOTE: This formula should not be taken by patients with fevers of the deficient qi type, or by those whose lesions have ulcerated.

MODIFICATIONS: For furuncles that arise due to summerheat, add Herba Agastaches seu Pogostemi *(huo xiang)*, Herba Eupatorii Fortunei *(pei lan)*, Six-One Powder (see below) and Semen Coicis Lachryma-jobi *(yi yi ren)*. For extreme accumulation of heat-toxin, add dry-fried Rhizoma Coptidis *(huang lian)*, Radix Scutellariae Baicalensis *(huang qin)* and dry-fried Fructus Gardeniae Jasminoidis *(chao zhi zi)*. For lesions that are slow to suppurate, add Spina Gleditsiae Sinensis *(zao jiao ci)* and Radix Ligustici Chuanxiong *(chuan xiong)*. For scanty and deep yellow urine, add Semen Plantaginis *(che qian zi)*, Sclerotium Poriae Cocos Rubrae *(chi fu ling)* and Herba Lophatheri Gracilis *(dan zhu ye)*. For constipation, add Fructus Citri Aurantii *(zhi ke)*, wine-fried Radix et Rhizoma Rhei *(jiu chao da huang)* and Mirabilitum Purum *(xuan ming fen)*. For extreme deficiency of qi and blood, add Radix Astragali Membranacei *(huang qi)*, Radix Codonopsitis Pilosulae *(dang shen)* and Radix Cynanchi Baiwei *(bai wei)*. For cases with slight yin deficiency, add Six-Ingredient Pill with Rehmannia *(liu wei di huang wan)*.

❧ Six-One Powder
六一散
liù yī sǎn

Talcum *(hua shi)* 60g
Radix Glycyrrhizae Uralensis *(gan cao)* 10g

PREPARATION & DOSAGE: Grind the ingredients together into a fine powder. Wrap 9g in cloth and add to recommended decoction.

EXTERNAL

For acute lesions, the strategy is to reduce the swelling and alleviate the pain. For such cases, either Jade Dew Powder (see herpes simplex in Chapter 8), Golden-Yellow Powder, or Three-Yellow Wash is recommended.

❧ Golden-Yellow Powder
金黄散
jīn huáng sǎn

Radix et Rhizoma Rhei *(da huang)* 25g
Cortex Phellodendri *(huang bai)* 25g
Rhizoma Curcumae Longae *(jiang huang)* 25g
Radix Angelicae Dahuricae *(bai zhi)* 25g
Rhizoma Arisaematis *(nan xing)* 10g
Pericarpium Citri Reticulatae *(chen pi)* 10g

Rhizoma Atractylodis *(cang zhu)* 10g
Cortex Magnoliae Officinalis *(hou po)* 10g
Radix Glycyrrhizae Uralensis *(gan cao)* 10g
Radix Trichosanthis Kirilowii *(tian hua fen)* 50g

PREPARATION & DOSAGE: Grind the ingredients together into a fine powder. Prior to application, mix the powder with commercially available chrysanthemum flower essence or honeysuckle flower essence (water may be substituted) to form a paste. Apply once daily. Store the extra powder in a glass container with a tight-fitting lid.

Three-Yellow Wash
三黄洗剂
sān huáng xǐ jì

Radix et Rhizoma Rhei *(da huang)*
Cortex Phellodendri *(huang bai)*
Radix Scutellariae Baicalensis *(huang qin)*
Radix Sophorae Flavescentis *(ku shen)*

PREPARATION & DOSAGE: Grind equal amounts of the herbs together into a fine powder. For every 10-15g of powder, mix with 100ml of distilled water and 1ml of carbolic acid (for medicinal use). Apply with sterile gauze or cotton swab 4-5 times daily.

For Jade Dew Powder (see herpes simplex in Chapter 8), mix the powder with chrysanthemum or honeysuckle flower essence to form a paste. Apply once daily.

For suppurated lesions, the strategy is to promote the discharge of pus. The formula recommended in such cases is Red Cloth Plaster.

Red Cloth Plaster
红布膏
hóng bù gāo

Magarita *(zhen zhu)* 90g
Calomelas *(qing fen)* 15g
Realgar *(xiong huang)* 15g
Mimium *(qian dan)* 15g
Resina Pini *(song xiang)* 150g

PREPARATION & DOSAGE: Grind all ingredients together into a fine powder, then mix with castor seed oil to form a paste. Apply 1-2 times daily, and cover with a dressing.

CLINICAL NOTE: Because of the toxicity of some of the ingredients (Minium, Calomelas, Realgar), long-term use should be avoided.

Following suppuration, to promote generation of flesh and closure of the wound, apply Borneol and Gypsum Powder (see herpes zoster in Chapter 8) directly to the affected area, followed by Coptis Ointment (again see herpes zoster), which is first applied onto a dressing to cover the affected area. Apply once daily.

ACUPUNCTURE

In treating furuncles, the primary acupoint for needling is GV-10 *(ling tai)*, as it clears heat from the qi and blood. Use even manipulation and retain the needle for 10-15 minutes. After removing the needle, squeeze 2-3 three drops of blood from the needle hole. For furuncles on the head and face, add LI-4 *(he gu)* and LI-11 *(qu chi)*; for furuncles on the chest and stomach, add ST-36 *(zu san li)* and SP-6 *(san yin jiao)*; for furuncles on the back, add BL-40 *(wei zhong)*. Treat once daily, with ten sessions considered one course of therapy. Improvement is usually apparent within one course.

EMPIRICAL REMEDIES

[A] For early stage furuncles, stir-fry 3g of dried raw ginger until brown. Grind into a powder and mix with vinegar to form a paste. Apply to the affected area, leaving the head of the lesion clear.[6]

[B] For multiple lesions, bake ripened chili peppers in an iron skillet until crisp. Grind into a powder and sprinkle on the lesions once daily. Or mix the powder with sesame oil to form a paste and apply on the lesions once daily.[7]

[C] For early stage furuncles, Modified Golden-Yellow Powder According to One's Wishes[8] is recommended.

❦ Modified Golden-Yellow Powder According to One's Wishes
如意金黄散加减
rú yì jīn huáng sǎn jiā jiǎn

Rhizoma Paris Polyphyllae *(zao xiu)*	1.5g
Tuber Dioscoreae Bulbiferae *(huang yao zi)*	1.5g
Rhizoma Coptidis *(huang lian)*	0.5g
Realgar *(xiong huang)*	0.5g
Borneol *(bing pian)*	0.3g

PREPARATION & DOSAGE: Grind the ingredients together into an extremely fine powder. Store in a container in a dry, cool and dark place. When ready to use, mix with honey, tea, wine or petroleum jelly to form a paste. Apply 1-2 times daily. It has been suggested that healing usually occurs in 2-5 days.[9]

Traditional vs. Biomedical Treatment

Traditional treatment of the occasional furuncle may be no more effective than biomedical treatment, which recommends applying intermittent moist heat to the lesion to allow it to point and drain spontaneously. However, for cases of furunculosis (multiple and recurrent furuncles), traditional treatment may prove superior to biomedical intervention, which consists of administering systemic antibiotics. Often, prior to starting such therapy, it is necessary to have culture and sensitivity tests performed so that the correct antibiotic is prescribed. Once antibiotics are started, the problems of undesirable side effects and recurrence after the medication is discontinued must be considered. With traditional treatment, if the root of the condition is resolved, and modifications in diet and living habits are undertaken, recurrence should not take place.

Prevention

Because furuncles may become recurrent under unsanitary conditions, good personal hygiene is essential. Patients should be advised not to pick or squeeze the lesions.

According to Chinese medicine, this condition is more common during hot weather when attack by summerheat is most likely. Measures to dispel summerheat should be undertaken, such as drinking plenty of fluids and eating foods that are cool in nature, such as watermelon, mung bean soup or chrysanthemum tea. Foods and beverages that are spicy or warm/hot in nature, such as lamb, shrimp, capon and alcohol, should be avoided.

Carbuncles
疽
jū

A carbuncle is a cluster of interconnected furuncles that have several heads from which they drain. The condition is often slow to heal and leaves a large scar. In Chinese medicine the word *jū* means a blockage of qi and blood by toxin. Early Chinese texts such as the *Yellow Emperor's Inner Classic* did not differentiate precisely between abscesses *(yōng)* and carbuncles, and these types of conditions were simply referred to by a combined term of "abscesses-carbuncles" *(yōng jū)*. Modern medical historians, however, have reviewed the ancient literature pertaining to the signs and symptoms of abscesses and carbuncles and concluded that there are, in fact, distinctions between the two.

Abscesses occur in soft tissues. Prior to suppuration the skin is somewhat opaque and soft, with redness and swelling, and clear demarcation of the lesion. The abscess resolves easily before pus formation. Following pus formation, the lesion points and discharges easily; and after suppuration, healing is usually swift and without scarring. Abscesses are similar to the biomedical condition of cutaneous abscesses and lymphadenitis. Carbuncles, on the other hand, develop quickly into pustules with heads. The infection spreads easily beneath the skin, resulting in deep suppuration, necrosis and a large scar.

Biomedically, *Staphylococcus aureus* is almost always the causative agent.

Signs & Symptoms

In traditional Chinese medicine there are two types of carbuncles: those due to excess and those due to deficiency.

Carbuncles due to excess break out as nodules with millet-sized, pus-filled heads with pain and itching. As the infection progresses the swelling increases and more pustules appear, and the lesions become red, with burning and more acute pain. This progression usually takes place over one week and may be acompanied by fever, aversion to cold, headache, loss of appetite, a sticky white or yellow tongue coating, and a slippery, rapid or flooding, rapid pulse.

During the suppuration phase the heads of the lesions necrotize and the affected area is honeycomb-like. By the third week, if pus has drained and the necrotized tissue has sloughed, the infection has stopped progressing. If, however, the condition continues to deteriorate, the generalized symptoms worsen into high fever, thirst, constipation, a yellow sticky tongue coating, and a wiry, slippery and rapid pulse. Once suppuration occurs the generalized symptoms ameliorate.

Carbuncles of the deficiency type generally occur in the elderly, or in patients with diabetes mellitus or other debilitating diseases. In individuals with deficient fluids and extreme fire toxin, the lesion is cyanotic in appearance and somewhat depressed, with a diffuse base. The lesion is very painful, does not suppurate easily, and the discharge is thin and scanty, and may be streaked with blood. The necrotized tissue does not slough easily. Generalized symptoms may include high fever, dry lips and mouth, constipation, scanty and deep yellow urine, loss of appetite, a red tongue with a yellow coating, and a thin, rapid pulse.

In patients with deficiency of qi and blood with stagnant toxin, the lesion is slightly depressed with a diffuse base because there is insufficient qi to discharge the pus, thus it spreads—or oozes—into the surrounding tissues. The lesion is dull gray because of insufficient blood to nourish the skin. There is either very little or no pain because the insufficient normal qi is unable to combat the pathogenic factor. The lesion suppurates slowly because deficiency of yang results in slowed pus formation and sloughing of necrotized tissue. The pus is thin, scanty and grayish green. The lesion may ulcerate. Generalized symptoms may include low fever, semiliquid stools, frequent and copious urination, thirst but without a desire to drink, lackluster skin, apathy, a pink tongue with a sticky white coating, and a rapid and forceless pulse.

Differential Diagnosis

Carbuncles should be differentiated from folliculitis and furuncles. Folliculitis is an infection that involves the superficial openings of the hair follicles. A furuncle is inflammation and necrosis of the entire hair follicle. If the inflammation progresses and involves a cluster of hair follicles with subcutaneous spreading of infection and deep suppuration, the condition is known as a carbuncle.

Traditional Chinese Etiology

Carbuncles may be caused by external and/or internal factors. External pathogenic factors include attack by wind-warm or damp-heat toxin disrupting the flow of qi and blood, resulting in the accumulation of toxin in the skin and tissues. Internal causes include pent-up emotions leading to qi stagnation, sexual indulgence causing depletion of essence and Kidney water, resulting in yin deficiency and preponderance of fire; and overeating of spicy or greasy foods, inducing dysfunction of the Spleen/Stomach's transportive and transformative mechanisms and resulting in formation of damp-heat fire toxin.

Patients whose physical constitutions are already compromised, such as diabetics, or those who are suffering from yin deficiency, or qi and blood deficiency, are especially prone to developing carbuncles under the above circumstances.

Treatment

Treatment of carbuncles should be based on the presenting pattern, the stage and location of the condition, the severity of the heat toxin, the degree of deficiency or excess of qi and blood, and the patient's age.

INTERNAL

Excess condition. During the acute stage the causative factor is usually damp-heat toxin or wind-heat toxin attacking and accumulating in the skin and tissues, leading to blockage of the flow of qi and blood. The strategy is to scatter wind, clear heat and resolve dampness, and harmonize the nutritive level and support the normal qi to expel pus. The formula recommended for this pattern is Sublime Formula for Sustaining Life.

❧ Sublime Formula for Sustaining Life
仙方活命饮
xiān fāng huó mìng yǐn

Flos Lonicerae Japonicae *(jin yin hua)*	9g
Radix Glycyrrhizae Uralensis *(gan cao)*	3g
Bulbus Fritillariae Thunbergii *(zhe bei mu)*	3g
Radix Trichosanthis Kirilowii *(tian hua fen)*	3g
Radix Angelicae Sinensis *(dang gui)*	6-12g
Radix Paeoniae Rubrae *(chi shao)*	3g
Gummi Olibanum *(ru xiang)*	3g
Myrrha *(mo yao)*	3g
Radix Ledebouriellae Divaricatae *(fang feng)*	3g
Radix Angelicae Dahuricae *(bai zhi)*	3g
Squama Manitis Pentadactylae *(chuan shan jia)*	3g
Spina Gleditsiae Sinensis *(zao jiao ci)*	3g
Pericarpium Citri Reticulatae *(chen pi)*	9g

PREPARATION & DOSAGE: Decoct the herbs in one part water and one part wine to strengthen the blood-invigorating action of the formula. Administer in two doses daily.

MODIFICATIONS: For fever and chills, add Herba seu Flos Schizonepetae Tenuifoliae *(jing jie)* and Radix Ledebouriellae Divaricatae *(fang feng)*. For constipation, add Radix et Rhizoma Rhei *(da huang)* at end of decoction (cook for no more than 10 minutes) and Fructus Citri seu Ponciri Immaturus *(zhi shi)*. For deep yellow urine, add Rhizoma Dioscoreae Hypoglaucae *(bei xie)*, Rhizome Alismatis Orientalis *(ze xie)* and Semen Plantaginis *(che qian zi)* (wrapped).

For large areas of necrosis the strategy is to protect the tissues and the Heart, i.e., to prevent deepening of the toxin, and to invigorate the blood and relieve toxicity. In conjunction with Sublime Formula for Sustaining Life, the following formula may also be used.

❧ Succinum, Beeswax, and Alum Pill
琥珀蜡矾丸
hǔ pò là fán wán

Alumen *(ming fan)*	36g
Realgar *(xiong huang)*	3.6g
Succinum *(hu po)*	3g
Cinnabaris *(zhu sha)*	3g
White Honey	6g
Yellow Beeswax	30g

PREPARATION & DOSAGE: Grind the first four ingredients together into a fine powder. Combine with the white honey and yellow beeswax and cook over low heat until dissolved. Stir thoroughly and remove from heat. When the substance is congealed, make into small boluses the size of mung beans. Take 20 boluses once daily with warm water. For more severe cases, increase dosage to twice daily.

For the suppurating phase, add the following to Sublime Formula for Sustaining Life: Rhizoma Coptidis *(huang lian)*, Radix Scutellariae Baicalensis *(huang qin)* and Fructus Gardeniae Jasminoidis *(zhi zi)*.

CLINICAL NOTE: In cases where suppuration is slow, the lesion should be drained surgically by a dermatologist.

During the healing phase, no internal formula specifically for treating the lesion(s) is necessary. However, in cases of qi and blood deficiency, the strategy is to regulate and tonify the qi and blood. Formulas such as Eight-Treasure Decoction are recommended for this purpose.

❧ Eight-Treasure Decoction
八珍汤
bā zhēn tāng

Radix Ginseng *(ren shen)*	6-9g
Rhizoma Atractylodis Macrocephalae *(bai zhu)*	9-12g
Sclerotium Poriae Cocos *(fu ling)*	12-15g
Honey-toasted Radix Glycyrrhizae Uralensis *(zhi gan cao)*	3-6g

Radix Rehmanniae Glutinosae Conquitae *(shu di huang)*	15-18g
Radix Paeoniae Lactiflorae *(bai shao)*	12-15g
Radix Angelicae Sinensis *(dang gui)*	12-15g
Radix Ligustici Chuanxiong *(chuan xiong)*	6-9g

PREPARATION & DOSAGE: Cook with 3 slices of Rhizoma Zingiberis Officinalis Recens *(sheng jiang)* and 2 pieces of Fructus Zizyphi Jujubae *(da zao)*. Administer in two doses daily.

Deficiency condition. For insufficient yin fluids and extreme fire toxin, the strategy is to enrich the yin and generate fluids, and clear heat and support the normal qi to expel pus. The formula recommended for this pattern is Lophatherus and Astragalus Decoction.

❦ Lophatherus and Astragalus Decoction
竹叶黄芪汤
zhú yè huáng qí tāng

Radix Ginseng *(ren shen)*	2.5g
Radix Astragali Membranacei *(huang qi)*	2.5g
Calcined Gypsum *(duan shi gao)*	2.5g
Rhizoma Pinelliae Ternatae *(ban xia)*	2.5g
Tuber Ophiopogonis Japonici *(mai men dong)*	2.5g
Radix Paeoniae Lactiflorae *(bai shao)*	2.5g
Radix Glycyrrhizae Uralensis *(gan cao)*	2.5g
Radix Ligustici Chuanxiong *(chuan xiong)*	2.5g
Radix Angelicae Sinensis *(dang gui)*	2.5g
Radix Scutellariae Baicalensis *(huang qin)*	2.5g
Radix Rehmanniae Glutinosae *(sheng di huang)*	6g
Herba Lophatheri Gracilis *(dan zhu ye)*	6g

PREPARATION & DOSAGE: Decoct with 3 slices of fresh Rhizoma Zingiberis Officinalis *(gan jiang)* and 20 strands of Medulla Junci Effusi *(deng xin cao)*. Administer in one dose daily.

For cases of qi and blood deficiency, and stagnant toxin that does not easily transform, the strategy is to support the normal qi to expel pus. The formula recommended for this pattern is Support the Interior and Eliminate Toxin Decoction.

❦ Support the Interior and Eliminate Toxin Decoction
托里消毒散
tuō lǐ xiāo dú sǎn

Spina Gleditsiae Sinensis *(zao jiao ci)*	1.5g
Radix Glycyrrhizae Uralensis *(gan cao)*	1.5g
Radix Platycodi Grandiflori *(jie geng)*	1.5g

Radix Angelicae Dahuricae *(bai zhi)*	1.5g
Flos Lonicerae Japonicae *(jin yin hua)*	3g
Radix Ligustici Chuanxiong *(chuan xiong)*	3g
Radix Astragali Membranacei *(huang qi)*	3g
Radix Angelicae Sinensis *(dang gui)*	3g
Radix Paeoniae Lactiflorae *(bai shao)*	3g
Rhizoma Atractylodis Macrocephalae *(bai zhu)*	3g
Radix Ginseng *(ren shen)*	3g
Sclerotium Poriae Cocos *(fu ling)*	3g

PREPARATION & DOSAGE: Decoct and administer in one dose daily.

EXTERNAL

For the acute phase, use either Golden-Yellow Plaster, which is a combination of eight parts Golden-Yellow Powder (see furuncles) and two parts petroleum jelly; or Jade Dew Plaster (see herpes simplex in Chapter 8).

For the suppuration phase, in addition to applying one of the topical formulas above, Eight-Two Special Powder is recommended.

❧ Eight-Two Special Powder
八二丹
bā èr dān

Calcined Gypsum *(duan shi gao)*	8g
Mimium *(qian dan)*	2g

PREPARATION & DOSAGE: Grind the ingredients together into a fine powder. Apply directly to the lesion, or onto a cotton spill, which is then inserted into the open lesion in order to promote drainage.

CLINICAL NOTE: This formula should not be used long-term because of the lead (minium) content.

For scanty pus that is grayish green, Seven-Three Special Powder may be applied in addition to Golden Yellow Plaster or Jade Dew Plaster.

❧ Seven-Three Special Powder
七三丹
qī sān dān

Calcined Gypsum *(duan shi gao)*	7g
Mimium *(qian dan)*	3g

PREPARATION & DOSAGE: The ingredients of this formula are identical to those in Eight-Two Special Powder, but their amounts are different. Preparation and application is the same.

During the healing phase, Generate Flesh Powder is recommended.

❖ Generate Flesh Powder
生肌散
shēng jī sǎn

Smithsonitum *(lu gan shi)*	15g
Stalactitum *(e guan shi)*	9g
Talcum *(hua shi)*	30g
Succinum *(hu po)*	9g
Cinnabaris *(zhu sha)*	3g
Borneol *(bing pian)*	0.3g

PREPARATION & DOSAGE: Grind the ingredients together into a fine powder. Apply 1-2 times daily and then bandage.

CLINICAL NOTE: Because of the mercury content (cinnibaris), long-term use should be avoided. Daily application for seven days is recommended. If healing has not started, discontinue and consider other treatments.

ACUPUNCTURE

Treatment is the same as that for furuncles.

EMPIRICAL REMEDIES

[A] Thick-needle needling may be used to treat carbuncles in the following manner. Needle GV-11 *(shen dao)* through to GV-9 *(zhi yang)* with an acupuncture needle 1.0mm in diameter and 12.5cm in length. The needle is retained for 1-6 hours depending on the severity of the condition. Treat once daily, with 10 sessions constituting a course of therapy, and 3-5 days' rest between courses. Secondary points are GV-14 *(da zhui)* for conditions of short duration and in patients who do not present with deficiency, and GV-4 *(ming men)* for recalcitrant cases and in patients who do present with deficiency.

It has been suggested[10] that use of the thick needle clears the channels and collaterals of stagnation and regulates the yin and yang, inasmuch as carbuncles are attributed to an imbalance of yin-yang resulting in fire toxin, which causes stagnation of the qi and blood. The governing vessel is the meeting point of all of the yang channels of the body and thus controls these channels. By needling points on the governing vessel, the yin and yang (especially yang) are regulated such that the fire toxin is relieved and the normal qi is supported, thereby promoting suppuration and healing.

[B] Remove the seeds of fresh bitter melon and mash the melon into a paste. Apply to the affected area 1-2 times daily.[11]

Traditional vs. Biomedical Treatment

See furuncles.

Prevention

Recurrent carbuncles can often be controlled by improving hygiene. Lesions that are just breaking out should be treated promptly by using remedies that are cool or cold in nature, and by keeping the surrounding areas clean. In transmitted cases, it is important to find and treat family and friends who may be sources of reinfection for the patient. Individuals prone to carbuncles should avoid foods that are spicy, greasy or that are warm or hot in nature. Successful traditional treatment of carbuncles entails correct pattern differentiation, particularly in those cases that are chronic and/or recalcitrant.

Erysipelas
丹毒
dān dú, "red toxin"

Erysipelas is an acute inflammation of the dermis and subepidermal tissues. It is marked by flaming redness which extends rapidly in tongue-like patterns over the affected area. Records of this disease have been found in such early works as *Basic Questions* (Chapter 74), in which the condition is referred to as "red flare" *(dān piāo).* In *Discussion of the Origins of Symptoms of Diseases* (610), Chao Yuan-Fang made the following notation: "Red disease: the body suddenly becomes flaming red, like having put on rouge." And in *Thousand Ducat Formulas* (652), Sun Si-Miao observed that "[r]ed toxin is also known as heavenly fire. There is suddenly redness in the tissues, like the color of rouge." Different names have been used to describe the condition based on its location: erysipelas of the head was called "fire toxin covering the head" *(bāo tóu huǒ dān);* erysipelas of the thoracic region was known as "red toxin arising from the interior" *(nèi fā dān dú);* and erysipelas of the legs was referred to as "flowing fire" *(liú huǒ).* Erysipelas in infants was known as "red traveling rouge" *(chì yóu fēng).*

Biomedically, erysipelas is caused by group A ß-hemolytic streptococci.

Signs & Symptoms

The face (often bilaterally), an arm or a leg is most often involved. The affected skin initially feels uncomfortable and tense. Redness and edema soon follow, with the redness being sharply demarcated. The lesion is slightly raised, shiny, hot, and tender. The lesion is well demarcated, slightly elevated, shiny, hot to the touch and tender. With effective treatment, the condition subsides within 5-6 days with good prognosis. Bacteremia leading to septicemia may develop if erysipelas is not treated in a timely manner. Recurrent erysipelas may result in chronic lymphedema, and elephantiasis of the extremities, requiring long-term treatment.

Differential Diagnosis

The characteristic appearance of erysipelas usually simplifies its diagnosis. Erysipelas of the face must be differentiated from herpes zoster, either through the characteristic distribution of the herpes vesicles along a nerve route, or serologically. Contact dermatitis will have a history of contact with a chemical irritant; drug eruptions will have a history of drug exposure. Erysipeloid (a bacterial infection that affects the deeper tissues) develops slowly, and is caused by an animal pathogen, especially from swine. Infection in man is primarily occupational, and typically follows a penetrating hand wound in persons who handle fish or animal tissues (e.g., fishermen and butchers).

Traditional Chinese Etiology

Erysipelas is a manifestation of disharmony of the nutritive and protective levels, such that qi and blood stagnate and fire-heat toxin accumulates in the blood and sears the skin and tissues. The three primary sources of fire-heat toxin are wind-heat transforming into fire, Liver/Spleen damp-heat, and damp-heat transforming into fire. In addition, any of these or other patterns that becomes protracted may transform into the more serious condition of inward attack of fire-heat toxin.

Wind-heat transforming into fire. This pattern usually affects the the head. It may be due to attack by wind-heat that is not treated in a timely manner or treated improperly, such that the wind-heat transforms into fire, thus giving rise to erysipelas. Another cause is injury to the skin, which allows entry of wind-heat toxin that later transforms into fire and produces erysipelas.

Liver/Spleen damp-heat. The flanks, abdomen and genitals are affected in this pattern. The cause is usually fire in the Liver channel that contends with damp-heat in the Spleen channel. The struggle between the two pathogenic factors gives rise to erysipelas.

Damp-heat transforming into fire. This pattern is mainly caused by pre-existing conditions of dampness or damp-heat affecting the lower leg or foot (e.g., leg ulcers or toe web infections), such that the dampness or damp-heat transforms into fire, thus giving rise to erysipelas of the leg.

Treatment

INTERNAL

Wind-heat transforming into fire. Erysipelas of this pattern often begins on the face in front of the ears or adjacent to the nose. The skin at the affected site is flaming red, tender and edematous. The inflammation quickly spreads to other areas, such that the entire face and even the scalp may become involved. The erythema is sharply demarcated and small bullae and vesicles may develop near the advancing margin. Generalized symptoms include sudden onset of high fever, headache, malaise and vomiting. Severe cases may present with delirium. The tongue is red and the coating is yellow and sticky, and the pulse is floating and rapid. The strategy is to scatter wind, clear fire and relieve the toxin.

Formulas recommended for this pattern include Universal Benefit Decoction to Eliminate Toxin, or Arctium and Taraxacum Formula to Cool the Blood.

❦ Universal Benefit Decoction to Eliminate Toxin
普济消毒饮
pǔ jì xiāo dú yǐn

Wine-fried Radix Scutellariae Baicalensis *(jiu chao huang qin)* 15g
Wine-fried Rhizoma Coptidis *(jiu chao huang lian)* 15g
Fructus Arctii Lappae *(niu bang zi)* 3g
Fructus Forsythiae Suspensae *(lian qiao)* 3g
Herba Menthae Haplocalycis *(bo he)* 3g
Bombyx Batryticatus *(jiang can)* 1.5g
Radix Scrophulariae Ningpoensis *(xuan shen)* 6g
Fructificatio Lasiosphere seu Calvatiae *(ma bo)* 3g
Radix Isatidis seu Baphicacanthi *(ban lan gen)* 3g
Radix Platycodi Grandiflori *(jie geng)* 6g
Radix Glycyrrhizae Uralensis *(gan cao)* 6g
Pericarpium Citri Reticulatae *(chen pi)* 6g
Radix Bupleuri *(chai hu)* 6g
Rhizoma Cimicifugae *(sheng ma)* 1.5g

PREPARATION & DOSAGE: Decoct and administer in 1-2 doses daily.

❦ Arctium and Taraxacum Formula to Cool the Blood
牛公凉血方
niú gōng liáng xuè fāng

Fructus Arctii Lappae *(niu bang zi)* 10g
Herba Taraxaci Mongolici cum Radice *(pu gong ying)* 12g
Radix Isatidis seu Baphicacanthi *(ban lan gen)* 15g
Radix Scrophulariae Ningpoensis *(xuan shen)* 12g
Flos Chrysanthemi Indici *(ye ju hua)* 10g
Radix Scutellariae Baicalensis *(huang qin)* 6g
Flos Lonicerae Japonicae *(jin yin hua)* 12g
Fructus Forsythiae Suspensae *(lian qiao)* 10g
Cortex Moutan Radicis *(mu dan pi)* 6g
Radix Paeoniae Rubrae *(chi shao)* 10g
Bombyx Batryticatus *(jiang can)* 10g
Radix Glycyrrhizae Uralensis *(gan cao)* 3g

PREPARATION & DOSAGE: Decoct and administer in two doses daily.

Liver/Spleen damp-heat. This pattern exhibits erysipelas lesions that affect the flanks, abdomen and even genitals. Generalized symptoms may include fever, bitter taste in the mouth, pain in the hypochondria, scanty and yellow urine, a yellow and sticky tongue coating, and a wiry, slippery pulse. The strategy is to clear Liver fire and drain damp-heat. The formula recommended for this pattern is Bupleurum Decoction to Clear the Liver.

❦ Bupleurum Decoction to Clear the Liver
柴胡清肝汤
chái hú qīng gān tāng

Radix Bupleuri (*chai hu*)	4.5
Radix Rehmanniae Glutinosae (*sheng di huang*)	4.5g
Radix Angelicae Sinensis (*dang gui*)	6g
Radix Paeoniae Rubrae (*chi shao*)	4.5g
Radix Ligustici Chuanxiong (*chuan xiong*)	3g
Fructus Forsythiae Suspensae (*lian qiao*)	6g
Fructus Arctii Lappae (*niu bang zi*)	4.5g
Radix Scutellariae Baicalensis (*huang qin*)	3g
Fructus Gardeniae Jasminoidis (*zhi zi*)	4.5g
Radix Trichosanthis Kirilowii (*tian hua fen*)	3g
Radix Ledebouriellae Divaricatae (*fang feng*)	3g
Radix Glycyrrhizae Uralensis (*gan cao*)	3g

PREPARATION & DOSAGE: Decoct and administer in one dose daily.

Damp-heat transforming into fire. The legs are mainly affected in this pattern of erysipelas. In addition to the characteristic lesions, the tongue is red and the coating yellow and sticky, while the pulse is slippery and rapid. The strategy is to clear heat, drain dampness and relieve the toxin. The formula recommended for this pattern is Combined Coptis Decoction to Relieve Toxicity and Three-Marvel Pill.

❈ Combined Coptis Decoction to Relieve Toxicity and Three-Marvel Pill
黄连解毒汤合三妙丸
huáng lián jiĕ dú tāng hé sān miào wán

Rhizoma Coptidis (*huang lian*)	9g
Radix Scutellariae Baicalensis (*huang qin*)	6g
Cortex Phellodendri (*huang bai*)	6g
Fructus Gardeniae Jasminoidis (*zhi zi*)	6g
Rhizoma Atractylodis (*cang zhu*)	9g
Radix Achyranthis Bidentatae (*niu xi*)	6g

PREPARATION & DOSAGE: Decoct and administer in one dose daily.

Inward attack of fire-heat toxin. This is the result of improperly or untreated fire-heat toxin that turns inward. Generalized symptoms may include high fever, impaired consciousness, raving, restlessness, headache, nausea and vomiting, constipation, deep yellow urine, a scarlet tongue with a yellow coating, and a flooding, rapid pulse. (This pattern corresponds closely to the biomedical diagnosis of septicemia.) The strategy is to cool the nutritive level and relieve toxicity.

Formulas recommended for this pattern are Clear Epidemics and Overcome Toxin Decoction, or Clear the Nutritive Level Decoction.

Clear Epidemics and Overcome Toxin Decoction
清瘟败毒饮
qīng wēn bài dú yǐn

Gypsum *(shi gao)*	60-120g
Rhizoma Anemarrhenae Asphodeloidis *(zhi mu)*	6-12g
Radix Glycyrrhizae Uralensis *(gan cao)*	3-6g
Herba Lophatheri Gracilis *(dan zhu ye)*	3-6g
Cornu Rhinoceri *(xi jiao)*	9-12g
Radix Rehmanniae Glutinosae *(sheng di huang)*	9-15g
Cortex Moutan Radicis *(mu dan pi)*	6-12g
Radix Paeoniae Rubrae *(chi shao)*	6-12g
Radix Scrophulariae Ningpoensis *(xuan shen)*	6-12g
Rhizoma Coptidis *(huang lian)*	6-12g
Radix Scutellariae Baicalensis *(huang qin)*	3-9g
Fructus Gardeniae Jasminoidis *(zhi zi)*	6-12g
Fructus Forsythiae Suspensae *(lian qiao)*	6-12g
Radix Platycodi Grandiflori *(jie geng)*	3-6g

PREPARATION & DOSAGE: First decoct the Gypsum *(shi gao)* for 15-20 minutes before adding the other herbs. Administer in one dose daily.

CLINICAL NOTE: Ten times the amount of Cornu Bubali *(shui niu jiao)* is usually substituted for the Cornu Rhinoceri *(xi jiao)*, both because of expense and the fact that all species of rhinocerus are endangered. The substitute should be decocted along with the Gypsum *(shi gao)*.

Clear the Nutritive Level Decoction
清营汤
qīng yíng tāng

Cornu Rhinoceri *(xi jiao)*	9g
Radix Scrophulariae Ningpoensis *(xuan shen)*	9g
Radix Rehmanniae Glutinosae *(sheng di huang)*	15g
Tuber Ophiopogonis Japonici *(mai men dong)*	9g
Flos Lonicerae Japonicae *(jin yin hua)*	9g
Fructus Forsythiae Suspensae *(lian qiao)*	6g
Rhizoma Coptidis *(huang lian)*	4.5g
Herba Lophatheri Gracilis *(dan zhu ye)*	3g
Radix Salviae Miltiorrhizae *(dan shen)*	6g

PREPARATION & DOSAGE: Grind Cornu Rhinoceri *(xi jiao)* and take as a draft. Decoct the other herbs. It is reccommended that ten times the amount of Cornu Bubali *(shui niu jiao)* be substituted for the Cornu Rhinoceri *(xi jiao)*, both because of expense and the fact that all species of rhinocerus are endangered. The substitute should be decocted with the other herbs. Administer in one dose daily.

MODIFICATIONS: In addition to either of the above formulas, if the patient presents with impaired consciousness and raving, Calm the Palace Pill with Cattle Gallstone (dissolve one bolus) may also be administered.

❦ Calm the Palace Pill with Cattle Gallstone
安宫牛黄丸
ān gōng niú huáng wán

Calculus Bovis *(niu huang)*	30g
Cornu Rhinoceri *(xi jiao)*	30g
Secretio Moschus *(she xiang)*	7.5g
Rhizoma Coptidis *(huang lian)*	30g
Radix Scutellariae Baicalensis *(huang qin)*	30g
Fructus Gardeniae Jasminoidis *(zhi zi)*	30g
Realgar *(xiong huang)*	30g
Borneol *(bing pian)*	7.5g
Tuber Curcumae *(yu jin)*	30g
Cinnabaris *(zhu sha)*	30g
Magarita *(zhen zhu)*	15g

PREPARATION & DOSAGE: Grind the ingredients into a powder and form into pills with honey. The pills should weigh 3g each. It is recommended that five times the amount of Cornu Bubali *(shui niu jiao)* be substituted for the Cornu Rhinoceri *(xi jiao)*, both because of expense and the fact that all species of rhinocerus are endangered.

For more severe cases of high fever, delirium and impaired consciousness, Purple Snow Special Pill is recommended.

❦ Purple Snow Special Pill
紫雪丹
zǐ xuě dān

Gypsum *(shi gao)*	1500g
Calcitum *(han shui shi)*	1500g
Talcum *(hua shi)*	1500g
Cornu Rhinoceri *(xi jiao)*	150g
Cornu Antelopis *(ling yang jiao)*	150g
Secretio Moschus *(she xiang)*	37.5g
Radix Scrophulariae Ningpoensis *(xuan shen)*	500g
Magnetitum *(ci shi)*	1500g
Rhizoma Cimicifugae *(sheng ma)*	500g
Honey-toasted Radix Glycyrrhizae Uralensis *(zhi gan cao)*	240g
Radix Aristolochiae *(qing mu xiang)*	150g
Lignum Aquilariae *(chen xiang)*	150g

Flos Caryophylli *(ding xiang)*	30g
Cinnabaris *(zhu sha)*	90g
Mirabilitum *(mang xiao)*	5000g
Niter *(xiao shi)*	96g
Gold *(huang jin)*	3000g

PREPARATION & DOSAGE: Crush the mineral ingredients into small pieces and boil in 60 liters of water until 24 liters remain, then discard the dregs. Ten times the amount of Cornu Bubali *(shui niu jiao)* is usually substituted for the Cornu Rhinoceri *(xi jiao)*, both because of expense and the fact that all species of rhinocerus are endangered. Then boil the herbal ingredients in the remaining liquid until 9 liters are left, and discard the dregs. Add powdered Mirabilitum *(mang xiao)* and Niter *(xiao shi)* into this liquid and bring to a boil over low heat. Stir occasionally with a wooden spatula. When 4.2 liters remain, pour the decoction into a wooden container. At this point, the decoction will be a syrup. Allow to cool before adding powdered Cinnabaris *(zhu sha)* and Secretio Moschus *(she xiang)*; stir well with a wooden spatula. Allow the mixture to thoroughly dry, then render into a powder. Administer 1.5-3.0g, 1-2 two times daily, with boiled lukewarm water. Once the symptoms of impaired consciousness improve, the formula should be discontinued to avoid injuring the source qi and exhausting the yin.

EXTERNAL

For the acute initial stage of erysipelas, either Jade Dew Plaster (see herpes simplex in Chapter 8) or Rheum Powder may be administered.

Rheum Powder
大黄散
dà huáng sǎn

Radix et Rhizoma Rhei *(da huang)*
Rhizoma Atractylodis *(cang zhu)*
Cortex Phellodendri *(huang bai)*

PREPARATION & DOSAGE: Grind equal amounts of the herbs together into a fine powder. To form a paste, mix either with a decoction of Flos Lonicerae Japonicae *(jin yin hua)*, or a decoction of Flos Chrysanthemi Morifolii *(ju hua)*, or with vegetable oil or boiled water (cooled). Apply 3-5 times daily.

When the redness and swelling have improved, Golden Yellow Powder (see furuncles) or Flush and Harmonize Plaster may be applied.

Flush and Harmonize Plaster
冲和膏
chōng hé gāo

Dry-fried Cortex Cercis Chinensis *(chao zi jing pi)*	150g
Radix Angelicae Pubescentis *(du huo)z*	90g
Radix Paeoniae Rubrae *(chi shao)*	60g
Radix Angelicae Dahuricae *(bai zhi)*	30g
Rhizoma Acori Graminei *(shi chang pu)*	45g

PREPARATION & DOSAGE: Grind the ingredients into a fine powder and mix with onion juice and fermented vinegar (a special type of Chinese vinegar; ordinary rice vinegar or distilled vinegar may be substituted) to form a paste. Apply 2-3 times daily.

ACUPUNCTURE

The primary acupoints include LI-4 *(he gu)*, LI-11 *(qu chi)*, BL-40 *(wei zhong)*, SP-10 *(xue hai)* and SP-6 *(san yin jiao)*. Auxilliary points: for high fever, add GV-14 *(da zhui)*; for headache, add M-HN-9 *(tai yang)* and GB-20 *(feng chi)*; for nausea and vomiting, add PC-6 *(nei guan)* and ST-36 *(zu san li)*; for constipation, add ST-25 *(tian shu)* and ST-44 *(feng long)*; for impaired consciousness and raving, add GV-26 *(shui gou)*, PC-7 *(da ling)* and K-1 *(yong quan)*. Use draining method. Treat once daily, retaining the needles for 30 minutes. BL-40 *(wei zhong)* may be bloodlet in order to drain blood toxin. Improvement should be evident after three treatments.

EMPIRICAL REMEDIES

Acute erysipelas may be treated with the following external remedy.

❧ Erysipelas Plaster[12]

丹毒膏

dān dú gāo

Semen Ricini Communis *(bi ma zi)*	40-50 seeds
Semen Croton Tiglii *(ba dou)*	7-8 seeds
Dry-fried Semen Strychni *(chao ma qian zi)* (powdered)	2g
Radix Glycyrrhizae Uralensis *(gan cao)* (powdered)	2g

PREPARATION & DOSAGE: Mash the ingredients together and mix with sesame oil to form a paste. Spread onto sterile gauze, then apply to the affected area and bandage. The redness and swelling should improve within a few hours. The plaster may remain in place for 10-20 hours. Generally, two applications are sufficient to effect complete alleviation. Local itching or hot sensation may be felt, but there are no other side effects. Internal formulas aimed at clearing heat and relieving toxicity, and invigorating the blood and unblocking the channels, will expedite healing.

CLINICAL NOTE: This formula is extremely toxic and is not for internal use. It is contraindicated during pregnancy. The plaster should be prepared in a non-metallic container.

BLOODLETTING WITH CUPPING[13]

Bloodletting is utilized by first using a tri-ensiform needle to gently prick the area just inside the border of the inflammation several times until drops of blood appear. Cupping is then applied for one minute to the same area. After the bleeding stops, the area is swabbed with alcohol to prevent infection. Avoid pricking too deeply. If bleeding is only slight from pricking, then cupping may be applied for a longer period in order to increase the bleeding. Individuals who are prone to bleeding should not undergo this treatment. The prognosis is good if for every 10mm, about 1-2ml of blood is let, thus achieving the goal of draining heat-toxin through bloodletting.

Traditional vs. Biomedical Treatment

In acute erysipelas the response time of traditional treatment is slightly longer than that of biomedical therapy. Traditional treatment can take anywhere from 3-10 days to effect signs of improvement, whereas biomedical treatment with antibiotics can often produce rapid relief within a couple days. Traditional treatment may be preferred for recurrent erysipelas, especially by using a combined internal and external approach in order to eliminate the root of the condition.

Prevention

Bedrest is essential to ensure timely healing. To prevent recurrent erysipelas, sources of infection should be treated, e.g., toe web infections. Foods that are hot in nature should be avoided, including items that are spicy, and those that produce heat, such as lamb, capon, shrimp and some vitamins and minerals.

Lupus Vulgaris
鸦啖疮
yā dàn chuāng, "crow's food sores"

Lupus vulgaris is the most common form of skin tuberculosis. The disease was first described in the Song dynasty work, *Complete Book of External Medicine,* by Dou Han-Qing:

> Individuals suffering crow's food sores have long-term pathogenic heat, deficient cold of the yin and yang Organs, insufficiency of blood and qi, so that the interstitial tissues are not tight; thus this disease arises on the skin, at first resembling coin holes [of ancient Chinese coins], then rotting into sores that resemble crow's food [probably indicating the pockmarks that crows leave when feeding on animal flesh]. If prolonged, the injury is not easily treated.

Biomedically, lupus vulgaris is caused by the bacteria *Mycobacterium tuberculosis.*

Signs & Symptoms

The lesions of lupus vulgaris commonly affect the face, mainly the median line and the nose. Mucous membranes may be involved. The primary lesion is a red or brown spot; the spots typically coalesce. Upon pressure with a glass spatula or slide, the blood of the lesions is displaced and the lesions resemble apple jelly, a telltale sign of lupus vulgaris. As the disease progresses, connective tissue is destroyed, such that upon moderate pressure a probe may break through the epidermis. As the tubercles grow, they form lesions with central scarring and contraction of fibrous tissue; scaling may also be present. Ulcer formation is common, with involvement of cartilage and bone the most frightening development, especially the rather swift destruction of the nose. Generalized symptoms may include low fever, night sweats, malaise, a red tongue with thin coating, and a thin, rapid pulse.

Differential Diagnosis

Flat lesions of tertiary syphilis may be distinguished from lupus vulgaris through serological tests. Superficial spreading basal cell epithelioma may be distinguished through biopsy. In contrast to psoriasis, mycosis and dermatitis, atrophy is a characteristic sign of lupus vulgaris.

Traditional Chinese Etiology

This condition is due to an originally weak constitution, with yin deficiency of the Lung and Kidney leading to internal heat. Internal heat transforms into fire that condenses the essence and transforms it into phlegm. Fire-phlegm accumulates in the skin, blocking the flow of qi and thus forming the lesions.

Treatment

INTERNAL

For the acute stage, the strategy is to relieve accumulation and transform phlegm, and dispel pathogens and dissipate the clumps. The formula recommended for this pattern is Modified Rambling Powder [A].

❦ Modified Rambling Powder [A]
逍遥散加减
xiāo yáo sǎn jiā jiǎn

Radix Bupleuri *(chai hu)*	6g
Charcoaled Cortex Moutan Radicis *(mu dan pi tan)*	6g
Radix Rehmanniae Glutinosae *(sheng di huang)*	10g
Dry-fried Radix Paeoniae Lactiflorae *(chao bai shao)*	10g
Pericarpium Citri Reticulatae Viride *(qing pi)*	10g
Rhizoma Atractylodis Macrocephalae *(bai zhu)*	10g
Bulbus Fritillariae Thunbergii *(zhe bei mu)*	12g
Fructus Forsythiae Suspensae *(lian qiao)*	12g
Spica Prunellae Vulgaris *(xia ku cao)*	12g
Gecko *(ge jie)*	1
Pericarpium Arecae Catechu *(da fu pi)*	30g

PREPARATION & DOSAGE: Decoct the ingredients. Administer in three doses daily.

For chronic lupus vulgaris, with recurrent lesions, the strategy is to benefit qi and nourish yin, and transform phlegm and dissipate the clumps. The formula recommended for this pattern is Cyperus and Fritillaria Decoction to Nourish the Nutritive Level.

❧ Cyperus and Fritillaria Decoction to Nourish the Nutritive Level
香贝养营汤
xiāng bèi yǎng yíng tāng

Dry-fried Rhizoma Atractylodis Macrocephalae *(chao bai zhu)*	6g
Radix Ginseng *(ren shen)*	3g
Sclerotium Poriae Cocos *(fu ling)*	3g
Pericarpium Citri Reticulatae *(chen pi)*	3g
Radix Rehmanniae Glutinosae Conquitae *(shu di huang)*	3g
Radix Ligustici Chuanxiong *(chuan xiong)*	3g
Radix Angelicae Sinensis *(dang gui)*	3g
Rhizoma Cyperi Rotundi *(xiang fu)*	3g
Bulbus Fritillariae *(bei mu)*	3g
Radix Paeoniae Lactiflorae *(bai shao)*	3g
Radix Platycodi Grandiflori *(jie geng)*	1.5g
Radix Glycyrrhizae Uralensis *(gan cao)*	1.5g
Rhizoma Zingiberis Officinalis *(gan jiang)*	3 slices
Fructus Zizyphi Jujubae *(da zao)*	2 pieces

PREPARATION & DOSAGE: Decoct and administer once daily.

EXTERNAL

The following herbal preparations may be applied topically.

[A] Mash into a paste 30g each of fresh Radix Dioscoreae Oppositae *(shan yao)* and Semen Ricini Communis *(bi ma zi)*, then apply once daily to the affected areas.

[B] Grind into a fine powder 30g each of Radix Sophorae Tonkinensis *(shan dou gen)* and Fructus Schisandrae Chinensis *(wu wei zi)*, and mix with vegetable oil to form a paste. Apply once daily to the affected areas.

[C] For lesions that have not ulcerated, either Exuvia Serpentis Plaster or Golden Plain Plaster is recommended.

❧ Exuvia Serpentis Plaster
蛇蜕膏
shé tùi gāo

Exuviae Serpentis *(she tui)*	3g
Scolopendra Subspinipes *(wu gong)*	2
Nidus Vespae *(lu feng fang)*	3g

PREPARATION & DOSAGE: Stir-fry the ingredients in sesame oil until crisp. Discard the dregs. Then mix the oil with corn starch to form a paste. Spread onto porous paper (e.g., filter paper) and allow to dry. Before applying, peel the plaster from the paper. Apply once daily.

CLINICAL NOTE: Because of this formula's toxicity, long-term use is discouraged. It is recommended that the formula be administered daily for 7-10 days. If symptoms do not improve, discontinue and consider other remedies.

❦ Golden Plain Plaster
金素膏
jīn sù gāo

Alumen Praeparatum *(ku fan)*	6g
Realgar *(xiong huang)*	10g
Petroleum Jelly	84g

PREPARATION & DOSAGE: Grind the first two ingredients together into a fine powder. Mix with the petroleum jelly to form an ointment. Apply once daily.

CLINICAL NOTE: Because of this formula's toxicity, long-term use is discouraged. It is recommended that the formula be administered daily for 7-10 days. If symptoms do no improve, discontinue and consider other remedies.

[D] For ulcerated lesions, apply Red Ointment.

❦ Red Ointment
红油膏
hóng yóu gāo

Nine-One Special Powder (see herpes zoster)	30g
Mimium *(qian dan)*	4.5g
Petroleum Jelly	300g

PREPARATION & DOSAGE: Dissolve the petroleum jelly in a non-metallic pot over low heat. Slowly add the Nine-One Special Powder and Mimium *(qian dan),* stirring thoroughly, to form an ointment. Spread onto sterile gauze and apply once daily.

CLINICAL NOTE: Because of this formula's toxicity, long-term use is discouraged. It is recommended that the formula be administered daily for 7-10 days. If symptoms do not improve, discontinue and consider other remedies.

Traditional vs. Biomedical Treatment

The treatment of tuberculosis in general is complex because of the resistance of *Mycobacterium tuberculosis* to destruction. Furthermore, because of the constant evolution of mycobactericidal resistant strains of the organism, biomedical treatment often requires the simultaneous use of two or more drugs for a long period lasting anywhere from 6-9 months. Such a long course of treatment poses patient compliance problems, especially in unreliable individuals.

Moreover, even if the course is completed, there is always a possibility of relapse. Additionally, the use of antituberculous drugs can lead to toxicity, especially of the liver. For these reasons, in China they are now encouraging a combined traditional and biomedical approach to therapy to improve response time, so that the course of treatment can be shortened to about 4-6 months; to strengthen the immune system with traditional therapy; and to offset the toxicity of the pharmaceuticals.

Prevention

Individuals who suspect possible previous exposure to tuberculosis should undergo tuberculin screening. Those exhibiting early signs of tuberculosis should be treated immediately.

Leprosy
麻风
má fēng, "numb wind"

Leprosy is an infectious disease that has been chronicled for centuries. Called "pestilence wind" *(lì fēng)* among other names by the ancient Chinese, it was described thusly in Chapter 42 of *Basic Questions:*

> Pestilence wind [is due to] heat in the nutritive and protective levels; blood and qi are not pure so that the nose is injured, the color of the face becomes bad, and the skin rots. Because wind-cold is lodged in the channels and cannot be removed, it is therefore called pestilence wind.

Through the ages, other terms for the disease have included "big wind" *(dà fēng),* "malevolent disease" *(è jí)* and "malevolent wind" *(lài fēng).* In the Ming dynasty, the disease came to be known by its present name—"numb wind"—because of the numbness that accompanies the disease.

Biomedically, leprosy is caused by the bacteria *Mycobacterium leprae,* which has a predilection for cooler regions of the body, such as the skin, mucous membranes and peripheral nerves.

Signs & Symptoms

The incubation period for leprosy is anywhere between one and thirty years. The disease evolves slowly and, depending on the immunologic status (cell-mediated immune capacity) of the patient, is classified into one of five types: tuberculoid, borderline-tuberculoid, midborderline, borderline-lepromatous, and lepromatous.

TUBERCULOID LEPROSY

Lesions associated with tuberculoid leprosy are characterized by macules or plaques that appear to be single or few in number. The small number of lesions is the main characterstic of this type of leprosy. The edges are well-demarcated with apparent central healing. The surface of the lesion is irregular in texture, and either hypopigmented, erythematous, or coppery in color. There is often reduction in or complete absence of sensation to temperature, pain, and light touch. A thickened peripheral nerve can often be felt nearby, or a thickened cutaneous nerve may be palpated entering or leaving the lesion. Skin scrapings usually are negative for bacteria.

BORDERLINE-TUBERCULOID LEPROSY

The lesions from this type of leprosy resemble those of tuberculoid leprosy, but are more numerous, numbering at least five, and frequently 10-20 or more. In addition, the edges are not as well-defined. The lesions are larger, sometimes affecting an entire extremity or other wide area. They vary in size, shape, and texture on the same patient. The lesions are distributed asymmetrically with involvement of several peripheral nerves, and sensation is moderately to markedly reduced. Skin scrapings are either negative or weakly positive.

MIDBORDERLINE LEPROSY

Midborderline leprosy is characterized by a considerable number of lesions that appear bilaterally and in varying forms. The lesions are greater in number than borderline-tuberculoid leprosy, but fewer than borderline-lepromatous leprosy (below). The plaques show unique geographic features, with poorly demarcated edges and punched-out centers. Sensation is slightly to moderately reduced. Peripheral nerve damage is variable since midborderline leprosy is an unstable form of the disease that is considered to be a transitional stage from either a borderline-tuberculoid or borderline-lepromatous type. Therefore, disease progression from borderline-tuberculoid leprosy will exhibit widespread and asymmetric peripheral nerve involvement, while improvement from the borderline lepromatous type (often under the influence of chemotherapy) will show more peripheral nerve involvement, symmetrically with little evidence of sensory or motor damage. Skin scrapings reveal moderate numbers of bacteria.

BORDERLINE-LEPROMATOUS LEPROSY

With this type of leprosy, there are many skin lesions that are widely distributed. These are macular in the early stages, followed by progression to papules, nodules, and plaques, with symmetrical involvement. Most lesions are small with central involvement, unlike those of midborderline leprosy, which show central "hole-in-cheese" centers. Peripheral nerve involvement is extensive and symmetrical, and sensory and motor damage may be marked. Skin scrapings are positive.

LEPROMATOUS LEPROSY

This form of the disease is generalized and systemic with continuous bacteremia, meaning that the M. leprae bacteria can be found in a very wide range of body tissues. In the early stages the lesions are macular, numerous, widespread, and symmetrical. They are poorly demarcated, and as the disease progresses, the lesions coalesce and affect the entire body surface except for the scalp, axillae, groin, perineum, and midline of the back (the "immune" areas). At this point, sensation is unaltered from the previous stage. If untreated, the lesions progress to formation of nodules, particularly on the forehead, ears, and face. Skin scrapings are invariably positive, even from apparently normal skin in between lesions. Perhaps the most disconcerting aspect of lepromatous leprosy is the insidious involvement of other systems: some patients may present with ocular, renal, or other clinical manifestations before the diagnosis of leprosy is suspected by examination of the skin, peripheral nerves, or through skin scrapings.

Differential Diagnosis

The lesions of other skin diseases which can resemble leprosy include ringworm and tinea versicolor. Ringworm presents with round lesions that usually itch, but with no neural involvement. Tinea versicolor is characterized by multiple, frequently asymptomatic patches of lesions varying in color from white to brown. Scaling of ringworm and tinea versicolor lesions is common upon scratching, whereas lepromatous lesions do not scale. Also, ringworm and tinea lesions do not involve loss of sensation. Diagnosis of leprosy is established by skin scrapings for the bacilli, especially in the later stages, as well as by taking a thorough history of the patient, assessing for travel to or residence in endemic areas.

Traditional Chinese Etiology

Leprosy is caused by invasion of wind and dampness which takes advantage of an already weak constitution (e.g., one with insufficient original qi). Blood and qi then stagnate, and the nutritive and protective levels are in disharmony, as are the yin and yang Organs.

The Chinese recognized early on that this disease was contagious. A passage in *Golden Mirror of the Medical Tradition* (1742) notes that "[o]ne cause [of leprosy] is through infection or contact with others who have leprosy."

Treatment

Early stages of leprosy may be considered conditions of excess, and treatment should be focused on the Liver and Lung. Advanced stages may be considered conditions of deficiency, and treatment should be aimed at the Heart and Kidney.

INTERNAL TREATMENT

Early stage. Included here are indeterminate and tuberculoid leprosies, as well as borderline leprosy with a tendency toward tuberculoid. The strategy is to disperse wind and resolve dampness, warm the channels and clear the collaterals, and invigorate the blood and relieve the toxicity.

Formulas recommended for this stage include Ten Thousand Efficacies Special Pill, Change Flesh Powder, or Drunken Fairy Powder.

❧ Ten Thousand Efficacies Special Pill
万灵丹
wàn líng dān

Rhizoma Atractylodis *(cang zhu)* 240g

Radix Polygoni Multiflori *(he shou wu)* 30g
Radix Angelicae Pubescentis *(du huo)* 30g
Herba seu Flos Schizonepetae Tenuifoliae *(jing jie)* 30g
Radix Aconiti *(wu tou)* 30g
Radix Linderae Strychnifoliae *(wu yao)* 30g
Radix Ligustici Chuanxiong *(chuan xiong)* 30g
Radix Glycyrrhizae Uralensis *(gan cao)* 30g
Herba Dendrobii *(shi hu)* 30g
Buthus Martensi *(quan xie)* 30g
Radix Ledebouriellae Divaricatae *(fang feng)* 30g
Herba cum Radice Asari *(xi xin)* 30g
Radix Angelicae Sinensis *(dang gui)* 30g
Herba Ephedrae *(ma huang)* 30g
Rhizoma Gastrodiae Elatae *(tian ma)* 30g
Realgar *(xiong huang)* 18g

PREPARATION & DOSAGE: Grind the ingredients together into a fine powder, combine with honey to form boluses, then coat with Cinnabaris *(zhu sha)*. Each bolus should weigh 9g. Administer one bolus 2-3 times daily with warm soup made from fermented black beans and onions, or with warm wine.

CLINICAL NOTE: Because of the mercury (Cinnabaris) content, long-term use of this formula is discouraged. Daily administration for 14 days is recommended; then reduce dosage to one bolus 1-2 times daily. If symptoms do not improve after 30 days, discontinue and consider other remedies.

❧ Change Flesh Powder
换肌散
huàn jī sǎn

Zaocys Dhumnades *(wu shao she)* 30g
Agkistrodon seu Bungarus *(bai hua she)* 30g
Lumbricus *(di long)* 30g
Herba cum Radice Asari *(xi xin)* 9g
Semen Momordicae Cochinchinensis *(mu bie zi)* 9g
Radix Angelicae Dahuricae *(bai zhi)* 9g
Rhizoma Gastrodiae Elatae *(tian ma)* 9g
Radix Paeoniae Rubrae *(chi shao)* 9g
Fructus Viticis *(man jing zi)* 9g
Radix Angelicae Sinensis *(dang gui)* 9g
Radix Clematidis *(wei ling xian)* 9g
Herba seu Flos Schizonepetae Tenuifoliae *(jing jie)* 9g
Flos Chrysanthemi Morifolii *(ju hua)* 9g
Asbestos *(shi hui mu)* 9g
Radix Salviae Miltiorrhizae *(dan shen)* 9g

Radix Sophorae Flavescentis *(ku shen)* 9g
Radix Adenophorae seu Glehniae *(sha shen)* 9g
Radix Polygoni Multiflori *(he shou wu)* 9g
Herba Equiseti Hiemalis *(mu zei)* 9g
Rhizoma Acori Graminei *(shi chang pu)* 9g
Tuber Asparagi Cochinchinensis *(tian men dong)* 9g
Radix Ligustici Chuanxiong *(chuan xiong)* 9g
Fructus Tribuli Terrestris *(bai ji li)* 9g
Radix Glycyrrhizae Uralensis *(gan cao)* 9g
Rhizoma Atractylodis *(cang zhu)* 9g
Radix Aconiti Kusnezoffii Praeparata *(zhi cao wu)* 9g

PREPARATION & DOSAGE: Grind the ingredients together into a fine powder. Administer 15g as a draft, or mix in warm wine, 2-3 times daily.

❧ Drunken Fairy Powder

醉仙散

zùi xiān sǎn

Dry-fried Fructus Arctii Lappae *(chao niu bang zi)* 30g
Semen Sesami Indici *(hei zhi ma)* 30g
Fructus Lycii *(gou qi zi)* 30g
Fructus Viticis *(man jing zi)* 30g
Radix Sophorae Flavescentis *(ku shen)* 15g
Fructus Tribuli Terrestris *(bai ji li)* 15g
Radix Ledebouriellae Divaricatae *(fang feng)* 15g
Radix Trichosanthis Kirilowii *(tian hua fen)* 15g

PREPARATION & DOSAGE: Grind the ingredients together into a fine powder. Administer in 3g doses, three times daily. Prior to each dose, mix in thoroughly 0.3g of Calomelas *(qing fen)*. Administer with warm, weak tea. The source for this formula is the *Golden Mirror of the Medical Tradition,* where it is observed:

> Five to seven days [after starting this formula], malodorous and yellow saliva will appear from between the teeth. At the same time, there will be pain of the entire body and restlessness. Then there will be passage of blood and pus in the stools, as well as malodorous material, indicating that the root of the condition has been eliminated.

Advanced stage. Included here are lepromatous leprosy and borderline leprosy tending toward lepromatous. The strategy is to nourish the nutritive level and relieve toxicity, support the normal qi and expel the pathogenic factor, and dispel wind and clear the channels.

Formulas recommended for this stage include Polygonum Wine, or Number One Sweep the Wind Powder.

Polygonum Wine
何首乌酒
hé shǒu wū jiǔ

Radix Polygoni Multiflori (he shou wu)	120g
Corpus Radicis Angelicae Sinensis (dang gui tou)	30g
Extremitas Radicis Angelicae Sinensis (dang guiwei)	30g
Prepared Squama Manitis Pentadactylae (chuan shan jia)	30g
Radix Rehmanniae Glutinosae (sheng di huang)	30g
Radix Rehmanniae Glutinosae Conquitae (shu di huang)	30g
Rana Limnocharis (xia ma)	30g
Cacumen Biotae Orientalis (ce bai ye)	120g
Folium Pini (song zhen)	120g
Cortex Acanthopanacis Gracilistylus Radicis (wu jia pi)	120g
Radix Aconiti Carmichaeli Praeparata (zhi chuan wu)	120g
Radix Aconiti Kusnezoffii Praeparata (zhi cao wu)	120g

PREPARATION & DOSAGE: Combine the ingredients and grind coarsely. Wrap in gauze. Soak in one liter of rice or millet wine in a non-metallic container that has a lid. The liquid is ready to use in seven days. Administer once daily an amount that will make the patient feel a bit tipsy, and cause slight sweating. Avoid drafts and wind at this time.

Number One Sweep the Wind Pill
一号扫风丸
yī hào sǎo fēng wán

Semen Hydnocarpi Anthelminticae (da feng zi)	1750g
Herba seu Flos Schizonepetae Tenuifoliae (jing jie)	240g
Semen Coicis Lachryma-jobi (yi yi ren)	240g
Radix Sophorae Flavescentis (ku shen)	120g
Fructus Tribuli Terrestris (bai ji li)	120g
Semen Sesami Indici (hei zhi ma)	120g
Fructus Xanthii Sibirici (cang er zi)	120g
Radix Ledebouriellae Divaricatae (fang feng)	120g
Agkistrodon seu Bungarus (bai hua she)	30g
Rhizoma Atractylodis (cang zhu)	60g
Rhizoma Typhonii Gigantei (bai fu zi)	60g
Ramulus Cinnamomi Cassiae (gui zhi)	60g
Radix Angelicae Sinensis (dang gui)	60g
Radix Gentianae Qinjiao (qin jiao)	60g
Radix Angelicae Dahuricae (bai zhi)	60g
Radix Aconiti Kusnezoffii Praeparata (zhi cao wu)	60g
Radix Clematidis (wei ling xian)	60g
Radix Ligustici Chuanxiong (chuan xiong)	60g
Ramulus cum Uncis Uncariae (gou teng)	60g

Fructus Chaenomelis Lagenariae *(mu gua)*	60g
Semen Cuscutae Chinensis *(tu si zi)*	60g
Cortex Cinnamomi Cassiae *(rou gui)*	60g
Rhizoma Gastrodiae Elatae *(tian ma)*	60g
Radix Cyathulae Officinalis *(chuan niu xi)*	60g
Radix Polygoni Multiflori *(he shou wu)*	60g
Rhizoma Homalomenae Occultae *(qian nian jian)*	60g
Lapis Micae seu Chloriti *(meng shi)*	60g
Radix Aconiti Carmichaeli Praeparata *(zhi chuan wu)*	60g
Rhizoma Anemarrhenae Asphodeloidis *(zhi mu)*	60g
Fructus Gardeniae Jasminoidis *(zhi zi)*	60g

PREPARATION & DOSAGE: Grind the ingredients together into a fine powder and mix with water to form a paste. Make into small boluses. Administer 6g twice daily for the first three days. If there are no side effects (such as nausea and vomiting), then the dose may be increased by 1.5 grams per dose, twice daily, until the eighth day, after which the dose should remain constant, and the frequency of administration increased to three times daily.

EXTERNAL

The following formula may be used as a wash to treat leprosy lesions.

Sophora Decoction
苦参汤
kŭ shēn tāng

Radix Sophorae Flavescentis *(ku shen)*	60g
Fructus Cnidii Monnieri *(she chuang zi)*	30g
Radix Angelicae Dahuricae *(bai zhi)*	15g
Flos Lonicerae Japonicae *(jin yin hua)*	30g
Flos Chrysanthemi Morifolii *(ju hua)*	60g
Cortex Phellodendri *(huang bai)*	15g
Fructus Kochiae Scopariae *(di fu zi)*	15g
Rhizoma Acori Graminei *(shi chang pu)*	9g

PREPARATION & DOSAGE: Decoct the herbs and remove the dregs. Apply wash once or twice daily.

While using Sophora Decoction as a wash, one of the following formulas may also be applied:

[A] Grind Radix Stellerae seu Euphorbiae *(lang du)* into a powder and mix with water to form a paste. Apply once daily. Because of this herb's toxicity, long-term use is discouraged.

[B] Apply Seven-Three Special Powder (see carbuncles) or Red Ointment (se lupus vulgaris) 2-3 times daily.

[C] After the necrotic tissue sloughs, apply Generate Flesh Powder (see carbuncles) and Red Ointment (see lupus vulgaris) 2-3 times daily.

ACUPUNCTURE

The strategy is to disperse wind and drain toxicity, and to invigorate the blood and clear the collaterals. The primary acupoints are LI-11 *(qu chi)*, LI-4 *(he gu)*, LU-10 *(yu ji)*, GB-34 *(yang ling quan)*, ST-36 *(zu san li)*, KI-2 *(ran gu)* and KI-1 *(yong quan)*. Treat once every other day. Needle manipulation is first draining then tonifying, retaining the needles for 20 minutes. Ten sessions are considered one course of therapy, and there should be two weeks' rest between courses.

MODIFICATIONS: For numbness of the fingers, add M-UE-22 *(ba xie)* and SI-3 *(hou xi)*, needling through to LI-3 *(san jian)*. For numbness of the toes, add M-LE-8 *(ba feng)*, LR-2 *(xing jian)* and GB-41 *(zu lin qi)*. For headache, add GB-20 *(feng chi)* and M-HN-9 *(tai yang)*.

EMPIRICAL AND FOLK REMEDIES

Omissions from the Grand Materia Medica by Zhao Xue-Min (1765) contains the following passage:

> Bananas collect leprosy toxin. The regions of Guangdong and Guangxi are damp and hot; many people are tainted with leprosy. Places that are to be inhabited, people do not dare contact; a banana tree must first be planted and bear fruit within the courtyard. One to two years later, all the toxin will have entered into the tree. Then people will dare to inhabit.

In fact, leprosy is endemic in the southern region of China, which includes Guangdong and Guangxi provinces. Perhaps, too, there is some truth to Zhao Xue-Min's statement about bananas and leprosy.

Traditional vs. Biomedical Treatment

In general, treatment of leprosy is rather difficult and prolonged. Biomedical treatment of lepromatous leprosy lasts the entire lifetime of the patient, and treatment of the other forms between six months and ten years. Usually 2-3 drugs are used to avoid mycobacterial resistance. Traditional treatment is also protracted, requiring active therapy of upwards to six months for indeterminate and tuberculoid forms, and 1-2 years for other forms. Thereafter, the patient should remain under observation for reactivation of the disease, upon which treatment should be repeated. In China, traditional practitioners who specialize in the treatment of leprosy suggest a regimen consisting of different formulas, rather than use of a single formula, to avoid mycobacterial resistance. Traditional treatment is also used in conjunction with chemotherapy to address drug side effects and the symptoms of nerve damage caused by the organism.

Prevention

Control requires early treatment. Other people who come into contact with patients should be examined every 6-12 months. Fastidious, long-term follow-up of exposed children is important. Cure by immediate active therapy can be expected if a lesion is found early.

CHAPTER NOTES

1. Yang, Q.S., "Fresh Herba cum Radice Houttuyniae Cordatae in the Treatment of Impetigo of the Scalp in Children," *Zhejiang Journal of Traditional Chinese Medicine,* 25(7): 304; 1990.

2. Luo, H.F., "Experience in Treating Impetigo, *Sichuan Journal of Traditional Chinese Medicine* 8(5): 36, 1990.

3. Ye, J.Q. *Traditional Chinese Food Medicinals and Folk Prescriptions (Shi wu zhong yao yu pian fang).* Jiangsu: Jiangsu Science and Technology Press, 1980.

4. Dai, Y.F. and Liu, C.J. *Medicinal Uses of Fruits (Yao yong guo pin).* Nanning: Guangxi People's Publishing House, 1982.

5. Ibid.

6. Dou, G.X. *Guide to Food Therapy (Yin shi zhi liao zhi nan).* Jiangsu: Jiangsu Science and Technology Press, 1981.

7. Ibid.

8. Zhang, H., "Modified Golden-Yellow Powder According to One's Wishes in the Treatment of Furuncles," *Sichuan Journal of Traditional Chinese Medicine,* 8(5): 38; 1990.

9. Ibid.

10. Li, F.F., Ma, X.T., and Qian, B.R., "Use of the Thick Needle in the Treatment of Carbuncles," *Chinese Acupuncture and Moxibustion,* 9(4): 13-14; 1989.

11. Dou, *Guide to Food Therapy (Yin shi zhi liao zhi nan).*

12. Duan, P., "External Use of Erysipelas Plaster to Treat Erysipelas," *Sichuan Journal of Traditional Chinese Medicine,* 8(2): 39-40; 1990.

13. Zhu, Y.J., "Bloodletting and Cupping in the Treatment of Erysipelas," *Shanghai Journal of Acupuncture and Moxibustion,* 9(3): 49; 1990.

CHAPTER 8

Viral Infections

Herpes Simplex
热疮
rè chuāng, "heat sores"

Herpes simplex is a common viral disease characterized by clusters of blisters on the skin or mucous membranes. A condition like this known as "heat sores" was first described in *Emergency Formulas to Keep Up One's Sleeve* (341), and later in Liu Juan-Zi's *Formulas Passed Down From a Spirit* (Jin dynasty). The disease was called "heat sores" because the lesions usually appear following febrile conditions.

Biomedically, herpes simplex is caused by the herpes simplex virus.

Signs & Symptoms

The first infection begins with local tenderness lasting one to two days. Small clusters of vesicles then appear; at this time, the pain may be severe. Accompanying symptoms may include high fever and swelling or tenderness of the lymph nodes. Crusting of the lesions begins after three to four days of onset, and complete healing within three weeks.

With recurrent infections, there is burning or tingling and redness of the skin for several hours prior to the appearance of the first blister. Recurrences are usually not as painful and uncomfortable as the initial infection. These secondary eruptions are often triggered by high fever or other infection in the body, overexposure to the sun, physical trauma, menstruation, or emotional upset.

During the initial stage of both first and recurrent infections, in addition to the aforementioned symptoms, there may also be dryness of the mouth, thirst, dry stools, yellow urine, redness of the tongue, and a wiry, rapid pulse.

Differential Diagnosis

Herpes simplex should be distinguished from herpes zoster (shingles). The latter usually does not recur and is often more painful than the former. The hallmark of herpes zoster is the dermatomal distribution of the blisters, commonly in the thoracic dermatomes. Other conditions that should be differentiated from herpes simplex include chickenpox, impetigo, drug eruptions, and dermatitis. Confirmation of herpes simplex is through glass slide smear (Tzanck smear), or laboratory culture for the virus, and, in primary infections, through the finding of serum antibodies.

Traditional Chinese Etiology

Herpes lesions that appear on the upper part of the body are generally due to wind-heat toxin attacking and leading to a fuming upwards in the Lung and Stomach channels. Lesions on the lower part of the body are often caused by damp toxin lodged in the Liver and Gallbladder channels. Recurrent herpes is usually the result of dysfunction of the Spleen/Stomach's transportive and transformative mechanisms, causing accumulation of heat which then steams upward; or it may be due to heat injuring the fluids, and giving rise to deficiency heat which blazes outward into the tissue and skin, thus causing the herpes lesions.

Treatment

INTERNAL

Wind-heat affecting the upper body. The lesions appear at the corners of the mouth, or about the lips, or on the upper lip below the nostrils, or on the cheeks. Generalized symptoms may include dryness of the mouth, restlessness, dry stools, redness of the tongue with a thin white or yellow coating, and a wiry, slippery and rapid pulse. The strategy is to disperse the wind and clear the heat. The formula recommended for this pattern is Magnolia Flower Decoction to Clear the Lung.

❀ Magnolia Flower Decoction to Clear the Lung
辛夷清肺饮
xīn yí qīng fèi yǐn

Flos Magnoliae *(xin yi hua)*	1.8g
Radix Glycyrrhizae Uralensis *(gan cao)*	1.5g
Calcined Gypsum *(duan shi gao)*	3g
Rhizoma Anemarrhenae Asphodeloidis *(zhi mu)*	3g
Fructus Gardeniae Jasminoidis *(zhi zi)*	3g
Radix Scutellariae Baicalensis *(huang qin)*	3g
Folium Eriobotryae Japonicae *(pi pa ye)* (with fur removed)	3g
Rhizoma Cimicifugae *(sheng ma)*	0.9g
Bulbus Lilii *(bai he)*	3g
Tuber Ophiopogonis Japonici *(mai men dong)*	3g

PREPARATION & DOSAGE: Decoct and administer in three doses daily after meals.

Damp-heat lodged in the lower burner. Lesions of this pattern usually affect the genitalia. Generalized symptoms may include blood-tinged urine, dry stools or constipation, a red tongue with a sticky yellow coating, and a wiry, slippery and rapid pulse. The strategy is to resolve the dampness and clear the heat. The formula recommended for this pattern is Gentiana Longdancao Decoction to Drain the Liver.

❧ Gentiana Longdancao Decoction to Drain the Liver
龙胆泻肝汤
lóng dǎn xiè gān tāng

Radix Gentianae Longdancao *(long dan cao)*	3g
Radix Scutellariae Baicalensis *(huang qin)*	3g
Fructus Gardeniae Jasminoidis *(zhi zi)*	3g
Rhizome Alismatis Orientalis *(ze xie)*	3g
Caulis Mutong *(mu tong)*	1.5g
Semen Plantaginis *(che qian zi)*	1.5g
Radix Angelicae Sinensis *(dang gui)*	1.5g
Radix Rehmanniae Glutinosae *(sheng di huang)*	1.5g
Radix Bupleuri *(chai hu)*	1.5g
Radix Glycyrrhizae Uralensis *(gan cao)*	1.5g

PREPARATION & DOSAGE: Decoct and administer in two doses daily.

Accumulated heat in the Spleen/Stomach. Lesions are usually found on the face, especially the cheeks, and are recurrent. Generalized symptoms may include lack of appetite, dry stools or constipation, red lips, a red tongue with a dry yellow coating, and a flooding, rapid pulse. The strategy is to clear accumulated heat from the Spleen/Stomach. The formula recommended for this pattern is Lophatherus and Gypsum Decoction.

❧ Lophatherus and Gypsum Decoction
竹叶石膏汤
zhú yè shí gāo tāng

Herba Lophatheri Gracilis *(dan zhu ye)*	9-15g
Gypsum *(shi gao)*	30g
Radix Ginseng *(ren shen)*	6g
Rhizoma Pinelliae Ternatae *(ban xia)*	9-18g
Nonglutinous rice *(geng mi)*	12-15g
Honey-toasted Radix Glycyrrhizae Uralensis *(zhi gan cao)*	3-6g

PREPARATION & DOSAGE: Decoct and administer in two doses daily.

For mild cases of accumulated damp-heat in the Stomach/Spleen, Ledebouriella Powder that Sagely Unblocks is recommended.

Ledebouriella Powder that Sagely Unblocks
防风通圣散
fáng fēng tōng shèng sǎn

Radix Ledebouriellae Divaricatae *(fang feng)*	15g
Herba seu Flos Schizonepetae Tenuifoliae *(jing jie)*	15g
Fructus Forsythiae Suspensae *(lian qiao)*	15g
Herba Ephedrae *(ma huang)*	15g
Herba Menthae Haplocalycis *(bo he)*	15g
Radix Ligustici Chuanxiong *(chuan xiong)*	15g
Radix Angelicae Sinensis *(dang gui)*	15g
Dry-fried Radix Paeoniae Lactiflorae *(chao bai shao)*	15g
Rhizoma Atractylodis Macrocephalae *(bai zhu)*	15g
Fructus Gardeniae Jasminoidis *(zhi zi)*	15g
Radix et Rhizoma Rhei *(da huang)* (wine steamed)	15g
Mirabilitum *(mang xiao)*	15g
Gypsum *(shi gao)*	30g
Radix Scutellariae Baicalensis *(huang qin)*	30g
Radix Platycodi Grandiflori *(jie geng)*	30g
Radix Glycyrrhizae Uralensis *(gan cao)*	6g
Talcum *(hua shi)*	9g

PREPARATION & DOSAGE: Grind the ingredients together into a powder. Add water to form a paste, and make into small pills the size of mung beans. Administer 6g once daily.

Deficiency heat pattern. The herpes lesions are recurrent. Generalized symptoms may include dry throat, dry lips, thirst with a desire to drink, a scarlet tongue with no coating, and a thin, rapid pulse. The strategy is to nourish yin and clear heat. The formula recommended for this pattern is Anemarrhena, Phellodendron, and Rehmannia Decoction.

Anemarrhena, Phellodendron, and Rehmannia Decoction
知柏地黄丸
zhī bǎi dì huáng wán

Radix Rehmanniae Glutinosae Conquitae *(shu di huang)*	240g
Fructus Corni Officinalis *(shan zhu yu)*	120g
Radix Dioscoreae Oppositae *(shan yao)*	120g
Sclerotium Poriae Cocos *(fu ling)*	90g
Cortex Moutan Radicis *(mu dan pi)*	90g
Rhizome Alismatis Orientalis *(ze xie)*	90g
Rhizoma Anemarrhenae Asphodeloidis *(zhi mu)*	90g
Cortex Phellodendri *(huang bai)*	90g

PREPARATION & DOSAGE: Administer in one dose daily. When the acute outbreak is resolved, this formula may administered twice weekly for three months as a preventive measure. For mild cases, the pill form may be used instead.

For deficiency heat patterns accompanied by deficient qi, Modified Ginseng Pill to Stabilize the Root is recommended.

❦ Modified Ginseng Pill to Stabilize the Root
人参固本丸加减
rén shēn gù běn wán jiā jiǎn

Radix Adenophorae seu Glehniae (sha shen)	15g
Radix Rehmanniae Glutinosae (sheng di huang)	15g
Tuber Asparagi Cochinchinensis (tian men dong)	12g
Tuber Ophiopogonis Japonici (mai men dong)	12g
Semen Coicis Lachryma-jobi (yi yi ren)	12g
Radix Dioscoreae Oppositae (shan yao)	12g
Radix Astragali Membranacei (huang qi)	10g
Radix Glycyrrhizae Uralensis (gan cao)	10g
Dry-fried Radix Paeoniae Lactiflorae (chao bai shao)	10g
Rhizoma Cimicifugae (sheng ma)	6g
Radix Isatidis seu Baphicacanthi (ban lan gen)	6g

PREPARATION & DOSAGE: Administer in three doses daily.

MODIFICATIONS: For lesions affecting the eye, add Semen Celosiae Argenteae (qing xiang zi), Flos Chrysanthemi Morifolii (hang ju hua) and Folium Mori Albae (sang ye); for lesions affecting the genitals, add dry-fried Radix Gentianae Longdancao (chao long dan cao), Rhizoma Imperatae Cylindricae (bai mao gen) and Herba Plantaginis (che qian cao); for recalcitrant lesions, add Radix Ampelopsis Japonicae (bai lian), Radix Cynanchi Baiwei (bai wei), Radix Panacis Quinquefolii (xi yang shen) and Testa Phaseoli Radiati (lu dou yi); for severe itching and pain, add Radix Arnebiae seu Lithospermi (zi cao), Ramulus cum Uncis Uncariae (gou teng) and Concha Haliotidis (shi jue ming).

EXTERNAL

For papular or vesicular lesions that show erosion, Portulaca Wash is recommended.

❦ Portulaca Wash
马齿苋水洗剂
mǎ chǐ xiàn shuǐ xǐ jì

Herba Portulacae Oleraceae (ma chi xian)	120g

PREPARATION & DOSAGE: Decoct the herb in 1500ml of water down to 300ml. Apply as a warm, wet compress 3-5 times daily, 10-15 minutes each time.

As a general topical application for all patterns of herpes simplex, Jade Dew Plaster is recommended.

❧ Jade Dew Plaster
玉露膏
yù lù gāo

Folium Hibisci Mutabilis *(mu fu rong ye)*	1000g
Petroleum Jelly	5000g

PREPARATION & DOSAGE: Dissolve the petroleum jelly over low heat in a non-metallic pot. Stir in the herb. Cook over low heat until the herb turns black. Remove the dregs and add beeswax until the consistency thickens. Store in an airtight glass container. Apply directly to the affected area twice daily; or spread onto gauze and affix to the affected area, changing the dressing once daily.

ACUPUNCTURE
See herpes zoster.

EMPIRICAL REMEDIES
For outbreaks near the mouth and nose, the acupoint known as Ear Apex (at the tip of the fold on the superior aspect of the helix as the ear is bent toward the tragus) may be bloodlet.[1] After pricking the point, squeeze out about 8-10 drops of blood. Treat once daily. The lesions usually form scabs after 3-4 treatments. This method is especially effective for primary outbreaks.

Traditional vs. Biomedical Treatment
Treatment in general is aimed at shortening the course of disease. Traditional treatment may be more effective in preventing recurrences, provided of course that the correct pattern differentiation is reached and the appropriate treatment is administered. The biomedical treatment of choice for herpes simplex is acyclovir, which is effective for both primary and recurrent herpes. However, the drug's disadvantages are its ineffectiveness against latent herpes (particularly genital herpes infections) and its side effects, which can include nausea, vomiting, diarrhea, headache and rashes. Individuals undergoing acyclovir therapy should slowly discontinue the drug after starting traditional treatment in order to allow the latter to take hold.

Prevention
Primary outbreaks should be treated promptly and thoroughly to prevent recurrence. In recurrent cases, the cause(s) of the outbreaks should be determined and eliminated, e.g., certain foods, emotional stress and environmental factors.

Herpes Zoster
蛇串疮
shé chuàn chuāng, "snake cluster sores"

Herpes zoster, or shingles, is an infection of the nerves that supply certain areas of the skin. The condition is characterized by painful vesicular eruptions. It was first described in *Discussion of the Origins of Symptoms of Diseases* (610) where it was called "snake cluster sores" because of the often unilateral, chain-like distribution of the lesions on the body. Other names for this condition include "fire band sores" *(huǒ dài chuāng)*, "spider sores" *(zhī zhū chuāng)* and "snake burrow sores" *(shé kē chuāng)*. And because the lesions often break out in the thoracic area, it has also been called "waist-binding erysipelas" *(chán yāo dān)*.

Biomedically, herpes zoster is caused by the varicella-zoster virus, which also causes chickenpox.

Signs & Symptoms

The condition begins with fever and malaise. Within two to four days, deep aching pain, itching, and hyperasthesia develop on the trunk and sometimes the arms and legs of the affected dermatome. After between four to 14 days, the characteristic eruption appears as clusters of red papules that soon develop into virus laden vesicles and pustules. Within three days the blisters turn yellow and dry, although new lesions may continue to erupt for two to four days in the dermatome. Healing is ordinarily within 14 days or so. Occasionally, herpes zoster affects the cranial nerves, particularly the trigeminal and geniculate ganglia or the oculomotor nerve, which may lead to impairment of vision and hearing. The intractable pain of postherpetic neuralgia, the most common complication of shingles in the elderly, may last for years and even be disabling. Herpes zoster rarely recurs.

Differential Diagnosis

Diagnosis is often not possible before eruption, but is easily made once the vesicles appear in the characteristic dermatome distribution. Pain is also an outstanding feature of herpes zoster, especially post-zoster pain. However, if the pain is in the thoracic region, it must be differentiated from that of appendicitis, renal colic, gallstones or colitis. Trigeminal neuralgia and Bell's palsy must be ruled out if the face is affected. Herpes simplex lesions may be nearly identical to those of herpes zoster. Herpes simplex generally recurs, whereas zoster rarely does. Contact dermatitis will have a history of skin contact with a substance, and generally there is no associated pain.

Traditional Chinese Etiology

The two primary causes of herpes zoster are blazing fire in the Liver channel and damp-heat in the Spleen channel. A third pattern, associated with post-herpetic pain, is caused by stagnation of qi and blood.

Blazing fire in the Liver channel. This pattern is often caused by emotional disturbance such that the Liver qi becomes constrained. Longstanding constrained qi leads to transformation into fire, which blazes outward from the channel and collaterals into the skin, thus causing the herpes lesions.

Damp-heat in the Spleen channel. Spleen deficiency is usually the source of this pattern. The Spleen's transportive and transformative functions are disturbed, which leads to accumulation of dampness. Unresolved dampness transforms into and contends with heat. The herpes lesions are thus the product of the struggle between the pathogenic factors of heat and dampness.

Stagnation of qi and blood. This commonly seen pattern appears in individuals who have experienced the initial attack, and whose qi and blood are stagnant, such that the toxin is still present in the tissue and skin and continues to cause pain.

Treatment

INTERNAL

Golden Mirror of the Medical Tradition (1742) described the various patterns associated with herpes zoster:

> This pattern can be differentiated by dry and wet, red and yellow; all [both types] are [characterized by] continuous beads. The dry ones are red and formed as clouds, topped by wind-millets, with itching and heat; this is due to wind-heat in the Heart and Liver channels. The wet ones are yellowish-white vesicles of different sizes, which when they fester will ooze, and are more painful than dry ones; this is due to damp-heat in the Spleen and Lung channels.

Successful treatment thus depends on correct differentiation of the lesions.

Blazing fire in the Liver channel. Lesions of this pattern are red, with taut vesicle walls that are bright red and have a burning sensation. The pain resembles pin-pricks. Generalized symptoms usually include a bitter taste in the mouth, dry throat, thirst with preference for cold beverages, restlessness and propensity toward anger, dry stools or constipation, a red tongue tip with a yellow or dry coating, and a wiry, rapid pulse. The strategy is to clear the Liver and drain the heat.

One of the formulas recommended for this pattern is Gentiana Longdancao Decoction to Drain the Liver (see herpes simplex), with the following modifications: for dry stools, add Radix et Rhizoma Rhei *(da huang)* (at the end of the decoction); for vesicles filled with blood, add Cortex Moutan Radicis *(mu dan pi)* and Radix Paeoniae Rubrae *(chi shao);* for eruptions on the face, add Flos Chrysanthemi Morifolii *(ju hua)* and Concha Haliotidis *(shi jue ming).*

Another appropriate formula is Modified Daqingye and Forsythia Decoction.

❧ Modified Daqingye and Forsythia Decoction
大青连翘汤加减
dà qīng lián qiáo tāng jiā jiǎn

Folium Daqingye *(da qing ye)*	9g
Radix Scrophulariae Ningpoensis *(xuan shen)*	9g
Rhizoma Guanzhong *(guan zhong)*	9g
Radix Scutellariae Baicalensis *(huang qin)*	9g
Fructus Forsythiae Suspensae *(lian qiao)*	12g
Flos Lonicerae Japonicae *(jin yin hua)*	12g
Radix Rehmanniae Glutinosae *(sheng di huang)*	12g

Herba Portulacae Oleraceae *(ma chi xian)*	12g
Dry-fried Cortex Moutan Radicis *(chao mu dan pi)*	6g
Radix Paeoniae Rubrae *(chi shao)*	6g
Testa Phaseoli Radiati *(lu dou yi)*	15g

PREPARATION & DOSAGE: Decoct and administer in two doses daily.

Damp-heat in the Spleen channel. Herpes vesicles of this pattern are large and filled with yellowish white serous fluid. The vesicle walls are thin and easily broken, after which there may be festering or pus formation. In serious cases, necrosis will occur followed by formation of black scabs. Generalized symptoms may include poor appetite, bloating and unformed stools, a fat tongue with a yellow sticky coating, and a soggy, moderate and slippery pulse. The strategy is to strengthen the Spleen in order to resolve dampness and clear heat.

Formulas recommended for this pattern include Eliminate Dampness Decoction by Combining Calm the Stomach and Five-Ingredient Powder with Poria; or Modified Coix and Phaseolus Decoction.

❧ Eliminate Dampness Decoction by Combining Calm the Stomach and Five-Ingredient Powder with Poria
除湿胃苓汤
chú shī wèi líng tāng

Rhizoma Atractylodis *(cang zhu)*	3g
Cortex Magnoliae Officinalis *(hou po)*	3g
Pericarpium Citri Reticulatae *(chen pi)*	3g
Sclerotium Polypori Umbellati *(zhu ling)*	3g
Rhizome Alismatis Orientalis *(ze xie)*	3g
Sclerotium Poriae Cocos Rubrae *(chi fu ling)*	3g
Rhizoma Atractylodis Macrocephalae *(bai zhu)*	3g
Talcum *(hua shi)*	3g
Radix Ledebouriellae Divaricatae *(fang feng)*	3g
Caulis Mutong *(mu tong)*	3g
Fructus Gardeniae Jasminoidis *(zhi zi)*	3g
Radix Glycyrrhizae Uralensis *(gan cao)*	1g
Cortex Cinnamomi Cassiae *(rou gui)*	1g
Medulla Junci Effusi *(deng xin cao)*	3g

PREPARATION & DOSAGE: Decoct the herbs in 400ml of water until 320ml remain. Administer the decoction in one dose daily on an empty stomach.

❧ Modified Coix and Phaseolus Decoction
薏仁赤豆汤加减
yì rén chì dòu tāng jiā jiǎn

Semen Coicis Lachryma-jobi *(yi yi ren)*	15g
Semen Phaseoli Calcarati *(chi xiao dou)*	15g
Cortex Poriae Cocos *(fu ling pi)*	12g

Flos Lonicerae Japonicae *(jin yin hua)* 12g
Fructus Kochiae Scopariae *(di fu zi)* 12g
Radix Rehmanniae Glutinosae *(sheng di huang)* 12g
Semen Plantaginis *(che qian zi)* 9g
Herba Plantaginis *(che qian cao)* 9g
Radix Paeoniae Rubrae *(chi shao)* 9g
Herba Portulacae Oleraceae *(ma chi xian)* 9g
Radix Glycyrrhizae Uralensis *(gan cao)* 9g
Secretio Moschus *(she xiang)* 10g
Herba Eupatorii Fortunei *(pei lan)* 10g

PREPARATION & DOSAGE: Decoct and administer in two doses daily.

Stagnation of qi and blood. This pattern corresponds with post-herpetic pain, and often affects the elderly. The lesions are characterized by semi-erupted papules, pain that is sharp and like pin pricks, or soreness that is exacerbated by movement of the affected area. Generalized symptoms may include lack of appetite, disturbed sleep, restlessness, a red tongue with thin yellow tongue coating, and a thin, choppy pulse. The strategy is to disperse and regulate Liver qi, and clear the channel and stop pain. Formulas recommended for this pattern include Rambling Powder, or Modified Melia Powder.

❦ Rambling Powder
逍遥散
xiāo yáo sǎn

Radix Bupleuri *(chai hu)* 9g
Radix Angelicae Sinensis *(dang gui)* 9g
Radix Paeoniae Lactiflorae *(bai shao)* 9g
Rhizoma Atractylodis Macrocephalae *(bai zhu)* 9g
Sclerotium Poriae Cocos *(fu ling)* 9g
Honey-toasted Radix Glycyrrhizae Uralensis *(zhi gan cao)* 6g

PREPARATION & DOSAGE: Decoct and administer in one dose daily.

❦ Modified Melia Powder
金铃子散加减
jīn líng zǐ sǎn jiā jiǎn

Fructus Meliae Toosendan *(chuan lian zi)* 9g
Tuber Curcumae *(yu jin)* 9g
Radix Arnebiae seu Lithospermi *(zi cao)* 9g
Rhizoma Corydalis Yanhusuo *(yan hu suo)* 6g
Radix Bupleuri *(chai hu)* 6g
Pericarpium Citri Reticulatae Viride *(qing pi)* 6g
Dry-fried Radix Paeoniae Lactiflorae *(chao bai shao)* 12g
Radix Angelicae Sinensis *(dang gui)* 12g

Fasciculus Vascularis Luffae *(si gua luo)* 10g

PREPARATION & DOSAGE: Decoct and administer in one dose daily.

EXTERNAL

For early eruptions accompanied by extreme pain, Aloe, Borneol, and Magarita Paste may be applied.

❦ Aloe, Borneol, and Magarita Paste
芦荟冰珠外敷剂
lú huì bīng zhū wài fū jì

Herba Aloes *(lu hui)* (fresh) .... 1 leaf (a few inches long)
Borneol *(bing pian)* 0.3–1.0g
Magarita *(zhen zhu)* (powdered) .... a pinch

PREPARATION & DOSAGE: Mash the ingredients together and apply 1-2 times daily.

For taut vesicles that are about to break, accompanied by severe pain, Jade Dew Plaster (see herpes simplex) may be applied once daily.

For vesicles that have broken and are oozing, first spread a layer of Coptis Ointment (described below) on sterile gauze. Then sprinkle a thin layer of Borneol and Gypsum Powder (described below) on the layer of Coptis Ointment. Affix the gauze to the affected area. Reapply this combined remedy every 2-3 days. Avoid bathing the area during the course of treatment.

❦ Coptis Ointment
黄连膏
huáng lián gāo

Rhizoma Coptidis *(huang lian)* (powdered) 9g
Radix Angelicae Sinensis *(dang gui)* 15g
Cortex Phellodendri *(huang bai)* 9g
Radix Rehmanniae Glutinosae *(sheng di huang)* 30g
Rhizoma Curcumae Longae *(jiang huang)* 9g
Sesame Oil 440ml
Beeswax 120g

PREPARATION & DOSAGE: Decoct the Radix Angelicae Sinensis *(dang gui)*, Cortex Phellodendri *(huang bai)*, Radix Rehmanniae Glutinosae *(sheng di huang)* and Rhizoma Curcumae Longae *(jiang huang)* in the sesame oil until the herbs turn brown. Remove the dregs, continue cooking over low heat and add the beeswax. When the beeswax has completely melted, turn the heat off and allow the contents to cool to lukewarm. Add the powdered Rhizoma Coptidis *(huang lian)* and stir well. Store the remedy in an airtight glass container.

🌸 Borneol and Gypsum Powder

冰石散

bīng shí sǎn

Calcined Gypsum (duan shi gao)	30g
Borneol (bing pian)	0.6g

PREPARATION & DOSAGE: Grind the two ingredients separately into fine powders, then combine them and store in an airtight glass container.

For pustular and necrotic lesions that have not sloughed, spread a thin layer of Coptis Ointment (see above) onto sterile gauze. Then sprinkle a thin layer of Nine-One Special Powder (see below) onto the Coptis Ointment. Affix the gauze to the affected area. Reapply this combined remedy once every two days. Avoid bathing the area during the course of treatment.

🌸 Nine-One Special Powder

九一丹

jiǔ yī dān

Calcined Gypsum (duan shi gao)	27g
Mimium (qian dan)	3g

PREPARATION & DOSAGE: Grind the ingredients together into a fine powder. Store in an amber glass jar, with a tight-fitting lid, and away from sunlight.

CLINICAL NOTE: Because of the lead content of Mimium *(qian dan)*, long-term use of this formula is discouraged.

ACUPUNCTURE

The following acupuncture regimens may be used to treat herpes simplex or herpes zoster.

Body needling. The primary points are LI-11 *(qu chi)*, GV-12 *(shen zhu)*, GB-34 *(yang ling quan)* and SP-6 *(san yin jiao)*. The secondary points are M-HN-9 *(tai yang)*, ST-8 *(tou wei)* and GB-14 *(yang bai)* for lesions near the eye; ST-2 *(si bai)*, BL-1 *(jing ming)* and ST-7 *(xia guan)* for lesions on the cheek; ST-6 *(jia che)*, ST-4 *(di cang)* and ST-5 *(da ying)* for lesions on the jaw. In addition, use LI-4 *(he gu)* for lesions above the umbilicus, and ST-36 *(zu san li)* for lesions below the umbilicus. Treat once daily with strong, even needle manipulation, and retain needles for 20-30 minutes.

Local needling. This may be utilized alone or in conjunction with body needling, depending on the patient's tolerance. Four needles (30-32 gauge, 3-4 units in length) are inserted radially at 15-30° angles (toward a central point) surrounding a cluster of lesions. Needles are retained for 30 minutes, with needle manipulation every 10 minutes. Treat once daily, with ten treatments constituting one course of therapy.

MOXIBUSTION

Apply moxa roll moxibustion to healthy areas between lesions. Extreme itching will occur due to the heat. Continue moxibustion until the itching stops and becomes a sensation of extreme heat, then cease treatment. Treat once daily. Lesions will usually show evidence of healing after 3-4 sessions.

CUPPING

Cupping may be used for early outbreaks. First apply one cup each at the two endpoints of a group of lesions (herpes zoster lesions are usually arranged linearly). Retain cups in place for about 15 minutes. Vesicles filled with serous fluid may appear during or following cupping. Cups are then applied consecutively along the path of the lesions. Treat once daily. Lesions will usually show evidence of healing after 4-5 sessions.

EMPIRICAL REMEDIES

[A] The following formula is directed at clearing heat and eliminating dampness, and relieving toxicity.

❧ Smilax and Rheum Decoction[2]
土茯苓大黄汤
tǔ fú líng dà huáng tāng

Rhizoma Smilacis Glabrae *(tu fu ling)*	120g
Radix et Rhizoma Rhei *(da huang)*	30g
Flos Lonicerae Japonicae *(jin yin hua)*	30g
Fructus Forsythiae Suspensae *(lian qiao)*	30g
Rhizoma Coptidis *(huang lian)*	10g
Cortex Phellodendri *(huang bai)*	10g
Radix Rehmanniae Glutinosae *(sheng di huang)*	10g

PREPARATION & DOSAGE: Decoct and administer in two doses daily. This formula should be administered only during acute outbreaks. It is very effective, with most patients experiencing relief of symptoms after 3-4 doses.

CLINICAL NOTE: Because this formula contains several herbs that are cold in nature, long-term use is discouraged.

[B] The following remedy is based on the classical formula known as Warming and Clearing Decoction *(wēn qīng yǐn)*, which is a combination of Four-Substance Decoction *(sì wù tāng)* and Coptis Decoction to Relieve Toxicity *(huáng lián jiě dú tāng)*. As applied to treating herpes zoster, the aim of this formula is to clear heat and eliminate dampness, and disperse Liver qi and alleviate pain.

❧ Modified Warming and Clearing Decoction[3]
温清饮加减
wēn qīng yǐn jiā jiǎn

Radix Rehmanniae Glutinosae *(sheng di huang)*	15g

Radix Angelicae Sinensis *(dang gui)*	12g
Radix Paeoniae Rubrae *(chi shao)*	15g
Radix Ligustici Chuanxiong *(chuan xiong)*	10g
Radix Scutellariae Baicalensis *(huang qin)*	15g
Fructus Gardeniae Jasminoidis *(zhi zi)*	10g
Rhizoma Coptidis *(huang lian)*	5g
Rhizoma Smilacis Glabrae *(tu fu ling)*	15g
Fructus Citri Aurantii *(zhi ke)*	10g
Fasciculus Vascularis Luffae *(si gua luo)*	10g
Radix Glycyrrhizae Uralensis *(gan cao)*	10g
Radix Sophorae Flavescentis *(ku shen)*	10g

PREPARATION & DOSAGE: Decoct and administer in one dose daily. Save some of the decoction and apply as a wash twice daily.

[C] The following needling method[4] may be applied to lesions at any stage. Use a 28 gauge, 0.5 unit needle to prick the healthy skin immediately adjacent to the herpes lesions. Plunge the needle perpendicularly to a depth of about 0.4 unit, then withdraw the needle quickly. Do not manipulate the needle. Each prick is separated by about 0.5 inch. Treat once daily, with five sessions constituting one course of treatment. Healing usually occurs after one course.

This type of needling is said to promote the flow of qi and blood, and to clear the channels and collaterals. In the specific case of herpes zoster, it clears constrained fire.

Traditional vs. Biomedical Treatment

Treatment in general is aimed at accelerating healing. Traditional therapy is perhaps more efficient than biomedical in that a single treatment can address both the herpetic lesions as well as the pain, with complete resolution (lesions and pain) within an average of ten days, often without post-herpetic neuralgia. Biomedical therapy, on the other hand, requires two separate medications: acyclovir to treat the lesions, and an analgesic or cortisone to manage the pain. However, even after such intervention, post-herpetic pain can still affect a number of patients.

Prevention

Herpes zoster rarely recurs. However, during the initial outbreak, precautions should be taken to avoid concurrent infections of the lesions. Patients should rest as much as possible during the outbreak to facilitate healing. Greasy, sweet or spicy foods, as well as alcohol, should be avoided during the outbreak.

Common Warts
千日疮
qiān rì chuāng, "thousand-day sores"

Warts are common, benign skin tumors. In Chinese medicine, warts are classified as *yóu,* which means an extraneous growth on the body. *Yóu* were first described in Chapter 10 of the *Divine Pivot*, but Chao Yuan-Fang's description in *Discussion of the Origins of Symptoms of Diseases* (610) more closely resembled warts. Chao called these growths "extraneous growth eyes" *(yóu mù)*: "Extraneous growth eyes arise on the sides of the hands or feet, and resemble beans or nodular sinews. Sometimes there are five and sometimes ten; they are connected and stronger [firmer] than [ordinary] tissue." In the Ming dynasty, Shen Dou-Yuan in *Profound Insights on External Diseases* termed these growths "thousand day sores":

> One name is extraneous growth sores, another is unlucky sores. These sores resemble fish scales, and grow on the hands and feet. . . . They grow for a thousand days, then drop off by themselves, thus the name thousand-day sores.

Biomedically, common warts are caused by at least thirty-five types of human papilloma virus.

Signs & Symptoms

Lesions can vary in shape depending on location and viral type. The most commonly affected sites include the fingers, elbows, knees, face, and scalp—areas that are subject to trauma. Warts can appear as a single lesion or in clusters. Common warts are generally painless, but plantar warts and those that grow into the finger or toenails can be exceedingly painful.

Common warts are nearly universal, and may appear at any age. They are most frequent in older children and are uncommon in the elderly. Complete regression after several months is typical with or without treatment, but warts may persist for years and may recur at the same or different sites.

Differential Diagnosis

Common warts should be distinguished from moles, which may resemble warts in shape, color and size. Other skin lesions that may be confused with warts are squamous cell carcinoma, keratoacanthoma and other keratoses (horny growths). Diagnosis of warts is made through laboratory demonstration of the presence of the human papilloma virus.

Traditional Chinese Etiology

Warts are usually due to dry blood of the Liver channel, such that blood is unable to nourish the sinews, whose qi then fails to flourish. Thus, when attacked by wind, blood and qi congeal, and give rise to warts.

Treatment

INTERNAL

Most cases of common warts do not require internal treatment. But for recurring and/or recalcitrant lesions, the internal formulas described below may be administered. Most formulas that treat warts are aimed at nourishing and invigorating the blood, calming the spirit and anchoring yang, and clearing heat and relieving toxicity. As such, they should be avoided or used only with caution in pregnant women.

❦ Lithospermum and Isatis Formula
紫蓝方
zǐ lán fāng

Herba Portulacae Oleraceae (ma chi xian)	60g
Radix Isatidis seu Baphicacanthi (ban lan gen)	30g
Folium Daqingye (da qing ye)	30g
Semen Coicis Lachryma-jobi (yi yi ren)	15g
Radix Arnebiae seu Lithospermi (zi cao)	15g
Radix Paeoniae Rubrae (chi shao)	15g
Flos Carthami Tinctorii (hong hua)	15g

PREPARATION & DOSAGE: Decoct and administer in a single daily dose for 7-10 days. If warts do not begin to disappear, discontinue the formula and consider other remedies.

❦ Modified Tangkuei, Peony, and Rehmannia Decoction
归芍地黄汤加减
guī sháo dì huáng tāng jiā jiǎn

Radix Rehmanniae Glutinosae Conquitae (shu di huang)	6g
Radix Angelicae Sinensis (dang gui)	6g
Radix Paeoniae Rubrae (chi shao)	6g
Radix Paeoniae Lactiflorae (bai shao)	6g
Radix Ligustici Chuanxiong (chuan xiong)	6g
Semen Persicae (tao ren)	6g
Flos Carthami Tinctorii (hong hua)	6g
Rhizoma Curcumae Ezhu (e zhu)	6g
Rhizoma Atractylodis Macrocephalae (bai zhu)	6g
Rhizoma Cyperi Rotundi (xiang fu)	6g
Radix Polygoni Multiflori (he shou wu)	15g
Spica Prunellae Vulgaris (xia ku cao)	15g
Radix Isatidis seu Baphicacanthi (ban lan gen)	15g
Concha Ostreae (mu li)	30g
Os Draconis (long gu)	30g

PREPARATION & DOSAGE: Decoct twice. Individuals who can take alcohol may add 30ml of rice wine at the end of each decoction. Administer the first decoction before bedtime, and the second the following morning. Continue taking the formula until the lesions have resolved.

EXTERNAL

According to Chinese medicine, the original lesion ("mother wart") should be treated first. After it is resolved, the remaining warts should resolve spontaneously. That having been said, it is probably more reliable to treat all of the lesions at the same time. The following external remedies may be used to treat warts.

❧ Thousand Ducat Powder
千金散
qiān jīn sǎn

Gummi Olibanum *(ru xiang)*	15g
Myrrha *(mo yao)*	15g
Calomelas *(qing fen)*	15g
Cinnabaris *(zhu sha)*	15g
Calcined Arsenic *(bai pi shuang)*	6g
Halloysitum Rubrum *(chi shi zhi)*	15g
Dry-fried Galla Rhois Chinensis *(chao wu bei zi)*	15g
Calcined Realgar *(duan xiong huang)*	15g
Pyritum Rotundum *(she han shi)*	15g

PREPARATION & DOSAGE: Grind each of the ingredients into a fine powder, then mix together well. Sprinkle on the wart, cover with sterile gauze, and afix with skin tape. Avoid wetting the area. Reapply the remedy every 2-3 days until the wart dissolves or drops off.

CLINICAL NOTE: This formula has a cauterizing action. Avoid contact with healthy skin, and do not use on the face. Because of the toxic nature of some of the ingredients, long-term use should be avoided. It is contraindicated during pregnancy.

❧ Brucea Poultice
鸦胆子敷贴
yā dǎn zǐ fū tiē

Fructus Brucae Javanicae *(ya dan zi)*	30g

PREPARATION & DOSAGE: Remove the shells and mash the kernals thoroughly. Swab the wart with alcohol, and lance the skin over the wart until a few drops of blood appear. Dab a small amount of the mashed herb on the wart. Cover with a sterile bandage, and affix with skin tape. Avoid wetting the area. Reapply the remedy every 3-4 days. The source text indicates that the wart usually drops off within ten days.

CLINICAL NOTE: This herb has a cauterizing action. Avoid contact with normal skin.

❧ Pinellia Poultice
生半夏敷贴
shēng bàn xià fū tiē

Untreated Rhizoma Pinelliae Ternatae *(sheng ban xia)*	1-3g
Table Sugar	0.3-1g

PREPARATION & DOSAGE: Grind the herb coarsely, add the sugar, then mix with a small amount of cold water to form a paste. Apply to the wart. Cover with a sterile bandage and affix with skin tape. Avoid wetting the area. Reapply the remedy every three days until the wart drops off. This formula is specifically for plantar warts.

CLINICAL NOTE: This remedy has a cauterizing action. Avoid contact with healthy skin. Untreated Rhizoma Pinelliae Ternatae *(ban xia)* is toxic and should never be taken internally.

The following external washes may be used to treat multiple warts.

❦ Cyperus and Equisetum Wash
香附木贼水洗剂
xiāng fù mù zéi shuǐ xǐ jì

Rhizoma Cyperi Rotundi *(xiang fu)*	50g
Herba Equiseti Hiemalis *(mu zei)*	50g

PREPARATION & DOSAGE: Decoct the herbs in one liter of water. When the decoction has cooled, wash the affected area for 20-30 minutes, 1-2 times daily. The source text indicates that the warts will drop off within one week.

❦ Portulaca, Atractylodes, and Wasp-nest Wash
马术蜂房水洗剂
mǎ zhú fēng fáng shuǐ xǐ jì

Herba Portulacae Oleraceae *(ma chi xian)*	30g
Rhizoma Atractylodis *(cang zhu)*	15g
Nidus Vespae *(lu feng fang)*	15g
Radix Angelicae Dahuricae *(bai zhi)*	15g
Pericarpium Citri Reticulatae *(chen pi)*	15g
Herba cum Radice Asari *(xi xin)*	10g
Fructus Cnidii Monnieri *(she chuang zi)*	12g
Radix Sophorae Flavescentis *(ku shen)*	12g

PREPARATION & DOSAGE: Decoct in 1.5-3.0 liters of water. When the decoction has cooled, wash the affected area for 20-30 minutes, 1-2 times daily. The source text indicates that the warts should drop off within ten days.

ACUPUNCTURE

The following two methods of acupuncture may be used alone or in conjunction with each other.

[A] Select channel points neighboring the lesions, and treat every other day.

[B] Piercing the original "mother wart": One method involves inserting a needle horizontally through the wart, and then removing the needle. The second method calls for inserting a needle perpendicularly through the tip of the wart to its base. In both cases the wart is first pinched tightly until it turns pale, then the needle is inserted swiftly. One or two drops of blood should be let. Use a 32-34 gauge, 0.5 unit needle. Treat every other day. The source text indicates that by the fourth treatment the wart will usually begin to resolve.

MOXIBUSTION

First sterilize the wart with alcohol. Then burn a small moxa cone about the size of a mung bean on the wart. Allow the cone to burn down to the base, at which time a popping noise will be heard. Treat twice daily, once at bedtime and once after getting up in the morning. After 2-3 days, the wart should be removable by tweezers or a scalpel.

EMPIRICAL REMEDIES

Reduce Wart Liquid[3] may be used to treat single or multiple warts.

❦ Reduce Wart Liquid
消疣液
xiāo yóu yè

Semen Coicis Lachryma-jobi *(yi yi ren)*	60g
Radix Isatidis seu Baphicacanthi *(ban lan gen)*	60g
Herba Equiseti Hiemalis *(mu zei)*	30g
Nidus Vespae *(lu feng fang)*	20g
Radix Clematidis *(wei ling xian)*	20g
Mirabilitum *(mang xiao)*	20g
Mimium *(qian dan)*	10g

PREPARATION & DOSAGE: Steep the ingredients in 0.5 liter of vinegar in an airtight glass container for five days. Shake the container once daily. Rub the liquid on the wart 3-5 times daily. The source text indicates that the wart will drop off within 7-10 days.

Traditional vs. Biomedical Treatment

Some methods of traditional treatment are probably just as effective and efficient as some biomedical methods. For example, Brucea Poultice and piercing the "mother wart" are just as simple as the biomedical methods of surgical excision, liquid nitrogen freezing, or the use of topical applications. Additionally, the more involved traditional formulas, especially the internal ones, should not be overlooked as a method of treating recurrent warts when biomedical modalities fail to control the problem.

Prevention

Trauma and irritation to existing warts should be avoided in order to prevent spread. The Chinese principle of eliminating the "mother wart" should be tried as both treatment and prevention of other warts.

Venereal Warts
尖锐湿疣
jiān ruì shī yóu, "pointed moist extraneous growths"

Venereal warts are papillomatous projections from the skin that affect the genitalia in men and in women. To our knowledge, there is no record of this condition in premodern Chinese medical texts.

Signs & Symptoms

Warts can appear on the penis and about the vagina and anus. The growths begin as small pink or red papules that eventually become pedunculated. Clusters of warts exhibit a cauliflower-like appearance. Genital warts can grow quickly during pregnancy or in immunosuppressed patients. Perspiration, poor hygiene, or accompanying infections may also induce rapid growth.

Biomedically, venereal warts are caused by human papilloma virus.

Differential Diagnosis

Venereal warts can ordinarily be identified by their appearance. They must be differentiated from the flat-topped hypertrophic areas typical of secondary syphylis. Atypical or persistent venereal warts should be biopsied to exclude carcinoma.

Traditional Chinese Etiology

Damp-heat lodged in the skin of the perineum is the source of this condition. When the damp-heat is unresolved and becomes protracted, it transforms into toxin, and gives rise to the lesions.

Treatment

INTERNAL

The strategy is to resolve dampness, clear heat and relieve toxicity. The formula recommended for internal treatment is Modified Dioscorea Decoction to Leach Out Dampness [B].

❦ Modified Dioscorea Decoction to Leach Out Dampness [B]
草薜渗湿汤加减
bèi xiè shèn shī tāng jiā jiǎn

Rhizoma Dioscorcae Hypoglaucae *(bei xie)*
Rhizoma Atractylodis *(cang zhu)*
Cortex Phellodendri *(huang bai)*
Semen Coicis Lachryma-jobi *(yi yi ren)*
Rhizoma Smilacis Glabrae *(tu fu ling)*
Cortex Moutan Radicis *(mu dan pi)*
Medulla Tetrapanacis Papyriferi *(tong cao)*

Rhizome Alismatis Orientalis *(ze xie)*
Folium Daqingye *(da qing ye)*
Herba Portulacae Oleraceae *(ma chi xian)*
Radix Arnebiae seu Lithospermi *(zi cao)*

PREPARATION & DOSAGE: The source text does not indicate amounts for the ingredients. Decoct and administer in one dose daily until the warts resolve.

EXTERNAL

In addition to the external washes described in the section on common warts, the following external remedies may be applied in the treatment of venereal warts.

❧ Portulaca and Daqingye Wash
马青水洗剂
mǎ qīng shuǐ xǐ jì

Herba Portulacae Oleraceae *(ma chi xian)*	60g
Folium Daqingye *(da qing ye)*	30g
Alumen *(ming fan)*	20g

PREPARATION & DOSAGE: Decoct the ingredients, then steam and wash the affected area. Steaming is accomplished by squatting over a large basin of the hot decoction for about 5-10 minutes. Treat 1-2 times daily using fresh decoction during each session. After each session, sterilize the basin, or use a large, disposable container each time.

❧ Brucea Liniment
鸦胆子油
yā dǎn zǐ yóu

Fructus Brucae Javanicae *(ya dan zi)* (shells removed)	3 parts
Vegetable Oil	1 part

PREPARATION & DOSAGE: Steep the herb in the vegetable oil for two weeks, shaking the mixture once daily. Apply the liniment twice daily.

CLINICAL NOTE: This remedy has a cauterizing action. Avoid contact with normal skin.

EMPIRICAL REMEDIES

The following remedy[4] is composed of two formulas, Psoralea Tincture Injection and Brucea Plaster.

❧ Psoralea Tincture Injection
补骨脂酊注射液
bǔ gǔ zhī dīng zhù shè yè

Fructus Psoraleae Corylifoliae *(bu gu zhi)* 10g
Radix Salviae Miltiorrhizae *(dan shen)* 10g
Herba Hedyotidis Diffusae *(bai hua she she cao)* 10g
Flos Carthami Tinctorii *(hong hua)* 5g

PREPARATION & DOSAGE: Grind the herbs together into a fine powder. Put into a glass jar with a tight-fitting lid, then cover the powder with 200ml of 75 percent grain alcohol. Steep the herbs for one week; shake the container three times daily. Filter the tincture into another jar that has been sterilized and has a tight-fitting lid. For injection, one part herbal mixture is combined with three parts procaine; 10-30cc are injected into the wart site. One injection per wart is usually sufficient to remove the wart.

After injection, apply Brucea Plaster.

❧ Brucea Plaster
鸦胆子膏
yā dǎn zǐ gāo

Fructus Brucae Javanicae *(ya dan zi)* 5g
Galla Rhois Chinensis *(wu bei zi)* 5g
Alumen *(ming fan)* 10g
Borneol *(bing pian)* 1g
Fructus Pruni Mume *(wu mei)* 20g
Vinegar 20ml

PREPARATION & DOSAGE: Grind all the ingredients into a paste. Apply this plaster to the wart following injection of Psoralea Tincture, then bandage with sterile gauze. Reapply the plaster every other day. The source text indicates that warts usually drop off within 10-30 days.

CLINICAL NOTE: Fructus Brucae Javanicae *(ya dan zi)* has a cauterizing action. Avoid contact with normal skin.

If local inflammation is present, use the following wash to first reduce the inflammation before applying the above treatment.

❧ Clear Heat and Reduce Toxin Wash
清热解毒洗剂
qīng rè jiě dú xǐ jì

Radix Stellerae seu Euphorbiae *(lang du)* 10g
Fructus Carpesii seu Daucusi *(he shi)* 10g
Radix Sophorae Flavescentis *(ku shen)* 15g
Fructus Cnidii Monnieri *(she chuang zi)* 15g
Radix Stemonae *(bai bu)* 15g
Herba Portulacae Oleraceae *(ma chi xian)* 15g
Fructus Zanthoxyli Bungeani *(chuan jiao)* 5g

PREPARATION & DOSAGE: Decoct the herbs, then steam and wash the affected area for 20-30 minutes, three times daily. The inflammation is generally resolved in 3-7 days.

As the warts drop off from the above injection/plaster therapy, the affected area may be steamed and washed with the following formula.

❧ Oldenlandia Wash
白花蛇舌草剂
bái huā shé shé cǎo xǐ jì

Herba Hedyotidis Diffusae *(bai hua she she cao)*	20g
Radix Isatidis seu Baphicacanthi *(ban lan gen)*	20g
Alumen *(ming fan)*	20g
Fructus Zanthoxyli Bungeani *(chuan jiao)*	5g

PREPARATION & DOSAGE: Decoct the ingredients, then administer the decoction as a sitz bath for 30 minutes, 1-2 times daily. Continue the baths until the scabs drop off.

Traditional vs. Biomedical Treatment

Traditional treatment of venereal warts is more involved than is biomedical intervention. However, if patience and persistence are exercised, traditional treatment is probably more effective in resolving the root of the problem. Except for laser treatment, with other biomedical methods, such as surgical procedures (which leaves scars) and podophyllum resin (which is toxic), the chance of recurrence still remains.

Prevention

Venereal warts will recur unless all the lesions are resolved. Some of the above formulas may be used periodically to prevent recurrence. Sexual partners of patients may also need to be treated and followed-up.

Measles
麻疹
má zhěn

Measles (rubeola) is an extremely communicable disease, occurring most often in the winter or spring, commonly affecting infants and childen, and characterized by a rash that covers the entire surface of the body. The ancient Chinese called this condition by several names, including "rash" *(zhěn zǐ* or *shā zǐ)*, "sugar sores" *(táng chuāng)* and "wheat bran sores" *(fū chuāng)*.

Biomedically, measles is caused by a paramyxovirus that is spread by contact or inhalation of airborne droplets of respiratory secretions from an infected individual. Measles spreads rapidly in populations that have not been immunized. Patients are contagious from two days prior to symptoms until four days after the rash appears.

Signs & Symptoms

The incubation period is approximately 10 to 14 days. This is followed by a prodromal phase, symptoms of which include malaise, fever (often reaching 40°C), sensitivity to light, conjunctivitis, nasal congestion, and hacking cough. The hallmark of measles, Koplik's spots, develop two to four days later on the oral mucosa opposite the first and second upper molars. The spots often look like grains of sand on a red base, and usually disappear once the rash erupts. Measles is contagious from shortly after exposure up to one week following the appearance of the symptoms.

About one to seven days after the prodromal onset, a somewhat itchy rash appears, commonly starting on the head and neck and spreading downward on the trunk and extremities. The rash fades in the same sequence as it developed, leaving a brown desquamation of minute, dust-like particles. At this time the symptoms subside as well.

Differential Diagnosis

Measles must be differentiated from rubella (German measles), atypical measles, scarlet fever, drug rashes, enteroviral infections and Rocky Mountain spotted fever. Atypical measles develops in persons who have been immunized with the heat-killed measles vaccine instead of the live attenuated vaccine; in these patients the lesions are located primarily on the arms and legs. Other disorders can be ruled out by clinical findings, appropriate laboratory tests, or by the patient's medical history. The combination of characteristic rash, prodromal signs and symptoms, and Koplik's spots is usually sufficient to make a clinical diagnosis of measles.

Traditional Chinese Etiology

Measles is caused by contraction of seasonal wind-heat toxin that invades and accumulates in the Lung and protective level, giving rise to fever, skin rash and the accompanying symptoms.

Treatment

In Chinese medicine, treatment of measles is based on the three stages of the condition: incipient heat (fever), expression and regression. This sequence, which results in resolution of the illness, i.e., release of heat through venting of the rash, is known as the progressive pattern *(shùn zhèng)* of measles. (Here, "progressive" connotes forward-moving, and should be distinguished from the biomedical meaning of a condition going from bad to worse.) If, during the course of disease, the heat toxin sinks inward and the condition deteriorates, this is known as the inversion-danger pattern *(nì xiǎn zhèng)*, a rather serious situation that requires immediate attention.

The overall treatment strategy of measles, therefore, is to draw out the heat by venting the rash. However, the stage of the condition should determine the actual remedy used. For each stage, particularly the incipient heat and expression patterns, treatment should continue until the rash is completely vented and the fever subsides. At this point, the strategy should turn toward enriching and nourishing the yin, which was injured due to the fever in the previous two stages.

PROGRESSIVE PATTERN

Incipient heat. During this stage, seasonal wind-heat toxin attacks the Lung and protective level and causes such symptoms as fever, slight aversion to cold, stuffy and runny nose, hacking cough, redness of the eyelids, aversion to light, watery eyes, malaise, redness of the lips and cheeks, pinpoint grayish white spots on the inner cheeks inside the mouth, and yellow and scanty urine. The tongue coating is often thin and white or yellow, or slightly yellow, and the pulse is usually floating and rapid. The treatment strategy is to disperse the wind and clear the heat. The formula recommended for this pattern is Honeysuckle and Forsythia Powder.

❧ Honeysuckle and Forsythia Powder
银翘散
yín qiáo sǎn

Flos Lonicerae Japonicae *(jin yin hua)*	9g
Fructus Forsythiae Suspensae *(lian qiao)*	9g
Radix Platycodi Grandiflori *(jie geng)*	3g
Fructus Arctii Lappae *(niu bang zi)*	9g
Herba Menthae Haplocalycis *(bo he)*	3g
Semen Sojae Praeparatum *(dan dou chi)*	3g
Herba seu Flos Schizonepetae Tenuifoliae *(jing jie)*	6g
Herba Lophatheri Gracilis *(dan zhu ye)*	3g
Rhizoma Phragmitis Communis Recens *(xian lu gen)*	15g
Radix Glycyrrhizae Uralensis *(gan cao)*	3g

PREPARATION & DOSAGE: Decoct for about 20 minutes, but do not overcook. Add the Herba Menthae Haplocalycis *(bo he)* about 5 minutes before the end. For children 1-3 years of age, the dosage should be one-quarter of the listed amount, administered 4-5 times daily. For children 4-6 years, the dosage should be about one-half of the listed amount, administered 4-5 times daily. For children 7-12 years, the amount listed may be administered 3-4 times daily. Continue the treatment until the rash is fully expressed and the fever has abated.

For incipient heat and expression pattern cases complicated by upper respiratory infection, Cimicifuga Combined Formula is recommended.

❧ Cimicifuga Combined Formula
升麻合剂
shēng má hé jì

Rhizoma Cimicifugae *(sheng ma)*	90g
Fructus Forsythiae Suspensae *(lian qiao)*	900g
Fructus Arctii Lappae *(niu bang zi)*	600g
Herba Ephedrae *(ma huang)*	90g

Radix Platycodi Grandiflori *(jie geng)* 120g

PREPARATION & DOSAGE: Decoct in about 1.5 liters of water until about 1.0 liter or slightly less remains (the decoction should be somewhat syrupy). For children 1-2 years of age, administer 10ml (about 1.5 teaspoons) daily, divided into six equal doses given at 4-hour intervals. For children 3-5 years, administer 10ml daily, divided into four equal doses, given at 4-hour intervals. For children 5-7 years, administer 10ml daily, divided into three equal doses, given at 4-hour intervals. For children 8-12 years, administer 20ml daily, divided into four equal doses, given at 4-hour intervals. Continue the treatment until the rash is fully expressed and the fever has abated.

Expression. During this stage, the heat toxin accumulates in the Lung and produces such symptoms as high fever (due to the conflict between the normal qi and the excess heat-toxin), thirst, worsening of the cough, irritability, sleepiness, or propensity for being startled, redness and crusting of the eyes, a red tongue with a yellow sticky or dry coating, and a flooding, or flooding and rapid pulse. The rash that appears during this time begins behind the ears and then affects the hairline at the nape, followed by the forehead and face, the chest and abdomen, the limbs and finally the palms and soles. Thus, the sequence of appearance of the rash is from upper to lower body, and from yang to yin. The treatment strategy is to clear heat and relieve toxicity, and disperse wind and vent the rash. The formula recommended for this stage is Vent the Rash Decoction.

❧ Vent the Rash Decoction
透疹汤
tòu zhěn tāng

Fructus Forsythiae Suspensae *(lian qiao)* 2.4g
Periostracum Cicadae *(chan tui)* 1.5g
Radix Arnebiae seu Lithospermi *(zi cao)* 3g
Fructus Arctii Lappae *(niu bang zi)* 2g
Radix Puerariae *(ge gen)* 6g
Radix Platycodi Grandiflori *(jie geng)* 2.4g
Flos Lonicerae Japonicae *(jin yin hua)* 2.4g
Radix Glycyrrhizae Uralensis *(gan cao)* 1.2g

PREPARATION & DOSAGE: Prepare as a decoction. The above dosage is for children 1-3 years of age. For children 4-6 years, increase the dosage by one-half, and for children 7-12 years, double the dosage. Administer in 4-5 doses daily until the rash is fully expressed and the fever has abated.

Regression. The fever during the incipient heat and expression stages has injured the yin. Thus, the primary symptom at this time is the fine bran-like scale affecting the skin. All other symptoms, such as fever and cough, should be resolved.

The tongue is usually red and the coating thin and sticky, and the pulse is often deficient and rapid. The strategy is to enrich and nourish the yin fluids and to clear and transform the residual heat-toxin. The formula recommended for this stage is Glehnia and Ophiopogonis Decoction.

❧ Glehnia and Ophiopogonis Decoction
沙参麦门冬汤
shā shēn mài mén dōng tāng

Radix Adenophorae seu Glehniae *(sha shen)*	9g
Tuber Ophiopogonis Japonici *(mai men dong)*	9g
Rhizoma Polygonati Odorati *(yu zhu)*	6g
Folium Mori Albae *(sang ye)*	4.5g
Radix Trichosanthis Kirilowii *(tian hua fen)*	4.5g
Semen Dolichoris Lablab *(bian dou)*	4.5g
Radix Glycyrrhizae Uralensis *(gan cao)*	3g

PREPARATION & DOSAGE: Prepare as a decoction. For children 1-3 years of age, use one-quarter of the listed dosage. For children 4-6 years, use one-half the listed dosage. For children 7-12 years, use the dosage listed above. Administer in 4-5 doses daily, until the yin deficiency signs (e.g., redness of the tongue) are resolved.

INVERSION-DANGER PATTERN

This pattern often appears during the expression stage and is the result of inward sinking of the toxin. The symptoms include high fever, severe coughing, panting, heaving of the chest, phlegm sounds in the throat, flaring of the nostrils, purple lips, scarlet tongue with a thin or thick yellow coating, and a floating and rapid or flooding and rapid pulse. The rash in this pattern is characterized by incomplete expression, or sudden expression and disappearance, or by dark purple rash that is unevenly distributed or that appears in patches. In severe cases, there is impaired consciousness and delirious speech, or even convulsions. The strategy is to open and disseminate the Lung, and vent the rash. The formula recommended for this pattern is Augmented Modified Five-Tiger Decoction.

❧ Augmented Five-Tiger Decoction
五虎汤加味
wǔ hǔ tāng jiā wèi

Herba Ephedrae *(ma huang)*	3g
Semen Pruni Armeniacae *(xing ren)*	10g
Gypsum *(shi gao)*	30g
Radix Peucedani *(qian hu)*	6g
Fructus Arctii Lappae *(niu bang zi)*	6g
Radix Platycodi Grandiflori *(jie geng)*	3g
Bulbus Fritillariae Thunbergii *(zhe bei mu)*	10g
Folium Eriobotryae Japonicae *(pi pa ye)*	10g
Rhizoma Belamcandae Chinensis *(she gan)*	3g

Fructus Perillae Frutescentis *(su zi)* 10g
Rhizoma Acori Graminei *(shi chang pu)* 5g
Green Tea 3g
Radix Glycyrrhizae Uralensis *(gan cao)* 5g

PREPARATION & DOSAGE: Decoct and administer in 2-3 doses daily. For children under the age of five, reduce the dosage by one-half. The source text indicates that improvement of symptoms, particularly in venting the rash, is accomplished after administering the formula for 1-2 days. Thereafter, formulas to address yin deficiency (e.g., Glehnia and Ophiopogonis Decoction, see above) and/or cough should be administered.

Because measles is often mistaken in the early stage for cold-induced disorders, formulas that are warming may be inadvertently prescribed, resulting in pent-up heat, the symptoms of which may include pain and swelling of the throat, sores on the tongue and in the mouth, and redness, pain and swelling of the eyes. For such cases, Green Robe Powder is recommended.

❧ Green Robe Powder
绿袍散
lù páo sǎn

Herba Menthae Haplocalycis *(bo he)* 15g
Indigo Pulverata Levis *(qing dai)* 7.5g
Borax *(peng sha)* 7.5g
Pasta Acaciae seu Uncariae *(er cha)* 9g
Radix Glycyrrhizae Uralensis *(gan cao)* 9g
Cortex Phellodendri *(huang bai)* 3g
Robigo Aeris (tong lü) 3g
Borneol *(bing pian)* 3g
Alumen *(ming fan)* 7.5g
Fermentatio Galla Rhois Chinensis *(bai yao jian)* 7.5g
Herba seu Flos Schizonepetae Tenuifoliae *(jing jie)* 15g

PREPARATION & DOSAGE: Grind all the ingredients together into a fine powder. Apply by placing on the tongue and allowing the powder to dissolve on the tongue before swallowing with warm water. For chldren 1-3 years of age, administer 250mg daily, divided into six approximately equal portions, and given at 4-hour intervals. For children 4-6 years, administer 500mg daily, divided into six approximately equal portions, and given at 4-hour intervals. For children 7-12 years, administer 750mg daily, divided into four approximately equal portions, and given at 6-hour intervals. Discontinue this remedy once the signs of pent-up heat are resolved, and treat with formulas to vent the rash.

EMPIRICAL REMEDIES

For slow eruption of measles rash, the following remedies are recommended.

[A] Decoct 30-60g of cilantro (Herba Coriandrum, *hú suī*) in 500ml of water to which 25ml of grain alcohol has been added. Strain the dregs and rub down the skin with the warm decoction; do not apply to the face and head. One application will usually promote full eruption; if not, a second application the following day should suffice. Do not use this remedy if eruption has already commenced.[5]

[B] Decoct 9g of crushed cherry pits in water for 20-30 minutes. Filter and discard the dregs. Administer one dose per day orally. A sponge bath made from a decoction of 150g of cherry pits may also be administered.[6]

[C] Crush 3-9g of raw sunflower seeds. Add 250ml of boiling water and steep for two hours. Filter and discard the dregs. Administer orally in two equal portions daily.[7]

Traditional vs. Biomedical Prognosis

Traditional treatment of measles is more effective than biomedical intervention, which is mainly palliative. If the pattern/stage is differentiated correctly and the appropriate formula is prescribed, the course of disease can be shortened by about 3-4 days. Patients who present with toxic signs, i.e., the inversion-danger pattern, should be monitored closely. If traditional formulas are administered and improvement is not evident within two days, such patients should be referred for biomedical treatment or even hospitalization, as encephalitis or respiratory tract bleeding and gastrointestinal bleeding, or sepsis, may ensue if immediate medical attention is not given.

Prevention

Measles is preventable by immunization with live attenuated measles virus vaccines. Exposed susceptible individuals may be protected if they are given the live vaccine within two days of exposure.

The symptoms associated with the early stage of measles can lead to a misdiagnosis of cold-induced disorder. To avoid prescribing the incorrect formula, practitioners should obtain a detailed patient history, e.g., ascertaining exposure to the virus, and should also look for the telltale sign of measles—Koplik's spots on the buccal mucosa inside the mouth—in order to differentiate between measles and cold-induced disorder.

Chickenpox
水痘
shuǐ dòu, "fluid pock"

Chickenpox (varicella) is an acute, highly contagious disease characterized by a generalized vesicular eruption. Because of the frequency with which children succumb to this disease, it is not surprising that several Chinese medical classics on childhood diseases describe this condition. Typical of these is the following passage from *A Hundred Questions About Infants and Children* (1506): "There is fever for one to two days, followed by eruption of vesicles which [then] disappear. This is known as fluid pock."

Biomedically, chickenpox is caused by the varicella-zoster virus, which is also responsible for herpes zoster (shingles). During the viremic phase the virus spreads on the skin, causing the characteristic symptoms of chickenpox. From the skin the virus travels to the peripheral nerves and dorsal root ganglia, where it remains latent until various factors, such as immunosuppression or trauma, reactivate it, causing herpes zoster.

Signs & Symptoms

Following an incubation period of two to three weeks, the symptoms begin with a slight fever and malaise. In young children, the fever is usually mild, while adolescents and adults may have more serious symptoms and complications, including pneumonia and encephalitis. Within 24-36 hours the first series of lesions appear, initially as itchy, erythematous macules that quickly evolve over a few hours into papules, and then into the typical "teardrop" vesicles. Crusting takes place within six to eight hours. Recurrent crops of new lesions appear during the first three to five days. Vesicles are concentrated on the upper trunk, although other areas such as the scalp, face, oral mucosa, larynx, or trachea may also be affected. Healing begins after six to eight days, with most crusts resolving in about 20 days after onset.

Differential Diagnosis

Chickenpox may be confused with impetigo, scabies, insect bites, hives, secondary syphilis, contact dermatitis and drug rashes. Usually, the characteristic teardrop vesicles of chickenpox, as well as the history, will confirm diagnosis.

Traditional Chinese Etiology

Chickenpox is caused by contraction of seasonal wind-heat combined with an accumulation of internal damp-heat, all of which gather in the exterior tissues, thus giving rise to the vesicular eruption and accompanying symptoms.

Treatment

The treatment strategy is to disperse wind and clear heat, and vent the exterior and relieve toxin.

CLINICAL NOTE: When administering the following formulas to children, use one-fourth or one-third of the listed amount for each herb.

INTERNAL

Formula selection is based on the severity of the condition, as defined by three distinct patterns.

Mild patterns are limited to heat in the qi level, and present with vesicles that are diffuse, contain clear fluid, and crust within 2-3 days. Generalized symptoms may include either low-grade or absence of fever, a thin white tongue coating, and a floating and rapid pulse (or, if dampness is present, a sticky white tongue coating, and slippery and rapid pulse). The strategy is to vent the exterior, disperse wind, and clear the qi level. The formula recommended for this pattern is Modified Honeysuckle and Forsythia Powder [A].

❦ Modified Honeysuckle and Forsythia Powder [A]
银翘散加减
yín qiáo sǎn jiā jiǎn

Flos Lonicerae Japonicae *(jin yin hua)*	10g
Fructus Forsythiae Suspensae *(lian qiao)*	6g
Herba seu Flos Schizonepetae Tenuifoliae *(jing jie)*	6g
Herba Lophatheri Gracilis *(dan zhu ye)*	6g
Testa Phaseoli Radiati *(lu dou yi)*	12g
Radix Platycodi Grandiflori *(jie geng)*	4.5g
Periostracum Cicadae *(chan tui)*	4.5g
Folium Daqingye *(da qing ye)*	4.5g
Radix Arnebiae seu Lithospermi *(zi cao)*	4.5g
Radix Glycyrrhizae Uralensis *(gan cao)*	4.5g

PREPARATION & DOSAGE: Decoct and administer in three doses daily.

MODIFICATIONS: For dampness, add Semen Coicis Lachryma-jobi *(yi yi ren)* and Sclerotium Poriae Cocos *(fu ling)*.

A moderately severe pattern with heat affecting the blood level presents with vesicles that are profuse, and contain reddish opaque fluid, with the surrounding skin flushed; crusting does not occur for about a week. Generalized symptoms may include fever, restlessness, a red tongue with a dry yellow coating, and a flooding and rapid pulse. The strategy is to cool the nutritive level and relieve toxicity. The formula recommended for this pattern is Modified Clear the Nutritive Level Decoction.

❦ Modified Clear the Nutritive Level Decoction
清营汤加减
qīng yíng tāng jiā jiǎn

Testa Phaseoli Radiati *(lu dou yi)*	10g
Radix Rehmanniae Glutinosae *(sheng di huang)*	10g
Radix Scrophulariae Ningpoensis *(xuan shen)*	10g
Folium Daqingye *(da qing ye)*	6g
Flos Lonicerae Japonicae *(jin yin hua)*	6g
Fructus Forsythiae Suspensae *(lian qiao)*	6g
Radix Arnebiae seu Lithospermi *(zi cao)*	4.5g
Flos Carthami Tinctorii *(hong hua)*	4.5g
Dry-fried Cortex Moutan Radicis *(chao mu dan pi)*	4.5g
Radix Glycyrrhizae Uralensis *(gan cao)*	4.5g

PREPARATION & DOSAGE: Decoct and administer in three doses daily.

Severe patterns present with vesicles that are deep purple. Generalized symptoms usually include high fever, extreme thirst, deep yellow and scanty urine, dry stools, a thick yellow tongue coating, and a flooding and rapid pulse. The strategy is to cool the blood and drain fire, and clear heat and relieve toxicity. The formula recommended for this pattern is Modified Clear Epidemics and Overcome Toxin Decoction.

❧ Modified Clear Epidemics and Overcome Toxin Decoction
清瘟败毒饮加减
qīng wēn bài dú yǐn jiā jiǎn

Gypsum *(shi gao)*	60g
Cornu Bubali *(shui niu jiao)*	30g
Radix Rehmanniae Glutinosae *(sheng di huang)*	12g
Cortex Moutan Radicis *(mu dan pi)*	9g
Radix Paeoniae Rubrae *(chi shao)*	9g
Rhizoma Anemarrhenae Asphodeloidis *(zhi mu)*	9g
Rhizoma Coptidis *(huang lian)*	9g
Radix Isatidis seu Baphicacanthi *(ban lan gen)*	6g
Fructus Gardeniae Jasminoidis *(zhi zi)*	9g
Radix Scutellariae Baicalensis *(huang qin)*	3g
Radix Scrophulariae Ningpoensis *(xuan shen)*	9g
Fructus Forsythiae Suspensae *(lian qiao)*	9g
Radix Glycyrrhizae Uralensis *(gan cao)*	6g

PREPARATION & DOSAGE: First cook the Gypsum *(shi gao)* and Cornu Bubali *(shui niu jiao)* for 15-20 minutes, then add the remaining ingredients and decoct. Administer one-half in the morning and the remainder at night. Discontinue the formula once the fever has broken and most of the lesions have formed crusts.

EXTERNAL

To treat ulcerated lesions, apply Portulaca Wash (see herpes simplex) as a wet compress 3-5 times daily. Follow each treatment with an application of Indigo Powder.

❧ Indigo Powder
青黛散
qīng dài sǎn

Indigo Pulverata Levis *(qing dai)*	60g
Gypsum *(shi gao)*	120g
Cortex Phellodendri *(huang bai)*	60g

PREPARATION & DOSAGE: Grind each of the ingredients into a fine powder, and then mix together well. For ulcerated chickenpox lesions, mix some of the powder together with sesame oil to form a paste, and then apply to the lesions.

EMPIRICAL REMEDIES

To treat ulcerated lesions, grind dry black beans into a fine powder, and sprinkle on the affected area.[8]

Traditional vs. Biomedical Treatment

Since the goal of medical therapy is to restore the patient to health as rapidly as possible, in the case of chickenpox, traditional treatment is probably superior to biomedical treatment methods. This is because traditional treatment through pattern differentiation is aimed at shortening the course of the disease, whereas biomedical treatment is only palliative.

Prevention

Chickenpox can be prevented by administering zoster immune globulin (ZIG). If given within three days after exposure, the subsequent disease can be ameliorated.

Because of the high incidence of bacterial superinfection of chickenpox vesicles, patients should bathe frequently with soap and water, and change their underclothing often. Hands should be kept clean, and nails clipped, because of the propensity to scratch the itching lesions.

CHAPTER NOTES

1. Zhai, X., "Bloodletting Ear Apex to Treat Herpes of the Mouth and Nose Area," *Chinese Acupuncture and Moxibustion,* 9(3): 53, 1989.

2. Song, X.X., "Smilax and Rheum Decoction in the Treatment of Herpes Zoster," *Sichuan Journal of Traditional Chinese Medicine,* 8(2): 41, 1990.

3. Qin, G.Z., "Warming and Clearing Decoction: New Application to Skin Diseases," *Yunnan Journal of Traditional Chinese Medicine,* 11(1): 31-32, 1990.

4. Sun, Q.L., "Pricking as a Treatment for Snake Cluster Sores," *Xinjiang Traditional Chinese Medicine,* 8(1): 37, 1990.

5. Lan, M.P., "External Application of Reduce Wart Liquid to Treat Warts," *New Journal of Traditional Chinese Medicine,* 22(2): 55, 1990.

6. Yan, S.W. and Huang, J.Y., "Psoralea Tincture Compound in the Treatment of Venereal Warts," *Zhejiang Journal of Traditional Chinese Medicine,* 25(3): 113, 1990.

7. Dou, G.X. *Guide to Food Therapy (Yin shi zhi liao zhi nan).* Jiangsu: Jiangsu Science and Technology Press, 1981.

8. Dai, Y.F. and Liu, C.J. *Medicinal Uses of Fruits (Yao yong guo pin).* Nanning: Guangxi People's Publishing House, 1982.

9. Ibid.

10. Dou, *Guide to Food Therapy (Yin shi zhi liao zhi nan).*

CHAPTER 9

Fungal Infections

Tinea Corporis
圆癣
yuán xuǎn, "round tinea"

Tinea is a common, noninvasive cutaneous infection. This disease was described in the sixth century work, *Discussion of the Origins of Symptoms of Disease,* in a chapter entitled "Symptoms of Sores," which contains a specific section on the symptoms of "round tinea": "The characteristics of round tinea are that its mark is raised, its four borders are red, and there is itching and pain." A more detailed description is found in another section of the same chapter dealing with the symptoms of tinea in general:

> The form of tinea disease is that the skin has a raised rash resembling a thread, that slowly enlarges [over time], and may be either round or angular, with itching and pain confined; within the border, parasites are produced, and scratching induces fluid.

Biomedically, tinea is caused by fungi that invade the cornified components of the skin. The genera of causative fungi are *Trichophyton, Epidermophyton* and *Microporum.*

Signs & Symptoms

Tinea lesions are disc-like with sharply defined, raised borders that expand peripherally and clear centrally. Often there is red scaling with varying degrees of itching. Blisters and pustules may appear on the border. Continuous scratching may result in lichenification. Lack of signs of central healing may result in misdiagnosis of eczema or dermatitis. Tinea tends to flare up during the summer and improves or resolves during the winter.

Tinea corporis is more common in adults. In humid, tropical parts of the world, much of the population is affected.

Differential Diagnosis

Tinea is confirmed by demonstrating the pathogenic fungi in scrapings of lesions, either by microscopic examination or by culture. During preliminary examination, tinea should be differentiated from chronic eczema, which has undefined borders. Localized scratch dermatitis (neurodermatitis) has marked lichenification, severe itching and lacks pustules. Pityriasis rosea has numerous lesions, but unlike tinea, the borders are not as neat, there is no centrally healing center, and once the acute lesions are healed they usually do not recur. Psoriasis has erythematous papules or plaques covered with overlapping, silvery or slightly opalescent, shiny scales, and lacks a centrally healing center.

Traditional Chinese Etiology

Tinea is caused by the invasion of wind and damp-heat into the skin. Individuals who are overweight and have pre-existing phlegm and dampness are prone to tinea. The condition may also be caused by transmission from other individuals or sources.

Treatment

Most of the methods for treating tinea are external, although some formulas may be taken internally.

INTERNAL

❧ Three-Miracle Pill
三神丸
sān shén wán

Dry-fried Fructus Tribuli Terrestris *(chao bai ji li)*	30g
Cortex Erythrinae *(hai tong pi)*	30g
Radix Aconiti Kusnezoffii *(cao wu)*	30g

PREPARATION & DOSAGE: The last ingredients should be fried in salt, which must be removed prior to use. Grind all the ingredients together into a fine powder. Mix with water to make a paste. Form into small pills the size of mung beans. Administer 10-15 pills daily with warm water.

❧ Spirodela Pill for Stubborn Tinea
顽癣浮萍丸
wán xuǎn fú píng wán

Herba Lemnae seu Spirodelae *(fu ping)*	60g
Rhizoma Atractylodis *(cang zhu)*	60g
Fructus Xanthii Sibirici *(cang er zi)*	60g
Radix Sophorae Flavescentis *(ku shen)*	120g
Radix Scutellariae Baicalensis *(huang qin)*	30g
Bombyx Batryticatus *(jiang can)*	30g
Ramulus cum Uncis Uncariae *(gou teng)*	45g
Wine-steamed Herba Siegesbeckiae *(jiu zhi xi xian cao)*	60g

PREPARATION & DOSAGE: Grind all the ingredients together into a fine powder and mix with wine to make a paste. Form into pills. Administer 6g daily with warm, unseasoned pork soup or with warm water.

❧ Disperse Wind and Clear Heat Decoction
疏风清热饮
shū fēng qīng rè yǐn

Radix Sophorae Flavescentis (ku shen)	6g
Buthus Martensi (quan xie) (fried)	3g
Spina Gleditsiae Sinensis (zao jiao ci)	3g
Fructus Gleditsiae Sinensis (zao jiao)	3g
Radix Ledebouriellae Divaricatae (fang feng)	3g
Herba seu Flos Schizonepetae Tenuifoliae (jing jie)	3g
Flos Lonicerae Japonicae (jin yin hua)	3g
Dry-fried Periostracum Cicadae (chao chan tui)	3g

PREPARATION & DOSAGE: Decoct in a mixture of 200ml of water plus 200ml of grain alcohol. Add about 10cm of scallion whites, and decoct until about 100ml of fluid remains. Strain the dregs and administer the decoction while hot. Administer in one dose daily. Patients should abstain from spicy foods while taking this formula.

EXTERNAL

❧ Number 1 Tinea Liniment
一号癣药水
yī hào xuǎn yào shuǐ

Cortex Pseudolaricis Kaempferi Radicis (tu jing pi)	300g
Semen Hydnocarpi Anthelminticae (da feng zi) (without the pericarpium)	300g
Fructus Kochiae Scopariae (di fu zi)	300g
Fructus Cnidii Monnieri (she chuang zi)	300g
Sulphur (liu huang)	150g
Cortex Dictamni Dasycarpi Radicis (bai xian pi)	300g
Alumen Praeparatum (ku fan)	150g
Radix Sophorae Flavescentis (ku shen)	300g
Camphora (zhang nao)	150g

PREPARATION & DOSAGE: Grind the Cortex Pseudolaricis Kaempferi Radicis (tu jing pi) into a coarse powder, crush the Semen Hydnocarpi Anthelminticae (da feng zi), grind the Sulphur (liu huang) into a fine powder, and break apart the Alumen Praeparatum (ku fan). Put these and the remaining ingredients into a glass container and add 8 liters of 50 percent alcohol; steep at room temperature for two days. Decant the clear liquid into another airtight glass container. Add 6 liters of 50 percent alcohol to the dregs and steep for another two days. Decant the clear liquid into the first liquid. Add yet another 6 liters of 50 percent alcohol to the dregs and steep again for two days. Decant the clear liquid into the two previous liquids. Dissolve the Camphora *(zhang nao)* in 90 percent alcohol, then mix in with the herbal liquid and allow to settle. Decant the clear portion of the liquid into an airtight container.

Apply the liniment 3-4 times daily. Do not apply to lesions that are blistered or pustulated; for these lesions, use Indigo Ointment (see below) until they are relieved, then use Number 1 Tinea Liniment.

❦ Indigo Ointment
青黛膏
qīng dài gāo

Indigo Pulverata Levis *(qing dai)*	60g
Gypsum *(shi gao)*	120g
Talcum *(hua shi)*	120g
Cortex Phellodendri *(huang bai)*	60g

PREPARATION & DOSAGE: Grind each of the ingredients into a fine powder and mix together. Take 75g of this mixture and slowly stir it in with 300g of petroleum jelly. Store the ointment in an airtight, amber glass container. Spread the ointment onto sterile gauze and apply to the affected area once daily.

For recalcitrant lesions, Clinopodium Powder or Miraculous Tinea Remedy is recommended.

❦ Clinopodium Powder
剪草散
jiǎn cǎo sǎn

Cortex Pseudolaricis Kaempferi Radicis *(tu jing pi)*	240g
Herba Clinopodii *(jian dao cao)*	120g
Rhizoma Bletillae Striatae *(bai ji)*	120g
Semen Croton Tiglii *(ba dou)* (with husk)	14

PREPARATION & DOSAGE: Grind all the ingredients together into a fine powder. Store in an airtight glass container. Before application, mix some of the powder together with water to form a paste, and spread a thick layer on the affected area. When the paste has dried, remove it and apply another layer (this is considered one application). The source text indicates that this remedy is immediately effective. Because of the toxicity of Cortex Pseudolaricis Kaempferi Radicis *(tu jing pi)* and Semen Croton Tiglii *(ba dou)*, this formula should not be applied more than once daily for three consecutive days.

❦ Miraculous Tinea Remedy

神效癣药
shén xiào xuǎn yào

Mylabris *(ban mao)*	15g
Radix Stemonae *(bai bu)*	60g
Semen Arecae Catechu *(bing lang)*	30g
Cortex Pseudolaricis Kaempferi Radicis *(tu jing pi)*	30g
Fructus Liquidambaris Taiwanianae *(lu lu tong)*	30g
Rhizoma Bletillae Striatae *(bai ji)*	30g
Fructus Zanthoxyli Bungeani *(chuan jiao)*	30g

PREPARATION & DOSAGE: Steep the ingredients in hot grain alcohol for 30 minutes. Apply as a wash to the affected area 6-7 times daily.

ACUPUNCTURE

Acupoints that should be needled include LI-15 *(jian yu)*, PC-3 *(qu ze)*, LI-4 *(he gu)*, GB-31 *(feng shi)*, SP-10 *(xue hai)*, SP-6 *(san yin jiao)* and BL-40 *(wei zhong)*. Use draining manipulation, and do not retain the needles. Treat twice weekly, with ten treatments as one course.

EMPIRICAL REMEDIES

[A] Decoct 60-150g of Pericarpium Punicae Granati *(shi liu pi)* in water to a concentrated liquid. Apply to lesions with sterile cotton swab, or as a wash, 2-3 times daily.[1]

[B] Grind into a paste 5-8 Arillus Euphoriae Longanae *(long yan rou)* seeds with 20ml of rice vinegar. Apply to the lesions 1-2 times daily.[2]

[C] Mash one whole lemon (with skin). Apply the juice to the lesions 3-4 times daily.[3]

[D] Mash one whole unripe papaya together with 30ml of rice vinegar and 30g table salt. Apply the juice to the affected areas 2-3 times daily.[4]

[E] Mulberry sap remedy:[5] Obtain the white sap from a mulberry tree by cutting deeply into its trunk or branch. Allow the sap to drain into a small glass receptacle. Sap may be stored for 2-3 days, although using the fresh sap is more effective. Apply to lesions 1-2 times daily; do not wash the area until just prior to the next application. Ten days are considered one course of therapy. Most cases experience complete disappearance of lesions within one course.

A passage in the *Grand Materia Medica* indicates that mulberry sap is capable of "relieving a hundred toxins," suggesting its broad therapeutic application. It is on this basis that the source text recommends this remedy in the treatment of tinea.

[F] The following remedy is recommended for tinea lesions that present with vesicles and pustules.

❦ Sophora and Allium Vinegar Soak[6]
苦蒜醋浸泡
kǔ suàn cù jìn pào

Radix Sophorae Flavescentis *(ku shen)* 30g
Bulbus Alli Sativi *(da suan)* 30g
Pericarpium Punicae Granati *(shi liu pi)* 30g
Fructus Quisqualis Indicae *(shi jun zi)* 20g
Radix Clematidis *(wei ling xian)* 20g
Table Vinegar .... 1 liter

PREPARATION & DOSAGE: In a glass container, steep the herbs in the vinegar for 48 hours. Then decoct over low heat for 20-30 minutes. Pour the liquid into another glass container, discarding the dregs. Wash or soak the affected area for 15-30 minutes once daily before bedtime. After applying the remedy, do not wash the area until just before the next application. Seven days are one course of treatment. Most cases experience marked improvement within one course.

[G] The following remedy is most effective for tinea lesions that show blisters. It should not be applied to lesions that are eroded and ulcerated, or that show fissures.

❧ Zanthoxylum and Allium Paste[7]

川椒大蒜泥

chuān jiāo dà suàn ní

Fructus Zanthoxyli Bungeani *(chuan jiao)* (without seed) 25g
Bulbus Alli Sativi *(da suan)* (purple skinned) 100g

PREPARATION & DOSAGE: First grind the Fructus Zanthoxyli Bungeani *(chuan jiao)* into a powder, then combine with the Bulbus Alli Sativi *(da suan)* and crush into a paste. Put into a glass container. Prior to application, wash the affected area with warm water and pat dry. Using a sterile cotton swab, apply a thin layer of the herbal paste and then rub the paste into the skin with a sterile cotton ball. Apply 1-2 times daily, with ten days as one course of therapy.

When the lesions are nearly healed, discontinue the herbal paste, and apply a wash made from a decoction of 50g of Radix Rumicis Madaio *(tu da huang)* 2-3 times per week. Continue applying the wash for 2-3 months in order to consolidate the therapeutic effect.

MODIFICATIONS: For lesions that are eroded or ulcerated, first use a decoction of Rhizoma Coptidis *(huang lian)* as a wet compress 1-2 times daily until the erosions or ulcers are healed. Then apply the herbal paste and Radix Rumicis Madaio *(tu da huang)* wash.

[H] Vinegar and Rheum Wash[8] may be applied to tinea lesions. The remedy is prepared by steeping 100g of Radix et Rhizoma Rhei (da huang) in 1 liter of rice vinegar for ten days. Store the herbal remedy in an airtight glass container.

Wash the affected area for 10-15 minutes, two times daily. One week is considered a course of therapy. Most cases experience improvement within 1-2 courses.

Traditional vs. Biomedical Treatment

The acute, inflammatory form of tinea is usually self-limited, and treatment, both traditional and biomedical, involves the use of topical remedies in order to accelerate healing. For the chronic, widespread form, however, biomedical intervention is less than satisfactory because recurrence is the rule. Traditional treatment may thus prove more effective in such cases because, through pattern differentiation, the root of the condition can be resolved.

Prevention

Prompt treatment is important once tinea is diagnosed. Personal hygiene is important in preventing spread of the disease, particularly among family members. Clothing and washcloths should be laundered frequently.

When applying any of the herbal washes, containers or basins used during treatment should be sterilized afterward, or disposable containers used in their place.

CHAPTER NOTES

1. Dai, Y.F. and Liu, C.J. *Medicinal Uses of Fruits (Yao yong guo pin)*. Nanning: Guangxi People's Publishing House, 1982.
2. Ibid.
3. Ibid.
4. Ibid.
5. Lou, J.H., "External Application of Mulberry Sap in the Treatment of Tinea," *Zhejiang Journal of Traditional Chinese Medicine,* 25(9): 400; 1990.
6. Guo, Y.J., "Sophora and Allium Vinegar Soak in the Treatment of Tinea," *Yunnan Journal of Traditional Chinese Medicine,* 11(1): 48; 1990.
7. Ruan, Y.M. and Ruan, R., "Zanthoxylum and Allium Paste in the Treatment of Tinea," *Chinese Journal of Integrated Traditional and Western Medicine,* 10(4): 211; 1990.
8. Liang, X.Z., "Dahuang Soaked in Vinegar as an External Wash in the Treatment of Tinea," *Shaanxi Journal of Traditional Chinese Medicine,* 12(11): 511; 1991.

CHAPTER 10

Spirochete Infections

Syphilis
杨梅疮
yáng méi chuāng, "bayberry flower sores"

Syphyilis is a contagious, chronic systemic disease that progresses through stages, each exhibiting characteristic skin lesions. The first record of syphilis in China is found in Shi Ji-Hong's *Lingnan Hygiene Formulas* (Song-Yuan dynasties), which describes the internal and external treatment methods of this condition. It is surmised that syphilis was brought into southern China by Portuguese sea merchants. Li Shi-Zhen observed in his *Grand Materia Medica* (1578): "There are no ancient remedies for bayberry flower sores, nor were there patients [with this disease previously]. It recently began in Lingnan, and has spread throughout the land."

In 1632, Chen Si-Cheng wrote *Secret Records on Bayberry Flower Sores,* the first Chinese medical work devoted solely to this disease. (The name bayberry flower sores refers to the resemblance of the second stage lesions to flower petals of the red bayberry tree). In his book, Chen indicates that syphilis is transmitted either through sexual contact or from mother to fetus. Treatment methods mentioned in the text include remedies containing mercury and arsenic.

Biomedically, syphilis is caused by the spirochete *Treponema pallidum.*

Signs & Symptoms

The disease is characterized by four stages: primary, secondary, latent and tertiary. Since the disease is systemic, and can affect any tissue or vascular organ of the body, and because its course is protracted, we describe here the symptoms of the skin lesions of each stage, rather than the involved systemic-wide symptomology.

Primary syphilis. The primary lesion, known as a chancre, usually appears within four weeks of infection and heals within 4-8 weeks in untreated individuals. At the site of inoculation, a red papule develops and quickly erodes into a painless ulcer with a lacquer-like base and hard walls. It does not bleed, but when scratched exudes a clear serum containing numerous *T. pallida*. A red areola may surround the lesion. Common sites include the penis, scrotum, anus, and rectum in men, and the labia, fourchette, urethra, posterior labial commissure, and cervix in women. The face, lips, breasts, or fingers may also be affected. Chancres may also be found on the lips, tongue, buccal mucosa, tonsils or fingers.

Secondary syphilis. The secondary stage develops six to 12 weeks after infection. In about one-quarter to one-third of the patients, the primary lesions are still present. The principal feature of the secondary stage is a rash that may be transient, recurrent, or last for months. At the outset of this stage, the lesions are generalized, usually nonpruritic, painless, bilateral, and symmetrically distributed. Later the palms and soles are involved. In moist skin regions, gray or pink patches known as condylomata lata (lesions resembling horny warts) may develop, and are extremely contagious.

Constitutional symptoms are often present: malaise, headache, nausea, loss of appetite, fever, fatigue, bone pain, anemia, neck stiffness. The hair often falls out in clumps.

Lesions affecting the mucous membranes often become eroded, forming circular mucous patches that are grayish-white with a red areola. These patches are usually found in the mouth, on the palate, pharynx, larynx, penis, or vulva, or in the anal canal and rectum. Papules developing at the mucocutaneous junctions and in moist areas of the skin are flattened, hypertrophic, dull pink or gray, and are known as *condylomata lata* (lesions resembling horny warts); these are extremely contagious.

Latent syphilis. Clinical symptoms are absent during latent syphilis, but the disease can still be detected serologically. The early latent period begins about one year after infection, during which time contagious lesions may reappear up until year four of infection. Late latent syphilis begins four years following infection. About two-thirds of patients remain symptom-free for the remainder of their lives, while the remainder progress onto the tertiary stage.

Tertiary or late syphilis. Untreated syphyilis during this stage can present a wide range of symptoms, from none to those reflecting destruction of one or more body systems. There are three disease subtypes, any or all of which may develop: late benign syphilis, cardiovascular syphilis, and neurosyphilis. Since the latter two do not involve skin symptoms, we describe below only late benign syphilis. (Practitioners are encouraged to find the pertinent information regarding the other two subtypes in other biomedical references.)

The characteristic lesion of late benign syphilis is the *gumma* (so named because of its rubbery consistency), which are granulomatous formations. Gummas are often solitary, although they may occur in multiples. Size ranges between microscopic to several centimeters in diameter. The lesions are indurated circles with a necrotic center surrounded by granulomatous tissue. The most commonly affected sites include the skin, mouth and upper respiratory tract, larynx, liver, stomach, and bones, although any organ may be involved. Tissue destruction from gummas can be severe. For example, in the upper respiratory tract, perforation of the nasal septum or hard palate may result from gumma formation.

Differential Diagnosis

Syphilis can mimic most skin diseases. Biomedically, diagnosis is established by demonstrating the causative microorganism, *T. pallidum,* in exudates taken from chancres in primary syphilis, or from lesions in secondary syphilis. Other serologic tests are also helpful in confirming the diagnosis.

Genital lesions of primary syphilis should be differentiated from genital herpes, secondarily infected scabies or other lesions, fungal conditions, and other diseases characterized by ulceration. Extragenital chancres should be examined with syphilis in mind, since these lesions are often misdiagnosed.

Secondary syphilitic rashes may resemble pityriasis rosea, rubella, drug eruption, infectious mononucleosis, erythema multiforme or fungal infection. Scalp lesions may be mistaken for ringworm or alopecia areata. Mucocutaneous lesions may simulate warts, hemorrhoids or pemphigus vegetans.

Traditional Chinese Etiology

The Chinese recognized early on that syphilis was transmitted mainly through sexual contact, through nonvenereal contact, and congenitally. In traditional medicine, transmission through sexual contact is termed essence transformation, and transmission through nonvenereal contact is known as qi transformation. Transmission from mother to fetus is called fetus tainted with toxin.

Qi transformation. Here, the toxin primarily attacks the Lung and Spleen. The lesions are small, and the condition is less severe, rarely involving the internal physiology, other Organs or bones.

Essence transformation. Lesions usually develop on the genitalia. The toxin attacks the Liver and Kidney. The condition can be severe, involving the other Organs, the bone and the marrow.

Treatment

INTERNAL

Primary and secondary syphilis. The strategy is to clear the blood and relieve toxicity. Formulas recommended for this stage include Smilax Combined Formula, or Five-Treasure Powder.

❦ Smilax Combined Formula
土茯苓合剂
tǔ fú líng hé jì

Rhizoma Smilacis Glabrae *(tu fu ling)*	30-60g
Flos Lonicerae Japonicae *(yin hua)*	12g
Radix Clematidis Radix *(wei ling xian)*	9g
Cortex Dictamni Dasycarpi Radicis *(bai xian pi)*	9g
Radix Glycyrrhizae Uralensis *(sheng gan cao)*	6g

Herba Xanthii Sibirici *(cang er cao)* 15g

PREPARATION & DOSAGE: Decoct the herbs in 8 liters of water until 4 liters remain. Divide into three portions and administer one in the morning, one at noon and one at night. Two months is considered one course of therapy.

❦ Five-Treasure Powder
五宝散
wǔ bǎo sǎn

Stalactitum *(e guan shi)* 12g
Cinnabaris *(zhu sha)* 3g
Magarita *(zhen zhu)* 6g
Borneol *(bing pian)* 3g
Succinum *(hu po)* 6g

PREPARATION & DOSAGE: First cook the Magarita *(zhen zhu)* with tofu for about 15-20 minutes. Remove the Magarita, grind it and the remaining herbal ingredients into a fine powder, and then mix together. Mix 6g of this powder with 24g of unbleached wheat flour to form Five-Treasure Powder. Administer 0.3g of this powder ten times each day mixed with the following decoction: decoct 500g of Rhizoma Smilacis Glabrae *(tu fu ling)* in 500ml of water until one-half of the liquid remains. Remove the dregs and divide the decoction into ten parts, each to be mixed with 0.3g of Five-Treasure Powder. Administer the ten portions throughout the day at evenly-spaced times.

CLINICAL NOTE: Spicy and greasy foods, as well as beef, lamb, goose, shrimp and alcohol, should be avoided during therapy.

Latent or tertiary syphilis. The strategy for this stage is to support the normal qi and expel the toxin. Formulas recommended for this stage are Modified Rehmannia Decoction, or Clear the Blood and Collect the Toxin Pill.

❦ Modified Rehmannia Decoction
地黄饮子加减
dì huáng yǐn zǐ jiā jiǎn

Radix Rehmanniae Glutinosae Conquitae *(shu di huang)* 12g
Fructus Corni Officinalis *(shan zhu yu)* 12g
Herba Cistanches Deserticolae *(rou cong rong)* 12g
Radix Lateralis Aconiti Carmichaeli Praeparata *(fu zi)* 6g
Rhizoma Smilacis Glabrae *(tu fu ling)* 30g
Radix Morindae Officinalis *(ba ji tian)* 9g
Cortex Cinnamomi Cassiae *(rou gui)* 3g

PREPARATION & DOSAGE: Decoct and administer in two doses daily.

🌸 Clear the Blood and Collect the Toxin Pill
清血搜毒丸
qīng xuè sōu dú wán

Sanguis Draconis *(xue jie)*	60g
Radix Aucklandiae Lappae *(mu xiang)*	30g
Radix Aristolochiae *(qing mu xiang)*	30g
Flos Caryophylli *(ding xiang)*	30g
Pasta Acaciae seu Uncariae *(er cha)*	30g
Semen Croton Tiglii Praeparata *(ba dou shuang)*	18g

PREPARATION & DOSAGE: Grind all the ingredients together into a fine powder. Mix with water to form a paste. Make into small pills the size of mung beans. Administer 5-10 pills twice daily, with warm water or with mung bean gruel.

EXTERNAL

For chancres and secondary syphilitic papules and rashes, Light-Yellow Powder is recommended.

🌸 Light-Yellow Powder
鹅黄散
é huáng sǎn

Calcined Gypsum *(duan shi gao)*
Dry-fried Cortex Phellodendri *(chao huang bai)*
Calomelas *(qing fen)*

PREPARATION & DOSAGE: Grind equal amounts of the ingredients together into a fine powder. Sprinkle onto lesions 2-3 times daily until ulcers are healed.

For condylomata lata and gummas that are not eroded or ulcerated, Flush and Harmonize Plaster (see erysipelas) may be applied 2-3 times daily. For ulcerated or eroded lesions, Five-Five Special Powder is recommended.

🌸 Five-Five Special Powder
五五丹
wǔ wǔ dān

Calcined Gypsum *(duan shi gao)*	5g
Mercuric Oxide *(sheng yao)*	5g

PREPARATION & DOSAGE: Grind the two ingredients together into a fine powder. Sprinkle liberally onto the lesions and cover with gauze that has first been spread with a layer of petroleum jelly. Apply 1-2 times daily until the lesions are dry (no longer weep exudate). Then use Generate Flesh Powder (see carbuncles in Chapter 7) to promote closure of the lesions.

ACUPUNCTURE

Acupuncture may help alleviate the generalized pain associated with secondary and tertiary syphilis. Primary acupoints include GV-14 *(da zhui)*, GB-21 *(jian jing)*, LI-11 *(qu chi)*, GB-34 *(yang ling quan)* and CV-6 *(qi hai)*. Secondary points include LI-15 *(jian yu)*, PC-6 *(nei guan)*, BL-40 *(wei zhong)*, GB-30 *(huan tiao)* and BL-60 *(kun lun)*. Draining manipulation should be used. Treat twice weekly, with ten treatments as one course of therapy.

Traditional vs. Biomedical Treatment

The modern Chinese medical literature reveals mixed reports regarding which modality is more effective. Some studies claim that herbal formulas are just as effective, or even more effective, than chemotherapy, while others indicate that traditional formulas lack the powerful antispirochetal effects of pharmaceuticals like penicillin, tetracycline and erythromycin— the biomedical drugs of choice. Furthermore, this latter camp believes that the side effects of some of the traditional formulas cause patient compliance problems.

For early stage syphilis (less than one year duration), biomedical rather than traditional treatment is perhaps the simplest for patients to undertake, since it involves a single, one-dose injection of penicillin that often effects cure within one week. (Penicillin-allergic individuals must undergo a longer, two-week regimen of an alternative drug.) Biomedical treatment of the other stages of syphilis require longer regimens, generally lasting between 2-4 weeks. Thus, for these stages, traditional treatment may be an alternative if the patient is interested in a non-chemotherapeutic approach. Traditional treatment may be most helpful for neurosyphilis as an adjunct to pharmaceuticals, in order to manage the symptoms of nerve involvement.

Whether treatment is traditional or biomedical, all patients should be monitored through laboratory tests to detect the efficacy of therapy.

Prevention

Individuals with syphilis should be closely monitored, especially those in the primary and secondary stages. All sexual contacts during the prior three months in cases of primary syphilis, and up to one year in cases of secondary syphilis, should be examined and treated. Patients should also be informed that they are potentially contagious and should not engage in any form of sexual relations until they and their sexual partners have been examined and have completed treatment.

CHAPTER 11

Dermatoses Caused by Arthropods

Scabies
疥疮
jiè chuāng, "scabies sores"

Scabies is a transmissible parasitic skin infection caused by the itch mite *Sarcoptes scabiei,* which is transmitted between infected human hosts. The female mite burrows into the outermost layer of the skin and lays its eggs there.

The ancient Chinese names for scabies include, among others, "damp scabies" *(shī jiè)* and "insect scabies" *(chóng jiè).* By the Sui dynasty (581-618) there was already an understanding about the cause of this condition and its contagiousness. Chao Yuan-Fang's *Discussion of the Origins of Symptoms of Diseases* (610) noted that "[i]nfants, often because the person who breast feeds [them] is ill with scabies, are thus tainted," indicating that scabies is transmitted by contact. The Qing dynasty work *Stone Chamber Secret Records* (1687) by Chen Shi-Duo further instructed that "[when one] has scabies, [one] cannot go to a public bathhouse. Bathing must be [done] with an herbal decoction in one's own house."

Signs & Symptoms

The most pronounced symptom of scabies is itching, which is aggravated by warmth in bed, meaning that the itching is usually most intense at night. The first lesions are the pathognomonic burrows, which appear as short, wavy, grayish-white lines. Most patients will present red papules with signs of scratching at the burrow sites. The itching is due to sensitivity to parasite. Lesions often begin on the hands, particularly in the finger webs. Other common sites of infestation include the wrists, waistline, nipples in women, and genitalia in men. In infants, the burrows may be found on the head, face, and neck. Inflammation generally follows infestation, and, in most individuals, is itself followed by secondary reactions such as excoriation, eczematous lesions, or secondary bacterial infections. In patients with impaired immunity, scabies may proliferate extensively, with the entire skin affected by psoriasis-like lesions known as crusted scabies, an exceedingly infectious type.

Differential Diagnosis

Scabies may be confused with any other pruritic skin disease such as insect bites, atopic dermatitis, and urticaria. During the initial stage of the condition, the telltale sign is the wavy burrows in the skin. However, due to the intense itching, scratch marks and other secondary lesions may mask the true disease. Thus, it is essential to confirm diagnosis of the mites, eggs, or fecal pellets through microscopic examination of skin scrapings taken from burrow sites and unscratched papules.

Traditional Chinese Etiology

According to Chinese medical theory, scabies results from the struggle within the skin among the insect toxin, wind and damp-heat. If not treated properly, the condition becomes protracted, with incessant itching—an indication that wind and damp-heat still remain.

Treatment

Scabies mainly responds to external treatment, although herbs may also be taken internally to relieve the wind and damp-heat, particularly in protracted cases.

INTERNAL

For longstanding conditions, Eliminate Wind Powder is recommended.

❧ Eliminate Wind Powder
消风散
xiāo fēng sǎn

Herba seu Flos Schizonepetae Tenuifoliae *(jing jie)*	3g
Radix Ledebouriellae Divaricatae *(fang feng)*	3g
Fructus Arctii Lappae *(niu bang zi)*	3g
Periostracum Cicadae *(chan tui)*	3g
Rhizoma Atractylodis *(cang zhu)*	3g
Radix Sophorae Flavescentis *(ku shen)*	3g
Caulis Mutong *(mu tong)*	1.5g
Gypsum *(shi gao)*	3g
Rhizoma Anemarrhenae Asphodeloidis *(zhi mu)*	3g
Radix Rehmanniae Glutinosae *(sheng di huang)*	3g
Radix Angelicae Sinensis *(dang gui)*	3g
Semen Sesami Indici *(hei zhi ma)*	3g
Radix Glycyrrhizae Uralensis *(gan cao)*	1.5g

PREPARATION & DOSAGE: Decoct and administer in three doses daily.

EXTERNAL

Any one of the following four formulas is appropriate for the external treatment of scabies.

❧ One Sweep Gone
一扫光
yī sǎo guāng

Radix Sophorae Flavescentis *(ku shen)*	500g
Cortex Phellodendri *(huang bo)*	500g
Alumen Praeparatum *(ku fan)*	90g
Semen Momordicae Cochinchinensis *(mu bie zi)* (husk removed)	90g
Semen Hydnocarpi Anthelminthicae *(da feng zi)* (husk removed)	90g
Fructus Cnidii Monnieri *(she chuang zi)*	90g
Fructus Zanthoxyli Bungeani *(chuan jiao)*	90g
Camphora *(zhang nao)*	90g
Sulphur *(liu huang)*	90g
Alumen *(ming fan)*	90g
Calomelas *(qing fen)*	90g

PREPARATION & DOSAGE: Grind the ingredients together into a fine powder. Dissolve 1.12kg of lard in a nonmetallic pot, and mix in the herbal powder. Store in a glass container. Rub the ointment onto the affected lesions twice daily, always preceding application by carefully bathing the area. Apply for at least 7-10 consecutive days.

CLINICAL NOTE: Because of the toxicity of some of the ingredients, long-term use of this formula is discouraged. If symptoms do not improve, discontinue use and consider other remedies.

❧ Sophora Decoction
苦参汤
kǔ shēn tāng

Radix Sophorae Flavescentis *(ku shen)*
Fructus Cnidii Monnieri *(she chuang zi)*
Radix Angelicae Dahuricae *(bai zhi)*
Flos Lonicerae Japonicae *(jin yin hua)*
Flos Chrysanthemi Indici *(ye ju hua)*
Cortex Phellodendri *(huang bai)*
Fructus Kochiae Scopariae *(di fu zi)*
Rhizoma Acori Graminei *(shi chang pu)*

PREPARATION & DOSAGE: The source text indicates that equal amounts of the ingredients should be decocted in river water (although tap water may be substituted), and before applying as a wash, 4-5 drops of pig bile should be mixed in with the decoction (pig bile may be omitted if unavailable). Wash with the decoction once a day. Symptoms should be relieved after 2-3 applications.

❧ Sophora and Zanthoxylum Decoction
苦椒汤
kǔ jiāo tāng

Radix Sophorae Flavescentis *(ku shen)* 30g
Fructus Zanthoxyli Bungeani *(chuan jiao)* 9g

PREPARATION & DOSAGE: Decoct in water that has been used to wash raw rice. After decocting, remove the dregs and wash the affected areas with the warm decoction for 5-10 minutes. After washing, avoid drafts and wind. Apply twice a day until symptoms are relieved.

❧ Zanthoxylum and Artemisia Decoction
川艾汤
chuān ài tāng

Rhizoma Acori Graminei *(shi chang pu)* 30g
Fructus Zanthoxyli Bungeani *(chuan jiao)* 7.5g
Folium Artemisiae Argyi *(ai ye)* 7.5g
Scallion Whites .... 7 pieces

PREPARATION & DOSAGE: Decoct the ingredients in 1.8 liters of water, remove the dregs, and wash affected areas with the warm decoction once or twice daily until symptoms are alleviated.

Traditional vs. Biomedical Treatment

Traditional treatment may be preferred over biomedical therapy for scabies, primarily because many of the topical drugs used are toxic, and there is a tendency for patients to apply these remedies more frequently and over longer periods than prescribed. With one exception (One Sweep Gone), all of the traditional formulas described above are not toxic and can be used for several consecutive days.

Prevention

Scabies is easily transmitted, but only under circumstances of skin-to-skin contact such as with family members sharing a bed, or through sexual contact. Therefore, in treating, asymptomatic family members or bed partners may need to be treated simultaneously. At the end of treatment, bedding, intimate articles of clothing, and towels should be machine washed and dried under the hot cycles. Fortunately, the scabies mite survives only briefly away from the human host. Cleaning outerwear or furniture is not necessary.

Pediculosis
虱疮
shī chuāng, "louse sores"

Pediculosis is the infestation of humans by lice. The Chinese folk name for this parasite is "eight-footed bug." As early as the Sui dynasty (581-618) there were records of pediculosis in the Chinese medical literature. The following passage about lice infestation in children appears in *Discussion of the Origins of Symptoms of Diseases:*

> If children's hair is not washed in a timely manner, lice [infestation] will occur. The more they [the lice] grow, the more they multiply. [They] bite the head, after which sores arise. At the site of the sores are gathered lice; this site is known as the nest.

Eventually, three kinds of lice were recognized, each associated with a specific site of infestation: head, clothing and pubis. The contagiousness of lice was described by Gu Shi-Deng in *Collection of Treatments for Sores* (1760):

> This insect is most easily transmitted. Those who get this [insect/disease], should best not be approached. If approached it will result in the wife also getting this insect. [One] cannot but be cautious.

Signs & Symptoms

Head lice (pediculosis capitis). The species of lice that infests the head is *Pediculosis humanus capitis*. This condition is transmitted by direct contact (not necessarily head-to-head). Inanimate objects are usually the vehicles of transmission, e.g., shared combs, brushes, hats, towels. All social classes are involved, with children being most commonly affected. The condition is confined to the scalp, especially the occipital region. Symptoms are severe itching with scratching. In severe cases, excoriation often results in secondary bacterial infection, with matted, lusterless, and foul-smelling hair from the exudate. A number of individuals present with fever and swelling of the cervical lymph nodes caused by sensitivity to lice bites. When infestation is suspected, the hair should be inspected with a magnifying glass. Preliminary diagnosis can be made by finding numerous grayish-white oval nits that do not easily slide off the hair shaft by pulling, with confirmation made by examining a hair under a microscope, observing for nits, egg casings, and the occasional adult parasite.

Body lice (pediculosis corporis). The species of lice that affects the body is *Pediculus humanus humanus*. This parasite lives and lays eggs on clothing next to the skin, and visits the body only to feed. Therefore, the condition commonly infests individuals who continuously wear the same unlaundered clothes for days at a time. The initial symptom consists of red macules or papules at the puncture sites where the lice feed on the skin. As the infestation worsens, long scratch marks due to intense itching are the common presentation, followed by pustules from secondary bacterial infection. Adult parasites are few; diagnosis is therefore made by inspecting for nits, which are frequently found in the seams of clothing, especially around the collar, waistline, and armpits.

Pubic lice (pediculosis pubis). While the name implies that the primary site affected is the pubic area, infestation with *Pthirus pubis* can extend to any hairy area, including the armpits, the eyelashes and eyebrows, beard and mustache, and hairs of the thighs and trunk. The usual mode of transmission is through sexual contact. Often the condition coexists with other venereal diseases.

The outstanding symptom is itching with excoriation, frequently leading to secondary bacterial infection. The characteristic sign of pubic lice are the bluish- or slate-colored macules that can be found on the thighs and upper body. Because adult organisms are few, diagnosis is often reached by removing hairs and finding, through microscopic examination, the attached nits.

Differential Diagnosis

Diagnosis is made by finding the adult parasite or ova. Intense itching may resemble that of urticaria or eczema. However, because of the specific sites of infestation by the three kinds of lice, practitioners should be alerted to the possibility of pediculosis when patients present with any of the above symptoms.

Traditional Chinese Etiology

Lice are understood in traditional Chinese medicine to arise from lack of personal hygiene.

Treatment

The primary method of treatment for lice is topical application of herbal remedies. For all three kinds of pediculoses, Coreopsis Tincture to Eliminate Insects is recommended.

❦ Coreopsis Tincture to Eliminate Bugs
除虫菊酊
chú chóng jú dīng

Folium Coreopsidis Lanceolatae *(xian ye jin ji ju)*	1g
Rice Wine	200ml

PREPARATION & DOSAGE: Soak the herb in the rice wine for seven days. Filter the dregs. Apply to affected areas once daily for 5-7 consecutive days.

For pediculosis of the head, Veratrum Powder or Stemona Tincture is recommended.

❦ Veratrum Powder
藜芦散
lí lú sǎn

Rhizoma et Radix Veratri *(li lu)*	0.3-0.9g

PREPARATION & DOSAGE: Grind into a fine powder. Part the hair on the head, and sprinkle the powder onto the scalp. Avoid breathing the powder or getting it in the eyes. Cover the head with a shower cap and wear continuously for 24 hours. The source text indicates that the head lice should be eliminated thereafter. If not, wash the hair and apply once again in the same manner.

Stemona Tincture
百部酊
bǎi bù dīng

Radix Stemonae *(bai bu)* 20-50g
Rice Wine or 75% Rubbing Alcohol .... 5-7 liters

PREPARATION & DOSAGE: Soak the herb in the wine or alcohol for seven days. Filter the dregs. Pour about 150ml into a separate container and make a 1:1 dilution by adding about 150ml of water. Wash the scalp with this 50 percent herbal solution (avoid the eyes), followed by a normal washing of the hair. Repeat once daily for four consecutive days.

For pubic pediculosis, Acorus and Stemona Wash is recommended.

Acorus and Stemona Wash
石菖蒲百部汤
shí chāng pǔ bǎi bù tāng

Rhizoma Acori Graminei *(shi chang pu)*
Radix Stemonae *(bai bu)*

PREPARATION & DOSAGE: Decoct equal amounts of the two herbs in water. Remove the dregs. Wash the anogenital area, including pubic hair, with the warm decoction once or twice a day for 2-3 consecutive days. The source text indicates that the pubic hair should be shaved or trimmed close to the skin prior to using this formula.

Traditional vs. Biomedical Treatment

Traditional remedies are probably just as effective as chemical pediculocides, although the herbal formulas take longer to prepare. The disadvantages of the pharmaceuticals are toxicity and eye irritation, as some of them contain refined kerosene or distillates.

Prevention

Lice infestation is widespread when there is overcrowding or inadequate facilities for personal hygiene or for washing clothes. Treatment should be repeated in 7-10 days to eliminate any nits that may have survived. Infestation of eyelashes is difficult to manage, and requires removal of parasites with forceps. Sources of infestation such as combs, hats, clothing or bedding should be decontaminated by thorough laundering with hot water, or by boiling. Dry-cleaning destroys lice on wool garments.

Pediculosis pubis has become epidemic in the United States and Western Europe. Because the condition is typically transmitted sexually, sexual partners should be treated simultaneously. In hairy individuals, application of medications (whether traditional or biomedical) should include the thighs, trunk and axillary regions because of frequent involvement of these areas. One reason for treatment failure is that only the pubic area is treated in these persons.

Because recurrence is common, strict adherence to therapy, and persistent efforts to eradicate the source of infestation, are both necessary to completely resolve the condition. In some cases, more fastidious and drastic measures, such as manual removal of the parasites and nits (literally "nit-picking"), or shaving of the hair, may be required.

Insect Stings and Bites
虫螫咬伤
chóng shì yǎo shāng

Through their bites or stings, insects can cause reactions in humans ranging from a small papule at the site of injury to the more serious anaphylaxis in hypersensitive individuals. Fatality from insect bites or stings is not uncommon. Several Chinese medical classics describe insect bites and stings. Among them is the following passage from *True Lineage of External Medicine* (1617):

> Evil insects are endowed with different poisons. When one encounters [them] do not touch their poison[-ous parts]; centipedes use [their] pincers, scorpions and bees [wasps] use [their] tails . . . to sting people. When injured in such manner, treatment should be in accord with the kind of [offending insect].

The number of insects that can inflict harm is vast; only the more common ones will be dealt with here.

Signs & Symptoms

Lesions are usually found on exposed parts of the body, and may vary from a papule to a large ulcer. Insects that are more venomous may cause lesions that result in local vesiculation, pustulation, rupture, ulceration and even necrotization; local pain and/or itching is common. Systemic reactions may include nausea, vomiting, malaise and swelling of the lymph nodes. In hypersensitive persons, the reaction can be intense, and may even result in anaphylactic shock. Thus, prompt treatment is of the utmost importance.

Differential Diagnosis

In most cases the affected individual has knowledge of having been stung or bitten by an insect. In instances where insect bite is suspected but cannot be confirmed by the patient, close questioning may be necessary to ascertain the origin of the skin lesion.

Traditional Chinese Etiology

Chinese medicine correlates the reaction of insect bites to toxin carried by the insect.

Treatment

The strategy of treatment is to clear heat and relieve toxicity. For more effective relief, internal and external modalities should be used in combination.

INTERNAL

❧ Five-Ingredient Decoction to Eliminate Toxin
五味消毒饮
wǔ wèi xiāo dú yǐn

Flos Lonicerae Japonicae *(jin yin hua)* 9g
Herba Taraxaci Mongolici cum Radice *(pu gong ying)* 3.6g
Herba cum Radice Violae Yedoensitis *(zi hua di ding)* 3.6g
Flos Chrysanthemi Indici *(ye ju hua)* 3.6g
Herba Begoniae Fimbristipulatae *(zi bei tian kui)* 3.6g

PREPARATION & DOSAGE: Decoct and administer in four equal portions throughout the day.

MODIFICATIONS: For severe fire toxin pattern, add Rhizoma Coptidis *(huang lian)*, Cortex Phellodendri *(huang bai)*, Radix Rehmanniae Glutinosae *(sheng di huang)*, Cortex Moutan Radicis *(mu dan pi)* and Testa Phaseoli Radiati *(lu dou yi)*; for signs of wind toxin, add Folium Perillae Frutescentis *(zi su ye)*, Periostracum Cicadae *(chan tui)*, Herba Artemisiae Annuae *(qing hao)* and Radix Angelicae Dahuricae *(bai zhi)*.

❧ Snake Bite Medicine Pills
蛇咬片
shé yǎo piàn

Herba seu Radix Cirsii Japonici *(da ji)*
Radix Sophorae Flavescentis *(ku shen)*
Radix Aucklandiae Lappae *(mu xiang)*
Radix Rubiae Cordifoliae *(qian cao)*
Herba Bidentis Bipinnatae *(gui zhen cao)*
Radix Aristolochiae Fangchi *(fang ji)*
Folium Rohdeae Japonicae *(wan nian qing ye)*

PREPARATION & DOSAGE: Grind equal amounts of the ingredients together into a fine powder. Mix with water to form a paste. Make into pills weighing 0.5g each. Administer 4-6 pills daily.

EXTERNAL
Bites or stings from certain insects have specific remedies for treatment.

Bees and wasps
[A] Extract the milky fluid from Herba Taraxaci Mongolici cum Radice Recens *(xian pu gong ying)* by pulling apart the leaves or breaking up the root. Rub this fluid on the lesion 3-5 times daily.

[B] Mash Folium Allii Tuberosi Recens *(xian jiu cai)* until a paste is formed, and apply to the affected area 1-2 times daily.

[C] Apply human breast milk 3-5 times daily.

[D] Grind dried Nidus Vespae *(lu feng fang)* into a fine powder. Mix thoroughly with lard to form an ointment. Apply to the affected area once daily.

Mosquitos, bedbugs and fleas
[A] Apply vinegar to the affected area 3-5 times daily.

[B] Decoct Folium Broussonetiae Papyriferae *(chu ye),* and apply as a warm compress or as a wash 2-3 times daily.

Centipedes

[A] Grind a small amount of Excrementum Trogopterori seu Pteromi *(wu ling zhi)* into a fine powder. Mix with cold water to form a paste. Apply to the lesion 1-2 times daily.

[B] Grind equal amounts of Radix Glycyrrhizae Uralensis *(gan cao)* and Realgar *(xiong huang)* together into a fine powder and mix with vegetable oil to form a paste. Apply 1-2 times daily.

[C] Grind Secretio Bufonis *(chan su)* with vinegar, and apply the fluid 2-3 times daily.

[D] Express the juice from Folium Mori Albae Recens *(xian sang ye)* and apply 2-3 times daily.

Spiders

[A] Drink one liter of goat's milk after being bitten.

[B] Mix together fresh Rhizoma Zingiberis Officinalis *(gan jiang)* and powdered Fructus Piperis Nigri *(hu jiao)* to form a paste. Apply to the affected area.

[C] Decoct Radix Gentianae Qinjiao *(qin jiao)* and drink the decoction slowly. Then apply to the affected area a water-based paste made from finely powdered Alumen *(ming fan)* and Realgar *(xiong huang),* in equal amounts, 1-2 times daily.

[D] Decoct Herba Xanthii Sibirici *(cang er cao)* and administer internally and apply externally 2-3 times daily.

Scorpions

[A] Grind together into a fine powder equal amounts of Realgar *(xiong huang)* and Alumen Praeparatum *(ku fan)*. Mix with tea and apply 1-3 times daily.

[B] Mash one large (live) snail into a paste. Apply one snail once a day.

[C] Grind Alumen *(ming fan)* into a fine powder. Mix with vinegar to form a paste. Apply 1-2 times daily.

MOXIBUSTION

For insect bites and stings, indirect moxibustion with a moxa roll may be applied for ten minutes, twice daily, in order to alleviate the pain.

Traditional vs. Biomedical Treatment

Traditional treatment may be more effective than biomedical intervention, which is primarily palliative through use of corticosteroids. Many of the traditional remedies are aimed at neutralizing the venom, or at countering the hypersensitivity reaction produced by the sting or bite.

Prevention

Persons with known hypersensitivity to insect stings or bites should be especially wary when in an environment that is endemic for the offending insect(s). Clothing should cover the arms and legs, and in the case of bees and wasps, avoid wearing brightly colored clothing and using scented soaps and shampoos, perfume and cologne.

CHAPTER 12

Dermatoses Due to Environmental Influences

Chilblain
冻疮
dòng chuāng, "freeze sores"

Chilblain is injury to the skin and tissues by cold. The degree of injury varies in relation to the extent of exposure, and ranges from mild itching and redness to bullae and ulceration. The more severe cases include gangrene and even loss of the affected area, both of which are characteristic of frostbite.

Several Chinese medical classics describe chilblain. Among them is the following passage from *Profound Purpose from the Heavenly Abode* (1694):

> Freeze sores arise in individuals who are attacked by cold wind and exposed to coldness. In the poor and lowly, the hands and feet are affected; in the rich, the ears and face. First swelling arises, then pain; protracted pain is followed by ulceration . . . Persons [exposed] to extreme cold may have dropping off of the fingers and toes.

Signs & Symptoms

The most commonly affected areas include the back of the hands and feet, the face and ears, and other exposed regions. Mild cases of exposure to damp cold (temperatures around freezing) can cause the area to become firm, cold and white; peeling or blistering may occur 24-72 hours later. In more severe cases, the area is pale, edematous, clammy, cold and numb; tissue degeneration and infection may ensue.

Exposure to dry cold (temperatures well below freezing) will cause the area to become cold, hard, white and numb—all symptoms of frostbite. On warming, the affected area will become blotchy red, swollen and painful. Depending on the extent of the injury, the area may either recover normally or deteriorate to gangrene.

Differential Diagnosis

History of exposure to cold will confirm diagnosis of chilblain.

Traditional Chinese Etiology

Exposure to toxic cold causes qi and blood to stagnate, resulting in loss of warmth and nourishment to the area.

Treatment

The treatment strategy is to dispel cold and unblock the channels and collaterals. Treatment should be started as soon as possible following exposure.

INTERNAL

Formulas recommended for internal use include Modified Tangkuei Decoction for Frigid Extremities [A], or Modified Cinnamon Twig Decoction Plus Tangkuei.

❧ Modified Tangkuei Decoction for Frigid Extremities [A]
当归四逆汤加减
dāng guī sì nì tāng jiā jiǎn

Radix Angelicae Sinensis *(dang gui)*	12g
Ramulus Cinnamomi Cassiae *(gui zhi)*	12g
dry-fried Radix Paeoniae Lactiflorae *(chao bai shao)*	12g
Herba cum Radice Asari *(xi xin)*	6g
Rhizoma Curcumae Longae *(jiang huang)*	6g
Honey-toasted Radix Glycyrrhizae Uralensis *(zhi gan cao)*	6g
Rhizoma Zingiberis Officinalis Recens *(sheng jiang)*	3 slices
Fructus Zizyphi Jujubae *(da zao)*	7 pieces

PREPARATION & DOSAGE: Decoct and administer one-half in the morning and the remainder at night.

MODIFICATIONS: For constitutional aversion to cold due to yang deficiency, add prepared Radix Lateralis Aconiti Carmichaeli Praeparata *(fu zi)*, Gelatinum Cornu Cervi *(lu jiao jiao)* and Radix Morindae Officinalis *(ba ji tian)*; for deficiency of qi and blood, add Radix Codonopsitis Pilosulae *(dang shen)*, Radix Astragali Membranacei *(huang qi)* and Gelatinum Cornu Cervi *(lu jiao jiao)*; for racalcitrant, unhealing ulceration, add Cortex Cinnamomi Cassiae *(rou gui)*, Radix Astragali Membranacei *(huang qi)*, Radix Codonopsitis Pilosulae *(dang shen)* and Radix Ampelopsis Japonicae *(bai lian)*.

For severe frostbite, Modified Cinnamon Twig Decoction Plus Tangkuei may be used. This remedy was developed by the Research Group on Cold Injury at

Shenyang Medical University in northeast China, a region that experiences frigid cold winters.

❧ Modified Cinnamon Twig Decoction Plus Tangkuei
桂枝加当归汤加减
guì zhī jiā dāng guī tāng jiā jiǎn

Ramulus Cinnamomi Cassiae *(gui zhi)*	30g
Radix Paeoniae Rubrae *(chi shao)*	6g
Rhizoma Zingiberis Officinalis *(gan jiang)*	15g
Radix Angelicae Sinensis *(dang gui)*	15g
Fructus Crataegi *(shan zha)*	15g
Flos Lonicerae Japonicae *(jin yin hua)*	15g
Fructus Forsythiae Suspensae *(lian qiao)*	15g
Flos Carthami Tinctorii *(hong hua)*	6g
Semen Persicae *(tao ren)*	6g
Radix Scrophulariae Ningpoensis *(xuan shen)*	15g
Radix Scutellariae Baicalensis *(huang qin)*	15g
Myrrha *(mo yao)*	6g
Gummi Olibanum *(ru xiang)*	6g

PREPARATION & DOSAGE: Decoct and administer one-half in the morning and the remainder at night for 10-15 consecutive days.

EXTERNAL

For mild cases without ulceration, the following external formulas are recommended.

❧ Ten Percent Ground Pepper Alcohol
10% 胡椒酒精浸液
10% hú jiāo jiǔ jīng jìn yè

Ground Pepper	10g
95% Isopropyl Alcohol	100ml

PREPARATION & DOSAGE: Put the pepper in a jar with a tight lid. Add the alcohol and steep for seven days, shaking the container twice daily. Before using, shake the container for about five minutes, then allow the pepper to settle. Use a sterile cotton ball to apply the clear liquid to the affected area, once or twice daily. The source text indicates that this remedy prevents weeping of the lesion, reduces swelling, stops pain and itching, and promotes healing.

❧ Cherry Tincture
樱桃酒
yīng táo jiǔ

Fructus Pruni Pseudocerasi *(ying tao)*	2 cherries

Rice Wine 500ml

PREPARATION & DOSAGE: Put the cherries and rice wine in a jar that has an airtight lid. Steep for several days prior to using. Store in a dark, cool location. Apply the tincture with a sterile cotton swab 1-3 times daily.

❧ Freeze Sore Ointment
冻疮油
dòng chuāng yóu

Dried Chili Peppers (the spicier, the better) 100g
95% Isopropyl Alcohol 250ml
Borneol *(bing pian)* 5g
Camphora *(zhang nao)* 15g
Glycerine 10g

PREPARATION & DOSAGE: First chop the peppers into small pieces and put into a large glass jar with an airtight lid. Steep the peppers in 250ml of hot water (80-90°C) for about ten hours with the lid on. Strain the dregs through cheesecloth and retain the liquid. Add the alcohol to the pepper liquid; a reddish precipitate will form. Filter and dispose of the precipitate. Grind the Borneol *(bing pian)* and Camphora *(zhang nao)* together into a fine powder and mix with the liquid. Finally, add the glycerine and mix all the ingredients well. Store in a glass jar with a tight lid.

Apply the ointment 3-4 times daily, washing the affected area each time before application. Do not apply to ulcerated lesions.

❧ Eggplant Vine Wash
茄子秸煎水
qié zǐ jiē jiān shuǐ

Caulis Solani Melongenae cum Radicis *(qie zi jie)* . . . . 1 vine

PREPARATION & DOSAGE: Clean one Japanese eggplant vine (with the roots) under running water to remove the soil. (The vine should have been pulled during the autumn after the fruit had been harvested.) Decoct the entire vine in water for 25-30 minutes. Wash the affected area with the decoction while it is still hot (as hot as can be tolerated). Apply once daily at bedtime for 25 minutes. Allow the skin to air dry; do not wash again until just before the next application. Do not use other topical remedies. Continue the treatment until the area is healed.

❧ Effective Scarlet Wine
红灵酒
hóng líng jiǔ

Radix Angelicae Sinensis *(dang gui)* 60g

Flos Carthami Tinctorii *(hong hua)* 30g
Fructus Zanthoxyli Bungeani *(chuan jiao)* 30g
Cortex Cinnamomi Cassiae *(rou gui)* (thin slices) 60g
Camphora *(zhang nao)* 15g
Herba cum Radice Asari *(xi xin)* (fine powder) 15g
Rhizoma Zingiberis Officinalis *(gan jiang)* (thin slices) 30g

PREPARATION & DOSAGE: Steep the ingredients in one liter of 95 percent isopropyl alcohol for seven days in a glass jar with a tight-fitting lid. Gently rub the affected area with a cotton ball dipped in the remedy. Apply for 10 minutes twice daily.

For cases presenting with ulceration, either Freeze Sore Plaster or Daphne and Glycyrrhiza Wash is recommended.

❦ Freeze Sore Plaster
冻疮膏
dòng chuāng gāo

Fructus Xanthii Sibirici *(cang er zi)* 10g
Radix Clematidis *(wei ling xian)* 10g
Camphora *(zhang nao)* ***5g
Petroleum Jelly 85g

PREPARATION & DOSAGE: Dissolve the petroleum jelly in a glass saucepan over low heat. Add the Fructus Xanthii Sibirici *(cang er zi)* and Radix Clematidis *(wei ling xian)* and stir until completely mixed. Steep for five days, and then dissolve the concoction over low heat and remove the dregs. Add the Camphora *(zhang nao)* and mix well. After congealing, the remedy may be applied with a sterile cotton swab to the ulcerated lesion. Treat once daily.

❦ Daphne and Licorice Wash
芫花甘草洗剂
yuán huā gān cǎo xǐ jì

Flos Daphnes Genkwa *(yuan hua)* 9g
Radix Glycyrrhizae Uralensis *(gan cao)* 9g

PREPARATION & DOSAGE: Decoct the herbs in 2 liters of water. Wash the affected area three times daily with the warm decoction and allow to air dry. Apply a sterile dressing after each application.

For lesions that are infected or necrotic, first apply Nine-One Special Powder (see herpes zoster in Chapter 8) until the degenerated tissue sloughs off, then apply Generate Flesh Powder (see carbuncles in Chapter 7).

ACUPUNCTURE

Filiform needling. Chilblain of the hands and/or feet may be treated by needling points proximal to the affected areas. For chilblain of the back of the hand, LI-4 *(he gu)*, M-UE-9 *(ba xie)* and TB-4 *(yang chi)* may be needled. For chilblain of the dorsum of the foot, needle BL-60 *(kun lun)*, LR-2 *(xing jian)* and GB-41 *(zu lin qi)*. Treat once daily, with even needle manipulation, retaining the needles for 15-20 minutes. Symptoms should be alleviated within three treatments.

Bloodletting. For severe itching in the affected areas, bloodletting may be performed with a plum-blossom or a filiform needle. After the procedure, a few drops of blood should be squeezed out. Treat once daily or once every other day until the itching is relieved.

MOXIBUSTION

For upper extremity chilblain, apply indirect moxibustion with a moxa roll to LI-11 *(qu chi)* and the affected area. For the lower extremity, apply to ST-36 *(zu san li)* and the affected area. Treat for 15-20 minutes, once or twice daily, for about one week immediately after exposure.

EMPIRICAL REMEDY

Crush 30g of pine seeds (without hulls), and mix with vegetable oil until a paste is formed. Spread a layer of the paste on the affected area, and cover with sterile gauze. Apply once daily.[1]

Traditional vs. Biomedical Treatment

Following exposure, and before administering any other form of therapy, rapid rewarming should be performed with baths or soaks using water heated to 105-108°F (40.6-42.2°C). Traditional treatment, in particular the combined use of internal and external remedies, may be more effective than biomedical intervention, which is primarily directed toward preventing infection of the exposed areas. There is probably some basis to using traditional formulas that warm and invigorate the blood and dispel stasis, since cold is an excess that causes congealing and stasis which, in the case of frostbite, can lead to loss of sensation, hardening of the tissues and cyanosis. Thus, administration of these formulas may help speed recovery with minimal sequelae.

Prevention

Clothing worn in layers, as well as minimizing wetness and wind, are the keys to preventing injury from cold. Since substantial warmth can be lost through the head, complete head covering is essential. Warm food and fluids should be taken, and physical activity increased, to maintain body warmth.

Sunburn
日晒疮
rì shài chuāng, "sunshine sores"

Sunburn is an acute reaction of the skin to overexposure to sunlight. The first Chinese medical classic to describe this condition is Shen Dou-Yuan's *Profound Insights on External Diseases* (1604):

> [During] the dog days of summer, hard-working persons as they labor do not cherish their lives, [and] are exposed intensely to the sun. First there is pain, followed by breaking [of the skin], then development of sores. [This] is not a [condition] of the qi or blood.

Signs & Symptoms

The skin will show progressively severe lesions depending on the amount of overexposure to the sun. Short overexposure results in redness, while longer overexposure may cause swelling, tenderness, and blistering, accompanied by pain. In severe cases, systemic symptoms such as vomiting, fever, and collapse may appear. After several days, the dead skin cells are shed through peeling.

Differential Diagnosis

The erythema of mild sunburn should be differentiated from contact dermatitis and drug eruptions. History of overexposure to sun will confirm the diagnosis of sunburn.

Traditional Chinese Etiology

Prolonged exposure to intense sunlight causes invasion of summerheat. The heat becomes overwhelming and develops into toxic heat that injures the skin and tissues.

Treatment

The treatment strategy is to clear summerheat and dispel heat.

INTERNAL

Either White Tiger Decoction or Artemisia Annua Decoction is recommended for this pattern.

❦ White Tiger Decoction
白虎汤
bái hǔ tāng

Gypsum *(shi gao)* 30g
Rhizoma Anemarrhenae Asphodeloidis *(zhi mu)* 9g
Honey-toasted Radix Glycyrrhizae Uralensis *(zhi gan cao)* 3g
Nonglutinous Rice *(geng mi)* 9-15g

PREPARATION & DOSAGE: Decoct the ingredients in water until the rice is cooked. Strain the dregs and administer in three doses daily.

MODIFICATIONS: For aversion to cold, add Radix Bupleuri *(chai hu)* and Cornu Bubali *(shui niu jiao)*; for impaired consciousness and delirium, add Succinum *(hu po)*, Rhizoma Acori Graminei *(shi chang pu)* and Radix Polygalae Tenuifoliae *(yuan zhi)*.

❧ Artemisia Annua Decoction
青蒿饮
qīng hāo yǐn

Herba Artemisiae Annuae Recens *(xian qing hao)*	30g

PREPARATION & DOSAGE: Prepare by mashing and then steeping in cold tap water for 10-15 minutes. Strain and save the dregs. Administer 4-5 tablespoons (15ml) of the liquid three times daily. Apply the dregs to the affected area for 10 minutes, 2-3 times daily.

If the fresh herb is not available, decoct 18g of the dried herb for 15 minutes. Administer in three doses daily and apply the dregs in the same manner as above.

EXTERNAL

For mild to moderate sunburn causing erythema, wheals and/or itching, Clearing and Cooling Powder is recommended.

❧ Clearing and Cooling Powder
清凉粉
qīng liáng fěn

Talcum *(hua shi)*	120g
Radix Glycyrrhizae Uralensis *(gan cao)*	20g
Borneol *(bing pian)*	12g

PREPARATION & DOSAGE: Grind the first two ingredients together to form Six-One Powder (see furuncles in Chapter 7). Grind 120g of Six-One Powder together with the Borneol *(bing pian)*. Sprinkle on the affected area 3-5 times daily until the symptoms are relieved.

For severe sunburn that results in blisters, swelling or erosion, decoct together Flos Chrysanthemi Indici *(ye ju hua)*, Herba Portulacae Oleraceae *(ma chi xian)*, Herba Artemisiae Annuae *(qing hao)* and Herba Solani Nigri *(long kui)*, and apply the decoction as a cold compress 2-3 three times daily. Then apply Jade Dew Powder.

❧ Jade Dew Powder
玉露散
yù lù sǎn

Folium Hibisci Mutabilis *(mu fu rong ye)*

PREPARATION & DOSAGE: Grind any amount of the herb into a fine powder. Mix with sesame oil to form a paste. Apply to the affected area 2-3 three times daily until the lesions heal.

Traditional vs. Biomedical Treatment

Traditional treatment may be more effective than biomedical intervention in promoting recovery. The latter merely involves applying cold tap-water compresses for confined areas of sunburn, or administration of systemic corticosteroids for extensive and severe sunburn, to relieve the discomfort. Such treatment, however, does not resolve the root of the condition, which in Chinese medicine is caused by summerheat toxin. Thus, traditional remedies are perhaps more beneficial because their function is to expel summerheat toxin, after which healing can begin.

Prevention

Sunburn is easily prevented by either avoiding, or not being exposed for more than 30 minutes to, bright midday summer sun between 10 a.m. and 4 p.m. Sunscreen preparations are useful to some degree in shielding the skin from ultraviolet light damage.

CHAPTER NOTES

1. Dai, Y.F. and Liu, C.J. *Medicinal Uses of Fruits (Yao yong guo pin)*. Nanning: Guangxi People's Publishing House, 1982.

CHAPTER 13

Dermatitis
湿疹
shī zhěn, "damp rash"

Dermatitis, or eczema, is an inflammation of the skin. While there are different forms, the skin changes are basically the same, progressing from acute to subacute to chronic. The acute stage is characterized by intensely pruritic, erythematous papules and vesicles on a red base, or by oozing erosions. Subacute dermatitis presents with red, excoriated, scaling papules or plaques; the scaling is sometimes so fine and diffuse that the lesions acquire a silvery sheen. Chronic dermatitis is marked by thickening of the skin and lichenification; peeling, chafing, and color changes are frequently present. Western dermatologists tend to use the terms "dermatitis" and "eczema" interchangeably.

Chinese names for eczematous conditions are confusing, and include terms such as "sores" *(chuāng),* "tinea" *(xuǎn)* and others that indicate diseases caused by wind. Also, eczematous conditions affecting different parts of the body were given distinct names, such as "sores attached to the eyebrows" *(liàn méi chuāng)* for eczema of the eyebrow area, and "damp toxin sores" *(shī dú chuāng)* for eczema affecting the ankles.

Contact Dermatitis
接触性皮炎
jiē chù xìng pí yán

Contact dermatitis is an acute or chronic inflammation caused by substances in direct physical contact with the skin. Classical Chinese medical texts describe three conditions that resemble contact dermatitis: "lacquer sores" *(qī chuāng),* which affect persons who come in contact with the lacquer tree, lacquer or lacquer vapor; "commode tinea" *(mǎ tǒng xuǎn)*, which is contracted after using a newly painted/varnished toilet seat; and "medicinal plaster wind" *(gāo yào fēng)*, which is contracted after application of medicinal plasters to the skin. Today, however, no distinction is made between these classical types of contact dermatitis and the condition as it is now known.

Signs & Symptoms

The skin changes in contact dermatitis may be attributable to a direct toxic effect of the substance, or to an allergic response. Acute symptoms can develop within seconds or minutes after contact and include reddening, blistering, and oozing. Severe cases may present with generalized symptoms such as swelling of the face and eyes. Skin changes in chronic cases range from mild itching, dryness, cracking, blistering, and erosion, to ulceration.

Differential Diagnosis

Contact dermatitis may resemble other types of dermatitis. The characteristics of the changes in the condition of the skin, and a history of exposure, will aid in diagnosis. Determining the offending agent is straightforward in some cases, e.g., metallic jewelry, cosmetics, or plants, while in other cases persistent detective work is required. Patch tests are sometimes helpful, although the results may be ambiguous, especially in identifying the precise agent.

Traditional Chinese Etiology

The loss of impermeability of the skin and interstices that results from low constitutional resistance is the condition underlying contact dermatitis. Upon contact, substances (toxins) to which the individual does not have resistance enter the skin. The resulting conflict between the toxin and the qi and blood gives rise to heat and dampness, which accumulate in the skin and produce the skin lesions.

Treatment

The first step in treatment is to remove the offending agent, after which either internal or external remedies—or both—may be administered. The treatment strategy for contact dermatitis is to clear heat and drain dampness, and relieve toxicity.

INTERNAL

Appropriate formulas for internal administered are Five-Ingredient Decoction to Eliminate Toxin, or Clear and Relieve Tablet.

❧ Five-Ingredient Decoction to Eliminate Toxin
五味消毒饮
wǔ wèi xiāo dú yǐn

Flos Lonicerae Japonicae *(jin yin hua)*	9g
Herba Taraxaci Mongolici cum Radice *(pu gong ying)*	3.6g
Herba cum Radice Violae Yedoensitis *(zi hua di ding)*	3.6g

Flos Chrysanthemi Indici *(ye ju hua)* 3.6g
Herba Begoniae Fimbristipulatae *(zi bei tian kui)* 3.6g

PREPARATION & DOSAGE: Decoct and administer in one dose daily.

MODIFICATIONS: For redness, swelling and burning pain, add Cortex Moutan Radicis *(mu dan pi)*, Radix Rehmanniae Glutinosae *(sheng di huang)* and Flos Carthami Tinctorii *(hong hua)*; for severe itching, add Fructus Kochiae Scopariae *(di fu zi)*, Cortex Dictamni Dasycarpi Radicis *(bai xian pi)* and Periostracum Cicadae *(chan tui)*; for ulcerated lesions, add Semen Coicis Lachryma-jobi *(yi yi ren)*, Cortex Poriae Cocos *(fu ling pi)* and Epicarpium Benincasae Hispidae *(dong gua pi)*.

❧ Clear and Relieve Tablet
清解片
qīng jiě piàn

Radix et Rhizoma Rhei *(da huang)* 500g
Radix Scutellariae Baicalensis *(huang qin)* 500g
Cortex Phellodendri *(huang bai)* 500g
Rhizoma Atractylodis *(cang zhu)* 500g

PREPARATION & DOSAGE: Grind all the ingredients together into a fine powder. Press into pills, each weighing 0.3g. Administer five pills, twice daily, with warm water.

EXTERNAL

For simple redness of the skin and/or papular eruption, Three-Yellow Wash (see furuncles in Chapter 7), applied twice daily until the symptoms are relieved, is recommended.

For vesicles that weep and/or ulcerate, either Indigo Powder (see impetigo in Chapter 7), or Jade Dew Powder (see sunburn in Chapter 12), mixed with vegetable oil to form a paste, is recommended. Apply once or twice daily until the lesions heal.

ACUPUNCTURE

Acupoints that may be needled in the treatment of contact dermatitis include LU-5 *(chi ze)*, LI-11 *(qu chi)*, LI-4 *(he gu)*, PC-3 *(qu ze)* and BL-40 *(wei zhong)*. Treat once daily with strong draining manipulation. BL-40 *(wei zhong)* may be bloodlet every other session. Five treatments constitute one course of therapy; symptoms are usually alleviated within one course.

EMPIRICAL REMEDIES[1]

[A] Decoct in water 150g of mango skin for about 15 minutes. Discard the dregs, and after suitable cooling wash the affected area with the liquid for 5-10 minutes, three times daily.

[B] Crush 250-500g of sour plum with the skin (remove the pit), and decoct in water for 10 minutes. Filter the dregs. After suitable cooling, wash the affected area with the liquid for 5-10 minutes, 3-5 times daily.

[C] Split open one coconut and drain the fluid. Break the hull into smaller pieces and decoct in water for 20-30 minutes. Remove the dregs, and after suitable cooling wash the affected area with the liquid for 5-10 minutes, 3-5 times daily.

An alternative remedy using coconut hull calls for five coconuts prepared as above and decocted in 3-4 liters of water until the liquid is concentrated into a gel. The dregs are removed and the gel transferred into a glass container. The gel is then applied to the affected area 2-3 times daily.

[D] Crush one unripe papaya (about 500g) and add 25ml of rice vinegar and 30g of table salt. Mix well, and squeeze the concoction through cheesecloth. Apply the resulting liquid to the affected area 2-3 times daily.

[E] Decoct 250g of fresh raspberries for 20 minutes. Remove the dregs, and after suitable cooling wash the affected area with the liquid for 5-10 minutes, 2-3 times daily.

❧ Myrrha and Lonicera Decoction[2]
没银煎液
mò yín jiān yè

Myrrha *(mo yao)* 50g
Flos Lonicerae Japonicae *(jin yin hua)* 50g

PREPARATION & DOSAGE: Decoct the ingredients in 1.0 liter of water until 500-700ml remains. Remove the dregs, pour the liquid into a glass container, and refrigerate. Apply as a wet compress to the affected area for 30 minutes, three times daily. For small areas, a cotton swab may be used. Healing should be apparent within five days.

Traditional vs. Biomedical Treatment

Traditional treatment is not necessarily more effective than biomedical treatment in accelerating healing. It is, however, a non-chemical approach, since biomedical treatment usually involves the use of corticosteroids which can lead to side effects and tolerance to the medication. The most effective treatment still remains removal of the cause of the skin eruption, after which recovery may occur spontaneously and rapidly without any sort of medical treatment.

Prevention

The best prevention is avoiding the offending agent(s). If this cannot be achieved, then protection against the cause(s) should be undertaken. This may include gloves, protective clothing, headgear and the like, particularly in the workplace, where the risk of exposure to industrial chemicals and other allergens is rather high. Even after exposure, simple measures such as hand and face washing, or showering, can be highly effective in preventing skin eruption.

During outbreaks, avoidance of foods that give rise to heat and dampness should be avoided. These include spicy or greasy foods, meats such as lamb, chicken, capon and duck, as well as alcohol.

Atopic Dermatitis
四弯风
sì wān fēng, "four bends wind"

Atopic dermatitis is a chronic, superficial inflammation of the skin that is characterized by itching. The Chinese name, "four bends wind," reflects the four skin sites that are commonly affected: the insides of the elbows and the backs of the knees (the antecubital and popliteal fossae).

Signs & Symptoms

The essential features include itching, a typical morphology and distribution of the lesions, and personal or family history of allergies. The condition usually begins in infancy and recurs at intervals into adulthood. In infants, lesions characteristically appear at first on the cheeks and scalp, eventually involving the entire face and the extensor surfaces of the elbows and knees. In severe cases the entire body may be involved. The lesions are red, and through scratching, begin to weep and become crusted. As the condition progresses, dryness of the skin, and lichenification due to rubbing, characterize the eczematous sites. Secondary bacterial and viral infections are common.

The cardinal symptom of the disease is the severe, intractable itching that may be aggravated by contact with wool or other scratchy materials, and by psychological or environmental stress. Changes in humidity and ambient temperature may also trigger itching.

Differential Diagnosis

Diagnosis of atopic dermatitis is primarily based on the distribution of lesions and its long duration. Patients should thus be followed carefully before a definitive diagnosis is made. In infants, seborrheic dermatitis and miliaria rubra (heat rash) may be confused with atopic dermatitis. In older children and adults, contact dermatitis is differentiated from atopic dermatitis by the history or by patch testing of the skin.

Traditional Chinese Etiology

Innate insufficiency causes dysfunction of the Spleen/Stomach's transportive and transformative mechanisms, resulting in a build-up of damp-heat. When the individual is exposed to wind, dampness and heat excesses in the summer, these all accumulate in the skin, thus leading to dermatitis. Protracted conditions can result in injury to the fluids, causing blood deficiency and wind-dryness, such that the skin loses its source of nourishment.

Treatment

In Chinese medicine, atopic dermatitis can be categorized into three major stages based on the pattern of each stage: fetal heat (dermatitis in infants which is thought to develop *in utero*); damp-heat (dermatitis mainly in older children); and blood dryness (dermatitis primarily in adults).

INTERNAL

Fetal heat. The treatment strategy is to clear Heart heat and guide out the red (heat as manifested in dark urine), and to protect the yin and stop the itching. In such cases, any one of three formulas is recommended: Five-Treasure Powder (0.3g administered three times daily—see syphilis in Chapter 10); Clear and Relieve Tablet (two tablets dissolved in warm water with a small amount of sugar, administered three times daily—see contact dermatitis in this chapter); and Modified Three-Pith Guide Out the Red Powder (see below).

❧ Modified Three-Pith Guide Out the Red Powder
三心导赤散加减
sān xīn dǎo chì sǎn jiā jiǎn

Semen Forsythiae Suspensae *(lian qiao xin)*	1g
Medulla Cinnamomi Cassiae *(gui zhi xin)*	1g
Plumula Nelumbinis Nuciferae *(lian zi xin)*	2g
Radix Scrophulariae Ningpoensis *(xuan shen)*	2g
Radix Rehmanniae Glutinosae *(sheng di huang)*	2g
Sclerotium Poriae Cocos Rubrae *(chi fu ling)*	2g
Sclerotium Poriae Cocos *(fu ling)*	2g
Radix Dioscoreae Oppositae *(shan yao)*	3g
Semen Plantaginis *(che qian zi)*	3g
Radix Adenophorae seu Glehniae *(sha shen)*	4g
Caulis Mutong *(mu tong)*	0.5g

PREPARATION & DOSAGE: Decoct and administer in three doses daily.

Damp-heat. The treatment strategy for this pattern is to clear heat and dispel dampness, and support the normal qi and stop the itching. For this pattern, the appropriate formula is Modified Eliminate Dampness Decoction by Combining Calm the Stomach and Five-Ingredient Powder with Poria.

❧ Modified Eliminate Dampness Decoction by Combining Calm the Stomach and Five Ingredient Powder with Poria
除湿胃苓汤加减
chú shī wèi líng tāng jiā jiǎn

Cortex Poriae Cocos *(fu ling pi)*	10g
dry-fried Cortex Phellodendri *(chao huang bai)*	10g
Pericarpium Citri Reticulatae *(chen pi)*	10g
Radix Sophorae Flavescentis *(ku shen)*	10g
Sclerotium Polypori Umbellati *(zhu ling)*	12g
Fructus Kochiae Scopariae *(di fu zi)*	12g
Cortex Dictamni Dasycarpi Radicis *(bai xian pi)*	12g
Radix Astragali Membranacei *(huang qi)*	12g

Semen Coicis Lachryma-jobi *(yi yi ren)* 15g
Semen Phaseoli Calcarati *(chi xiao dou)* 15g
Fructus Xanthii Sibirici *(cang er zi)* 6g
Periostracum Cicadae *(chan tui)* 6g

PREPARATION & DOSAGE: Decoct and administer in three doses daily.

Blood dryness. The treatment strategy for this pattern is to enrich the yin and eliminate dampness. Modified Enrich the Yin and Eliminate Dampness Decoction is recommended in such cases.

❧ Modified Enrich the Yin and Eliminate Dampness Decoction
滋阴除湿汤加减
zī yīn chú shī tāng jiā jiǎn

Radix Angelicae Sinensis *(dang gui)* 6g
Dry-fried Radix Paeoniae Lactiflorae *(chao bai shao)* 6g
Radix Bupleuri *(chai hu)* 6g
Radix Scutellariae Baicalensis *(huang qin)* 6g
Radix Rehmanniae Glutinosae Conquitae *(shu di huang)* 15g
Cortex Lycii Radicis *(di gu pi)* 15g
Herba Leonuri Heterophylli *(yi mu cao)* 15g
Dry-fried Rhizoma Anemarrhenae Asphodeloidis *(chao zhi mu)* 10g
Rhizome Alismatis Orientalis *(ze xie)* 10g
Radix Ledebouriellae Divaricatae *(fang feng)* 10g
Radix Polygoni Multiflori *(he shou wu)* 10g
Radix Glycyrrhizae Uralensis *(gan cao)* 10g

PREPARATION & DOSAGE: Decoct and administer in three doses daily.

MODIFICATIONS: For severe weeping of lesions, add 30g each of Radix Aristolochiae Fangchi *(fang ji)* and Epicarpium Benincasae Hispidae *(dong gua pi)*; for severe itching, add Fructus Xanthii Sibirici *(cang er zi)*, Radix et Rhizoma Notopterygii *(qiang huo)*, Zaocys Dhumnades *(wu shao she)* and Periostracum Cicadae *(chan tui)*; for accompanying asthma, add Fructus Schisandrae Chinensis *(wu wei zi)*, Flos Tussilagi Farfarae *(kuan dong hua)*, dry-fried Fructus Citri Aurantii *(chao zhi ke)* and Fructus Corni Officinalis *(shan zhu yu)*; for lichenification of the skin, increase the amount of Radix Angelicae Sinensis *(dang gui)* and add Radix et Caulis Jixueteng *(ji xue teng)*, Radix Salviae Miltiorrhizae *(dan shen)* and Halloysitum Rubrum *(chi shi zhi)*.

EXTERNAL

Infants. Administer any one of the following three formulas: Indigo Powder (see impetigo in Chapter 7) mixed with vegetable oil to form a paste, and applied twice daily; Dispel Dampness Powder; or Eczema Powder.

❧ Dispel Dampness Powder

祛湿散
qū shī sǎn

Rhizoma Coptidis *(huang lian)*	24g
Cortex Phellodendri *(huang bai)*	240g
Radix Scutellariae Baicalensis *(huang qin)*	144g
Semen Arecae Catechu *(bing lang)*	96g

PREPARATION & DOSAGE: Grind all the ingredients together into a fine powder. Mix with vegetable oil to form a paste, or sprinkle some of the powder directly on the affected area. Apply once or twice daily.

❦ Eczema Powder
湿疹散
shī zhěn sǎn

Radix Scutellariae Baicalensis *(huang qin)*	150g
Calcined Gypsum *(duan shi gao)*	150g
Calcitum *(han shui shi)*	250g
Galla Rhois Chinensis *(wu bei zi)*	125g

PREPARATION & DOSAGE: Grind all the ingredients together into a fine powder. Mix with vegetable oil to form a paste, or sprinkle some of the powder directly on the affected area. Apply once or twice daily.

CLINICAL NOTE: Infants should be carefully monitored when they are given these formulas, whether internal or external. If symptoms persist or worsen, discontinue the remedy. External remedies should not be applied to the face, since infants may accidentally rub them into the mouth, nose or eyes.

Older children. Older children may be given Black Ointment or Light-Yellow Powder.

❦ Black Ointment
黑油膏
hēi yóu gāo

Calcined Gypsum *(duan shi gao)*	30g
Alumen Praeparatum *(ku fan)*	30g
Calomelas *(qing fen)*	30g
Calcined Os Draconis *(duan long gu)*	30g
Galla Rhois Chinensis *(wu bei zi)*	60g
Calcitum *(han shui shi)*	60g
Conchae Pulvis Mactrae Quadrangularis *(ge li fen)*	6g
Borneol *(bing pian)*	6g
Menthol	45g

PREPARATION & DOSAGE: In a glass jar with an airtight lid, combine all of the ingredients together with petroleum jelly to form an ointment. Steep for two days before using. Apply a thin layer on the affected area 3-5 times daily.

❧ Light-Yellow Powder
鹅黄散
é huáng săn

Calcined Gypsum *(duan shi gao)*
Dry-fried Cortex Phellodendri *(chao huang bai)*
Calomelas *(qing fen)*

PREPARATION & DOSAGE: Grind equal amounts of the ingredients together into a fine powder. Mix with vegetable oil to form a paste, or sprinkle directly on the affected area. Apply 2-3 times daily.

Adults. For mild weeping of lesions, apply Succinum and Two-Aconite Paste, or Sanguisorba, Xanthium, and Atractylodes Paste.

❧ Succinum and Two-Aconite Paste
琥珀二乌糊膏
hŭ pò èr wū hú gāo

Galla Rhois Chinensis *(wu bei zi)*	45g
Succinum *(hu po)*	15g
Radix Aconiti Kusnezoffii Praeparata *(zhi cao wu)*	15g
Radix Aconiti Carmichaeli Praeparata *(zhi chuan wu)*	15g
Calcitum *(han shui shi)*	30g
Borneol *(bing pian)*	6g

PREPARATION & DOSAGE: Grind all the ingredients together into a fine powder and combine with petroleum jelly to form an ointment. Apply once or twice daily.

CLINICAL NOTE: Because of the toxicity of Radix Aconiti Kusnezoffii Praeparata *(zhi cao wu)* and Radix Aconiti Carmichaeli Praeparata *(zhi chuan wu)*, long-term use of this remedy is discouraged. If improvement of symptoms is not evident after five days, discontinue and consider other remedies.

❧ Sanguisorba, Xanthium, and Atractylodes Paste
地榆二苍糊膏
dì yú èr cāng hú gāo

Cortex Phellodendri *(huang bai)*	18g
Rhizoma Atractylodis *(cang zhu)*	18g
Fructus Xanthii Sibirici *(cang er zi)*	18g
Radix Sanguisorbae Officinalis *(di yu)*	36g
Borneol *(bing pian)*	1.5g
Calomelas *(qing fen)*	1.5g

Menthol..3g

PREPARATION & DOSAGE: Grind all of the ingredients together into a fine powder and combine with petroleum jelly to form an ointment. Store in an airtight glass jar. Apply 2-3 times daily.

For recurrent, severe itching without weeping, Cotton Cloth Rub is recommended.

❧ Cotton Cloth Rub
布绵擦剂
bù mián cā jì

Cortex Hibisci Syriaci Radicis *(jin pi)*	5g
Alumen Praeparatum *(ku fan)*	5g
Radix et Rhizoma Rhei *(da huang)*	5g
Realgar *(xiong huang)*	5g
Fructus Zanthoxyli Bungeani *(chuan jiao)*	5g
Radix Angelicae Dahuricae *(bai zhi)*	10g
Semen Arecae Catechu *(bing lang)*	7g
Radix Aconiti Kusnezoffii Praeparata *(zhi cao wu)*	8g
Camphora *(zhang nao)*	2g
Semen Hydnocarpi Anthelminticae *(da feng zi)*	15g
Herba Lophatheri Gracilis *(dan zhu ye)*	10g
Semen Pruni Armeniacae *(xing ren)*	6g
Rhizoma Picrorhizae *(hu huang lian)*	6g

PREPARATION & DOSAGE: Grind each ingredient into a fine powder, then mix together well. Add vegetable oil to make a paste and form into an egg-shaped mass weighing about 70g. Wrap the mass in a 15cm x 15cm piece of sterile gauze and tie the open ends with thread. Rub the affected area with the medicinal gauze three times daily. For areas that are lichenified, pressure may be applied while rubbing. If the medicinal ball dries, knead in a bit more vegetable oil. When not using, store the mass in an airtight glass container.

CLINICAL NOTE: Because of the toxicity of Realgar *(xiong huang)* and Radix Aconiti Kusnezoffii Praeparata *(zhi cao wu)*, this remedy should not be applied for more than five consecutive days. If longer use is required, the dosage may be reduced to 1-2 daily applications, or once every other day.

ACUPUNCTURE

The primary acupoints for this condition are GV-14 *(da zhui)*, LI-11 *(qu chi)*, SP-10 *(xue hai)*, ST-36 *(zu san li)*, SP-6 *(san yin jiao)* and HT-7 *(shen men)*. For severe itching, add HT-8 *(shao fu)*; for pronounced dampness, add SP-9 *(yin ling quan)*; for blood deficiency, add BL-17 *(ge shu)*. For best results, treat at least twice weekly for one month, then reduce frequency to once a week as needed. Other internal and/or external remedies may be used in conjunction with acupuncture treatment.

EMPIRICAL REMEDIES

❧ Asarum, Dahurica, Schizonepeta, Ledebouriella Powder[3]
辛芷荆防散
xīn zhǐ jīng fáng sǎn

Herba seu Flos Schizonepetae Tenuifoliae *(jing jie)*
Radix Ledebouriellae Divaricatae *(fang feng)*
Herba cum Radice Asari *(xi xin)*
Radix Angelicae Dahuricae *(bai zhi)*

PREPARATION & DOSAGE: Grind equal amounts of the herbs together into a fine powder, and store in an airtight glass jar. Prior to treating with the herbal powder, decoct 3g of Fructus Zanthoxyli Bungeani *(chuan jiao)* in water, and wash the affected area with the warm decoction for 5-10 minutes, then pat dry with a clean towel. Combine a portion of the herbal powder with rice vinegar to form a paste, and apply to the lesions. The entire procedure should be performed twice daily. Three days constitute one course of therapy, with 1-2 days' rest between courses. Most patients should experience improvement—if not healing—within three courses.

❧ Indigo, Alumen, and Zanthoxylum Powder[4]
青黛苦椒散
qīng dài kǔ jiāo sǎn

Indigo Pulverata Levis *(qing dai)*	30g
Alumen Praeparatum *(ku fan)*	30g
Fructus Zanthoxyli Bungeani *(chuan jiao)*	30g
Realgar *(xiong huang)*	6g
Calomelas *(qing fen)*	10g
Sulphur *(liu huang)*	20g
Rhizoma Coptidis *(huang lian)*	10g
Cortex Phellodendri *(huang bai)*	18g

PREPARATION & DOSAGE: Grind all the ingredients together into a fine powder and store in an airtight glass jar. Prior to application, wash the affected area with a dilute solution of saltwater, pat dry, and disinfect the skin with rubbing alcohol. Mix a portion of the herbal powder together with vegetable oil to form a paste. Apply to the lesions and cover with a sterile dressing.

If weeping from the lesions is severe, first prepare a decoction of 30g Fructus Zanthoxyli Bungeani *(chuan jiao)*, 10g Rhizoma Coptidis *(huang lian)* and 18g Cortex Phellodendri *(huang bai)* in 500ml of water. Wash the area with this warm decoction 2-3 times daily until the weeping stops (usually within two days). The herbal powder can then be applied according to the above procedure. Treat once daily until the lesions are healed, generally within 2-3 weeks.

CLINICAL NOTE: Because of the toxicity of some of the ingredients, this formula should not be taken orally.

❦ Mirabilitum Wash[5]
芒硝洗剂
mǎng xiāo xǐ jì

Mirabilitum *(mang xiao)* 150-300g

PREPARATION & DOSAGE: Dissolve the Mirabilitum *(mang xiao)* in cold tap water. Use a sterile gauze pad to apply the medicinal fluid as a cold compress on the affected sites for 30-60 minutes, 2-3 times a day. This formula is particularly suited for the acute beginning stage of dermatitis. Symptoms are usually relieved within 3-4 days, and healing occurs within one week.

Traditional vs. Biomedical Treatment

Traditional measures are probably more effective than biomedical treatment. As long as the correct pattern is differentiated and the appropriate treatment instituted, the root of the condition can be eliminated. Biomedical intervention is primarily aimed at relieving the itching through use of corticosteroids, antihistamines, tar preparations and other topical medications. However, once these are discontinued, the condition often recurs.

Prevention

Sufferers of atopic dermatitis should avoid as many triggering factors as possible. This includes reducing psychological and environmental stressors, as well as physical irritants. Since secondary infections of lesions are common, measures such as keeping fingernails short (to minimize excoriations), and avoiding individuals who have infectious diseases such as herpes simplex, should be observed.

Because itching is the primary symptom, treatment should be aimed first at relieving the itching to break the itch-scratch-itch cycle, and only then at strategies to address the root cause.

Foods that produce dampness and heat, such as spicy or greasy foods, and meats such as lamb, chicken, capon, duck and shrimp, should be minimized or avoided. Nutritional supplements such as vitamins also tend to be warming in nature, and should be discontinued or taken in moderation during treatment.

Lichen Simplex Chronicus
牛皮癬
niú pí xuǎn, "cow skin tinea"

Lichen simplex chronicus is also known biomedically as localized neurodermatitis. It is a chronic condition characterized by lichenified, itchy scaling, and frequently by slightly purple patches. The Chinese term "cow skin tinea" was described in the Ming dynasty text *True Lineage of External Medicine* (1617) as "resembling the skin on a cow's neck, dense and hard, [which upon] scratching resembles decayed wood." Another Chinese name for this condition is "nape-collar sore" *(niè lǐng chuāng),* since one of the common lesion sites is the back of the neck.

Biomedically, lichen simplex chronicus appears to be psychological in origin. Many affected patients have obsessive personalities and focus, either consciously or subconsciously, most of their attention on scratching the patches, especially when agitated or in stressful situations. Women are more affected than men.

Signs & Symptoms

Some patients are already prone to spontaneous itching, while in others, the condition begins with a small event such as a pimple, cut, or scratch that does not heal normally because it itches and is thus scratched persistently. Nervousness perpetuates the itching, as do other environmental factors, such as heat or cold. As the condition progresses, rubbing replaces scratching as the process by which the itch is relieved, perhaps a means by which the person tries to reduce the trauma of scratching.

The patch or patches of skin are marked by thickening, discoloration, and scaling. Lesions may be single or multiple, but they are always within reach of the fingers. Common sites include the palms and soles, the insides of the wrists and ankles, the anogenital region, the nape of the neck, the extensor surfaces of the elbows, and the outer ear canal.

Differential Diagnosis

The patches of lichen simplex chronicus are usually distinct enough that diagnosis can be made through questioning the patient and by examining the lesions. Conditions that should be differentiated from lichen simplex chronicus include lichenified patches of psoriasis and lichen planus. Psoriasis will present with heaped-up lesions with large silvery scales; the removal of the superficial scale will typically show tiny bleeding points, known as Auspitz's sign. Lichen planus lesions tend to be distributed symmetrically and are much less thick than those of lichen simplex chronicus.

Asians and Native Americans have a predisposition to lichen simplex chronicus.

Traditional Chinese Etiology

The onset of lichen simplex chronicus may be caused by external excesses such as wind, heat, dampness or insect-bite toxin that accumulate in the skin. If left untreated, the excess transforms into heat and produces wind-dryness. Wind-dryness in turn injures yin and blood, which become deficient and lose their moistening and nourishing properties, thus resulting in dryness and itching of the skin.

Deficiency of blood can also lead to exuberant Liver fire and an easily aroused emotional state. Liver fire produces wind-dryness, which results in itching of the skin. Therefore, if the individual's emotions are repeatedly stressed, Liver fire and wind-dryness will continue unabated, as will the skin itch.

Treatment

In Chinese medicine, two typical patterns characterize lichen simplex chronicus: wind-heat-dampness, and blood deficiency and wind-dryness.

INTERNAL

Wind-heat-dampness. Lesions of this pattern are dense with papules and are moist and red, or are eroded or have crusts. The tongue has a thin yellow or yellow greasy tongue coating, and the pulse is soggy and rapid. The treatment strategy is to scatter wind and clear heat, and transform dampness and stop the itching. The formula recommended for this pattern is Modified Eliminate Wind Powder [A].

❧ Modified Eliminate Wind Powder [A]
消风散加减
xiāo fēng sǎn jiā jiǎn

Herba seu Flos Schizonepetae Tenuifoliae *(jing jie)*	6g
Radix Ledebouriellae Divaricatae *(fang feng)*	6g
Radix Sophorae Flavescentis *(ku shen)*	6g
Dry-fried Fructus Arctii Lappae *(chao niu bang zi)*	10g
Radix Rehmanniae Glutinosae *(sheng di huang)*	10g
Dry-fried Cortex Moutan Radicis *(chao mu dan pi)*	10g
Gypsum *(shi gao)*	12g
Cortex Poriae Cocos *(fu ling pi)*	12g
Fructus Kochiae Scopariae *(di fu zi)*	12g
Cortex Dictamni Dasycarpi Radicis *(bai xian pi)*	12g

PREPARATION & DOSAGE: Decoct and administer in three doses daily.

Blood deficiency and wind-dryness. This pattern produces lesions that are thick (lichenified) and dry, with some scaling; itching is severe, especially at night. Persons with this pattern show a red tongue with a thin coating, and a soggy, thin pulse. The treatment strategy is to nourish blood and moisten the skin, and extinguish wind and stop the itching.

Formulas recommended for this pattern include Modified Moisten the Skin Decoction with the Four Substances, or Anchor the Yang and Extinguish the Wind Decoction.

❦ Modified Moisten the Skin Decoction with the Four Substances
四物润肤汤加减
sì wù rùn fū tāng jiā jiǎn

Radix Angelicae Sinensis *(dang gui)*	10g
Semen Sesami Indici *(hei zhi ma)*	10g
Radix Gentianae Qinjiao *(qin jiao)*	10g
Dry-fried Radix Paeoniae Lactiflorae *(chao bai shao)*	12g
Radix Rehmanniae Glutinosae *(sheng di huang)*	12g
Radix Polygoni Multiflori *(he shou wu)*	12g
Ramulus cum Uncis Uncariae *(gou teng)*	12g
Concha Margaritaferae *(zhen zhu mu)*	15g
Radix Adenophorae seu Glehniae *(sha shen)*	15g
Fructus Zizyphi Jujubae *(da zao)*	6g
Radix Dioscoreae Oppositae *(shan yao)*	30g

PREPARATION & DOSAGE: Decoct and administer in three doses daily.

❦ Anchor Yang and Extinguish Wind Decoction
潜阳熄风汤
qián yáng xī fēng tāng

Radix Rehmanniae Glutinosae *(sheng di huang)*	15g
Radix Rehmanniae Glutinosae Conquitae *(shu di huang)*	15g
Radix Angelicae Sinensis *(dang gui)*	9g
Radix Polygoni Multiflori *(he shou wu)*	9g
Concha Zibei *(zi bei)*	30g
Magnetitum *(ci shi)*	15g
Os Draconis *(long gu)*	15g
Concha Ostreae *(mu li)*	15g
Haematitum *(dai zhe shi)*	15g
Concha Margaritaferae *(zhen zhu mu)*	30g
Radix Paeoniae Lactiflorae *(bai shao)*	9g

PREPARATION & DOSAGE: Decoct and administer one-half in the morning and the remainder at night.

CLINICAL NOTE: Because of the toxicity of Haematitum *(dai zhe shi)*, long-term use of this formula is discouraged. Suggested administration is one dose per day for five consecutive days, followed by three days' rest before resuming the formula at a reduced dosage of one dose every other day. Alternatively, Haematitum *(dai zhe shi)* may be eliminated from the formula, which may then continue to be administered at one dose daily.

EXTERNAL

Wind-heat-dampness. External remedies recommended for this pattern are Black Ointment (see atopic dermatitis in this chapter), Three-Yellow Wash (see furuncles in Chapter 7), or Mylabris Tincture.

❧ Mylabris Tincture
斑蝥酊
bān máo dīng

Mylabris *(ban mao)*	10
75% Alcohol	200ml
75% Dimethyl Sulfoxide (DMSO)	20ml

PREPARATION & DOSAGE: First, soak the Mylabris *(ban mao)* in the DMSO for 24 hours in a glass jar with a lid. Then add the alcohol and steep for 3-5 days in warm weather, or 7-10 days in cooler temperatures. Decant the liquid into a sterile amber glass jar with a lid. Discard the dregs. Use a sterile cotton swab to apply the tincture to a small area of affected skin. Wait 24 hours. If there are no untoward effects, such as flaring of symptoms, then apply to other affected sites once or twice daily.

CLINICAL NOTE: Because of the toxicity of Mylabris *(ban mao)*, long-term use of this remedy is discouraged. Suggested administration is daily application for 5-7 days, followed by 2-3 days' rest before resuming application. If blistering occurs, discontinue use until the skin is healed. Do not apply to broken or eroded skin.

Blood deficiency and wind-dryness. For this pattern, Cotton Cloth Rub (see atopic dermatitis in this chapter) or Nervous Wind Ointment is recommended.

❧ Nervous Wind Ointment
疯油膏
fēng yóu gāo

Calomelas *(qing fen)*	4.5g
Mimium *(qian dan)*	3g
Cinnabaris *(zhu sha)* (refined with water)	2-3g
Sesame Oil	120g
Yellow Beeswax	30g

PREPARATION & DOSAGE: Grind the Calomelas *(qing fen)* and Mimium *(qian dan)* into fine powders. (Cinnabaris *(zhu sha)* is already in powder form.) Heat the sesame oil in a non-metallic saucepan until just boiling, and then add the beeswax. Continue boiling until the yellow froth disappears. Remove the saucepan from the heat and immediately transfer into a pre-heated amber glass jar with a lid. Slowly stir in the medicinal powders until well mixed. Allow to congeal.

Apply the ointment to the affected area. Then use a hand-held hair dryer to heat the area (use low or medium setting, taking care not to overheat the skin) for 10-20 minutes. The ointment may then be wiped off with a sterile cotton ball. Application is once daily; four weeks constitutes one course of therapy. Generally, after the first week the itching will be alleviated; after the second, lichenification will show regression; at the end of the third, normal skin will show through; and after the fourth week, lesions should have all but disappeared.

CLINICAL NOTE: Because of the toxicity of Cinnabaris *(zhu sha)*, long-term use of this remedy is discouraged. Recalcitrant lesions should be treated subsequently with another external formula such as Cotton Cloth Rub (see atopic dermatitis in this chapter), or an internal formula such as Modified Moisten the Skin Decoction with the Four Substances (see above).

ACUPUNCTURE

Filiform needling. The primary acupoints for this disorder include LI-11 *(qu chi)*, LI-4 *(he gu)*, SP-10 *(xue hai)*, SP-6 *(san yin jiao)* and GV-14 *(da zhui)*. Best results are obtained if treatment is performed once every other day, with draining manipulation.

Cutaneous needling. Plum blossom needling is applied by directly tapping lichenified lesions, or by tapping the surrounding skin of early stage lesions. Treatment is once every other day for 10-15 minutes, or until the area is flushed or begins to exude tiny drops of blood from the skin.

MOXIBUSTION

Moxa roll moxibustion may be applied to affected sites once daily for 15-20 minutes.

EMPIRICAL REMEDIES

[A] Crack open a fresh coconut and remove a piece of the flesh. Rub affected sites with the coconut flesh 3-5 times daily.[6]

[B] Wrap shavings from the green outer hull of an unripe walnut in gauze. Apply pressure while rubbing affected sites 2-3 times daily. Or sun-dry the shavings and then decoct in water, and apply the decoction as a wash.[7]

[C] Use a cotton swab to apply rice vinegar to lesions 3-4 times daily.[8]

❧ Eliminate Wind and Transform Stasis Decoction[9]
消风化瘀汤
xiāo fēng huà yū tāng

Herba seu Flos Schizonepetae Tenuifoliae *(jing jie)*	10g
Radix Ledebouriellae Divaricatae *(fang feng)*	10g
Rhizoma Sparganii Stoloniferi *(san leng)*	10g
Rhizoma Curcumae Ezhu *(e zhu)*	10g
Radix Glycyrrhizae Uralensis *(gan cao)*	10g
Periostracum Cicadae *(chan tui)*	5g

Nidus Vespae *(lu feng fang)*	3g
Radix Rehmanniae Glutinosae *(sheng di huang)*	15g
Rhizoma Paris Polyphyllae *(zao xiu)*	15g
Radix Arnebiae seu Lithospermi *(zi cao)*	20g

PREPARATION & DOSAGE: Decoct and administer one-half in the morning and the remainder in the evening. Save the dregs and decoct again, then use the fluid in a warm compress applied to the affected area for 10-15 minutes, once daily. After two weeks, the internal and external dosages may be reduced to once every other day.

MODIFICATIONS: For severe lichenification of the skin, add Semen Persicae *(tao ren)* and Semen Vaccariae Segetalis *(wang bu liu xing)*; for severe itching, add Zaocys Dhumnades *(wu shao she)*; for scaling of the skin, add Radix Angelicae Sinensis *(dang gui)*; for erosion and weeping of lesions, add Fructus Kochiae Scopariae *(di fu zi)*; for restless sleep, add Caulis Polygoni Multiflori *(ye jiao teng)*; for individuals prone to anger, add Fructus Schisandrae Chinensis *(wu wei zi)* and Radix Paeoniae Lactiflorae *(bai shao)*. For each of the preceding modifications, the amount is 10g.

Most patients experience improvement after two months. Since this formula treats recalcitrant conditions, patient compliance with the regimen is necessary to effect healing.

❦ Table Vinegar Paste[10]

食醋糊剂

shí cù hú jì

Rice Vinegar (preferably Shanxi Fermented brand)	1 liter
Radix Sophorae Flavescentis *(ku shen)*	20g
Fructus Zanthoxyli Bungeani *(chuan jiao)*	15g

PREPARATION & DOSAGE: In a cast iron sauce pan, boil the vinegar down to 100ml (the liquid will be thick and paste-like), and transfer to a wide-mouthed glass jar. Wash the Radix Sophorae Flavescentis *(ku shen)* and Fructus Zanthoxyli Bungeani *(chuan jiao)* and then add to the vinegar. Steep for at least one week (the longer the better). Before treating, wash the affected skin sites with warm water. Apply the remedy with a sterile cotton swab once in the morning and once at night. Improvement of symptoms is usually experienced after 4-5 days, and healing within two weeks.

ACUPUNCTURE[11]

Insert four or five 32-34 gauge filiform needles into the healthy skin surrounding the lesion. Needles should be inserted radially toward the center of the lesion. Then, with a dermal needle, tap the lesion itself a few times. Remove the filiform needles and immediately apply cupping on top of the lesion. Retain the cups for 30 minutes.

In addition to the needling technique described above, the following points should be needled during the same session, using draining manipulation: PC-6 *(nei guan)*, LI-4 *(he gu)*, SP-6 *(san yin jiao)* and ST-36 *(zu san li)*. Treat once every other day, with ten treatments constituting one course of therapy. If itching and lichenification improve, then dermal needling and cupping may be discontinued.

Most patients experience healing within three courses of treatment.

Traditional vs. Biomedical Treatment

Treatment in general is difficult because the scratching has often become a habit that is not easily broken. Thus, therapy should not only involve measures to relieve the itching, but also psychological counseling when necessary (see Prevention below). Since biomedical treatment for relieving the itching involves the use of topical corticosteroids or coal-tar preparations, patients may appreciate the non-pharmaceutical traditional approach.

Prevention

Lichen simplex chronicus tends to persist indefinitely, and controlling it requires a multi-pronged approach. Since lichen simplex chronicus is thought biomedically to be perpetuated by psychological factors after its onset, practitioners should attempt to converse with the patient about work and other aspects of life in general. Such conversation is often in itself a form of therapy. Vigorous exercise may be helpful to expend excess physical energy that may otherwise be directed toward rubbing. Eliminating a cause of nervous stress may produce positive results as well.

Patients should also be informed of the problems associated with secondary infections that can be caused by self-inoculation of bacteria through rubbing.

Seborrheic Dermatitis
面游风
miàn yóu fēng, "face traveling wind"

Seborrheic dermatitis is marked by an itchy, red, scaly rash that affects the face and scalp, and other areas. It is described in *Golden Mirror of the Medical Tradition* (1742):

> This condition arises on the face, and is produced by dryness, heat and dampness. [When it] first begins, the eyes and face swell, and the itching resembles moving insects; sometimes white scales are produced.

Biomedically, seborrheic dermatitis is thought to be genetically determined. Despite the name and the fact that the disorder occurs in seborrheic areas, sebaceous glands have no clear role in causation.

Signs & Symptoms

Despite its name, the sebaceous glands are not involved with the cause of this type of dermatitis. However, it is true that the condition is commonly distributed in seborrheic areas and is associated with increased greasiness of the skin. Adults develop this condition slowly; sometimes the only sign is diffuse greasy or dry dandruff of the scalp accompanied by some itching. Lesions at other sites are frequently marked by a yellow or orange hue. Itching is not a prominent symptom, although secondary bacterial or candidal infections can occur and must be treated promptly. Patients with AIDS and Parkinson's syndrome seem more likely to be affected.

Infants in the first month of life may develop seborrheic dermatitis, characterized by thick, yellow scales, a condition commonly known as "cradle cap."

Differential Diagnosis

The characteristic pattern of distribution of seborrheic dermatitis—predominantly on the scalp and face—usually determines the diagnosis. Psoriasis may be confused with seborrheic dermatitis. However, psoriasis is confirmed by removing the scales from lesions in order to produce the pinpoint bleeding sites known as Auspitz's sign. Some patients appear to have both diseases—at one time the classic lesions of psoriasis, and at another those of seborrheic dermatitis. Thus, treatment of these patients is particularly difficult, and requires careful pattern differentiation.

Traditional Chinese Etiology

Two pattern types characterize this disease: wind-heat/blood dryness, and damp-heat of the Intestines and Stomach.

Wind-heat/blood dryness is caused by the invasion of wind-heat that becomes longstanding and gives rise to blood dryness. Blood dryness causes insufficiency of blood and produces wind. Wind, dryness and heat accumulate in the skin, which then loses its source of nourishment and becomes dry and rough. This is considered the dry type of face-traveling wind.

Damp-heat of the Intestines and Stomach is due to a dietary excess of meat, greasy and/or spicy foods, or alcohol. The transportive and transformative functions of the Stomach and Intestines are injured, giving rise to dampness and heat. Longstanding damp-heat accumulates in the skin and causes the damp type of face-traveling wind.

Treatment

INTERNAL

Wind-heat/blood dryness seborrheic dermatitis is characterized by lesions that have a slightly erythematous base, and scales that are dry and powdery that may become quite thick on the scalp. The treatment strategy is to enrich yin, clear heat, and transform dampness.

Formulas recommended for this pattern include Nourish the Blood and Moisten the Skin Decoction, or Cool the Blood and Eliminate Wind Powder.

🌸 Nourish the Blood and Moisten the Skin Decoction
养血润肤饮
yǎng xuè rùn fū yǐn

Radix Angelicae Sinensis *(dang gui)*	9g
Radix Rehmanniae Glutinosae Conquitae *(shu di huang)*	12g
Radix Rehmanniae Glutinosae *(sheng di huang)*	12g
Radix Astragali Membranacei *(huang qi)*	12g
Tuber Asparagi Cochinchinensis *(tian men dong)* (pith removed)	6g
Tuber Ophiopogonis Japonici *(mai men dong)*	6g
Rhizoma Cimicifugae *(sheng ma)*	3g
Radix Scutellariae Baicalensis *(huang qin)*	3g
Semen Persicae *(tao ren)*	2g
Flos Carthami Tinctorii *(hong hua)*	2g
Radix Trichosanthis Kirilowii *(tian hua fen)*	4.5g

PREPARATION & DOSAGE: Decoct and administer while warm in one dose daily.

MODIFICATIONS: For dry stools, add 9-15g each of Semen Cannabis Sativae *(huo ma ren)* and Semen Pruni *(yu li ren)*; for patterns that are wind-dominant and present with severe itching, add 4.5g of Rhizoma Gastrodiae Elatae *(tian ma)*.

🌸 Cool the Blood and Eliminate Wind Powder
凉血消风散
liáng xuè xiāo fēng sǎn

Radix Rehmanniae Glutinosae *(sheng di huang)*	30g
Radix Angelicae Sinensis *(dang gui)*	9g
Herba seu Flos Schizonepetae Tenuifoliae *(jing jie)*	9g
Periostracum Cicadae *(chan tui)*	6g
Radix Sophorae Flavescentis *(ku shen)*	9g
Fructus Tribuli Terrestris *(bai ji li)*	9g
Rhizoma Anemarrhenae Asphodeloidis *(zhi mu)*	9g
Gypsum *(shi gao)*	30g
Radix Glycyrrhizae Uralensis *(gan cao)*	6g

PREPARATION & DOSAGE: Decoct and administer in one dose daily.

Damp-heat seborrheic dermatitis is characterized by lesions that are red, eroded and weeping. The scales and crusts are greasy, and often the lesions exude an unpleasant odor. Skin fissures may be present around and on lesions that affect the nasolabial folds and behind the ears.

Formulas recommended for this pattern include Astragalus and Atractylodes Decoction, or Chrysanthemum and Arctium Decoction.

Astragalus and Atractylodes Decoction
芪白汤
qí bái táng

Radix Astragali Membranacei *(huang qi)*	20g
Rhizoma Atractylodis Macrocephalae *(bai zhu)*	15g
Radix Ledebouriellae Divaricatae *(fang feng)*	15g
Radix Scutellariae Baicalensis *(huang qin)*	10g
Bombyx Batryticatus *(jiang can)*	10g
Periostracum Cicadae *(chan tui)*	10g
Concha Ostreae *(mu li)*	30g
Folium Daqingye *(da qing ye)*	30g
Radix Glycyrrhizae Uralensis *(gan cao)*	3g

PREPARATION & DOSAGE: Decoct and administer in one dose daily.

Chrysanthemum and Arctium Decoction
野菊牛子汤
yě jú niú zǐ tāng

Flos Chrysanthemi Indici *(ye ju hua)*	15g
Radix Rehmanniae Glutinosae *(sheng di huang)*	15g
Halloysitum Rubrum *(chi shi zhi)*	15g
Fructus Arctii Lappae *(niu bang zi)*	10g
Cortex Moutan Radicis *(mu dan pi)*	10g
Herba seu Flos Schizonepetae Tenuifoliae *(jing jie)*	9g
Radix Ledebouriellae Divaricatae *(fang feng)*	9g
Semen Coicis Lachryma-jobi *(yi yi ren)*	30g
Alumen *(ming fan)*	12g
Radix Glycyrrhizae Uralensis *(gan cao)*	6g

PREPARATION & DOSAGE: Decoct and administer in one dose daily.

MODIFICATIONS: For thirst, sensation of heat and lesions that consist of red papules with little exudate, add 15g Flos Lonicerae Japonicae *(jin yin hua)*, 10g Fructus Forsythiae Suspensae *(lian qiao)* and 15g Fructus Sophorae Japonicae Immaturus *(huai hua mi)*; for signs of severe dampness causing erosion of the lesions, add 9g Radix Sophorae Flavescentis *(ku shen)*, 12g Sclerotium Poriae Cocos *(fu ling)* and 20g Talcum *(hua shi)*; for intense itching, add 6g Periostracum Cicadae *(chan tui)*, 9g Bombyx Batryticatus *(jiang can)* and 15g Cortex Dictamni Dasycarpi Radicis *(bai xian pi)*; for lesions primarily affecting the head, add 6g Radix et Rhizoma Notopterygii *(qiang huo)*, 12g Fructus Viticis *(man jing zi)* and 6g Herba Menthae Haplocalycis *(bo he)*; for greasy scales, add 12g Rhizoma Atractylodis Macrocephalae *(bai zhu)* and 15g Fructus Crataegi *(shan zha)*; for dry stools, add 6g Radix et Rhizoma Rhei *(da huang)*.

EXTERNAL

For seborrheic dermatitis affecting the scalp, either Seborrhea Wash or Psoriasis Tincture is recommended.

❦ Seborrhea Wash
脂溢洗方
zhī yì xǐ fāng

Fructus Xanthii Sibirici *(cang er zi)*	30g
Semen Vaccariae Segetalis *(wang bu liu xing)*	30g
Radix Sophorae Flavescentis *(ku shen)*	15g
Alumen *(ming fan)*	9g

PREPARATION & DOSAGE: Decoct and remove the dregs and use a washcloth to repeatedly bathe the scalp with the warm decoction for 15 minutes. Apply twice a day every three days. For best results, first cut the hair short before using this remedy.

❦ Psoriasis Tincture
白屑风酊
bái xiè fēng dīng

Fructus Cnidii Monnieri *(she chuang zi)*	40g
Radix Sophorae Flavescentis *(ku shen)*	40g
Cortex Pseudolaricis Kaempferi Radicis *(tu jing pi)*	20g
Menthol	10g
75% Alcohol	1 liter

PREPARATION & DOSAGE: Grind together the Fructus Cnidii Monnieri *(she chuang zi)*, Radix Sophorae Flavescentis *(ku shen)* and Cortex Pseudolaricis Kaempferi Radicis *(tu jing pi)* into a fine powder. Put the powder in a large, amber glass jar that has an airtight lid. Pour 80ml of the alcohol over the powder, cover the lid, and steep for six hours. Add the remaining 920ml of alcohol slowly, permitting the liquid to settle into the herbal powder. Do not stir. As the final step, add the menthol.

Apply the tincture with a cotton swab, 3-5 times daily. Do not apply on lesions that are eroded and weeping.

For the dry-type of seborrheic dermatitis, either Rub the Wind Ointment, Moisten the Skin Ointment, or Rheum and Borneol Formula (see damp-type seborrhea below) is recommended.

❦ Rub the Wind Ointment
摩风膏
mó fēng gāo

Herba Ephedrae *(ma huang)*	15g
Radix et Rhizoma Notopterygii *(qiang huo)*	30g
Lignum Santali Albi *(tan xiang)*	3g
Rhizoma Cimicifugae *(sheng ma)*	6g
Radix Ledebouriellae Divaricatae *(fang feng)*	6g
Rhizoma Bletillae Striatae *(bai ji)*	3g
Radix Angelicae Sinensis *(dang gui)*	3g
Sesame Oil	150g
Yellow Beeswax	15g

PREPARATION & DOSAGE: Grind the ingredients together into a fine powder and put into an amber glass jar with an airtight lid. Pour in the sesame oil and steep for five days. Then transfer the concoction into a non-metallic saucepan and heat until the herbal ingredients turn brown. Remove the dregs and add the beeswax, which should be dissolved completely (reheat if necessary). Pour into the previously used amber glass jar and allow the herbal remedy to congeal. Apply 2-3 times daily by rubbing gently into the lesions.

❧ Moisten the Flesh Ointment
润肌膏
rùn jī gāo

Radix Angelicae Sinensis *(dang gui)*	15g
Radix Arnebiae seu Lithospermi *(zi cao)*	3g
Sesame Oil	120ml
Yellow Beeswax	15g

PREPARATION & DOSAGE: Heat the Radix Angelicae Sinensis *(dang gui)*, Radix Arnebiae seu Lithospermi *(zi cao)* and sesame oil in a non-metallic saucepan until the herbs turn brown. Filter the dregs, then add the beeswax to the herbal oil and reheat until the wax is dissolved. Pour into an amber glass jar with an airtight lid, and allow to congeal. Apply the ointment 2-3 times daily.

For damp-type seborrheic dermatitis, either Indigo Ointment (see tinea in Chapter 9), Rheum and Borneol Formula, or Pig Bile Wash is recommended.

❧ Rheum and Borneol Formula
大黄冰片方
dà huáng bīng piàn fāng

Radix et Rhizoma Rhei *(da huang)*	100g
Borneol *(bing pian)*	20g
Table Vinegar	250g

PREPARATION & DOSAGE: First grind the Radix et Rhizoma Rhei *(da huang)* into a coarse powder. Put all the ingredients into an airtight glass jar and allow to steep for seven days. When the fluid turns dark brown, it is ready to be used. Apply to affected sites with a sterile cotton swab three times daily.

CLINICAL NOTE: After application the skin may experience a tingling sensation, which dissipates after a few minutes.

❧ Pig Bile Wash
猪胆汁外洗方
zhū dǎn zhī wài xǐ fāng

Vesica Fellea Suis *(zhu dan)* 1

PREPARATION & DOSAGE: Cut open the pig gallbladder and empty the bile into a small basin half-filled with warm water. (Pig gallbladders may be available through a butcher.) Stir thoroughly. Use a sterile cotton ball or clean washcloth to repeatedly wash affected sites until the greasy scales have been removed. Then wash the area with clean, warm water (do not use soap). Pat dry. Administer once daily, i.e, use a fresh gallbladder each day. Most patients should experience alleviation of symptoms (itching and scaling) within ten treatments.

EAR ACUPUNCTURE

Points that should be needled include Liver, Endocrine, Spleen, Occiput, Adrenal and Kidney. Treat once daily, selecting 2-3 of these points for each session, and retaining the needles for 30 minutes.

Traditional vs. Biomedical Treatment

Traditional treatment is more effective than biomedical measures in eliminating the root cause. Biomedical methods usually consist of topical applications (e.g., corticosteroids or ketoconazole, among others) to control the condition, but once these are discontinued the problem usually recurs.

Prevention

According to Chinese medicine, diet plays an important role in controlling seborrheic dermatitis. Foods that produce dampness and heat, such as spicy and greasy foods, sweets, and meats such as lamb, chicken, capon, duck and shrimp, should be avoided during the course of treatment. Caffeinated beverages should also be discontinued. Even after the condition is controlled, these foods should either be avoided or eaten only rarely and in small amounts.

Mild soaps and shampoos should be used, and women whose faces are affected should avoid wearing makeup during the course of treatment.

Diaper Dermatitis
溻尻疮
yān kāo chuāng, "neglected tailbone sores"

Diaper dermatitis, or diaper rash, is a skin inflammation of the diaper area in infants and young children. It was described in *Discussion of Origins of Symptoms of Diseases* (610) and other early Chinese medical texts. A passage in *Profound Insights on External Diseases* (1604) includes the following observation:

> A suckling child within the month of confinement [has] the hands and feet swaddled and [suffers] damp-heat in the crotch. This often becomes neglected and erodes into sores.

Biomedically, the most frequent causes of diaper dermatitis are prolonged contact of diaper-area skin with urine or feces (which contain irritating chemicals such as urea and intestinal enzymes), and improper cleansing of this area.

Signs & Symptoms
Initially the skin becomes reddened; over time it becomes dry and scaly. Chronic, severe dermatitis will exhibit papules, blisters and erosions.

Differential Diagnosis
Diaper dermatitis should be differentiated from seborrheic dermatitis and atopic dermatitis, which may involve the diaper area. However, the two latter types of dermatites will usually present with similar lesions on other parts of the body. Severe diaper dermatitis may be confused with infections, such as those caused biomedically by *Candida albicans* (although in many cases of diaper dermatitis lasting over four days, the affected area does become colonized with *C. albicans*), *Staphylococcus aureus,* and even the *condylomata lata* of syphilis. Diagnosis should be confirmed by laboratory culture of skin scrapings.

Traditional Chinese Etiology
Diaper dermatitis is a damp-heat pattern that arises when urine or stools "soak" the skin, resulting in accumulation of dampness, which then transforms into heat, thus producing redness of the skin. When the condition persists, the skin develops erosion and sores.

Treatment
The treatment strategy for diaper dermatitis is to clear heat, relieve toxin, and drain dampness. Generally, external therapy is sufficient to treat diaper dermatitis, although severe cases that show erosion and/or weeping sores should also be treated with internal remedies.

INTERNAL
A formula recommended for both internal and external application is Pueraria, Scutellaria, and Coptis Decoction.

❧ Pueraria, Scutellaria, and Coptis Decoction
葛根芩连汤
gé gēn qín lián tāng

Radix Puerariae *(ge gen)*	5g
Radix Scutellariae Baicalensis *(huang qin)*	3g
Rhizoma Coptidis *(huang lian)*	2g
Radix Glycyrrhizae Uralensis *(gan cao)*	3g

PREPARATION & DOSAGE: Decoct and administer in four doses daily. Best results are obtained when this formula is also applied externally as a wash, three times daily after diaper changes.

EXTERNAL

Several formulas can be used for the topical treatment of diaper dermatitis. However, regardless of the choice of formula, it is important that it be used exclusively for several days so that its therapeutic effect can take hold (unless, of course, there is an immediate allergic reaction). External remedies should be applied only after thoroughly cleaning the area during diaper changes.

❧ Millet Soup
小米清汤
xiǎo mǐ qīng tāng

Semen Sentaniae Italicae *(qing liang mi)*	50g

PREPARATION & DOSAGE: Cook the millet in 1 liter of water over low heat until a gruel is produced. Draw off the top layer of soup and set aside until lukewarm. Using a sterile gauze pad or cotton ball, wash the affected area with the soup 3-4 times daily. Pat dry and then apply one of the herbal powders listed below.

For severe diaper dermatitis with reddened skin, erosion and weeping, Atractylodes, Phellodendron, and Achyranthes Formula is recommended.

❧ Atractylodes, Phellodendron, and Achyranthes Formula
苍柏牛膝方
cāng bó niú xī fāng

Rhizoma Atractylodis *(cang zhu)*	10g
Cortex Phellodendri *(huang bai)*	10g
Radix Achyranthis Bidentatae *(niu xi)*	10g
Herba Artemisiae Yinchenhao *(yin chen hao)*	10g
Rhizoma Anemarrhenae Asphodeloidis *(zhi mu)*	10g
Cortex Dictamni Dasycarpi Radicis *(bai xian pi)*	10g
Alumen *(ming fan)*	10g
Radix Sophorae Flavescentis *(ku shen)*	30g
Rhizoma Smilacis Glabrae *(tu fu ling)*	20g
Fructus Kochiae Scopariae *(di fu zi)*	20g
Flos Lonicerae Japonicae *(jin yin hua)*	20g

PREPARATION & DOSAGE: Decoct in water until about 200ml of fluid remain. Remove the dregs and use a sterile cotton ball or soft gauze to wash the affected area. Administer one dose daily, up to ten times, five minutes per session. Symptoms are usually alleviated after one week or so.

For reddened skin and pain, either Coptis Ointment (see herpes zoster in Chapter 8), Clearing and Cooling Ointment (see impetigo in Chapter 7), or Arnebia and Coptis Ointment may be applied after diaper changes.

❦ Arnebia and Coptis Ointment
紫连膏
zǐ lián gāo

Radix Arnebiae seu Lithospermi *(zi cao)*	30g
Rhizoma Coptidis *(huang lian)* (powdered)	15g
Sesame Oil	1 liter
Yellow Beeswax	50g

PREPARATION & DOSAGE: In a non-metallic saucepan, cook the Radix Arnebiae seu Lithospermi *(zi cao)* in the sesame oil until the herb turns brown. Filter out the dregs, then add the powdered Rhizoma Coptidis *(huang lian)* and yellow beeswax, reheating if necessary in order to dissolve the wax. Pour into a glass jar with an airtight lid, and allow to congeal. Apply to the affected area 3-5 times daily after diaper changes.

Powders that may be applied, either following treatment with any of the above formulas, or alone during diaper changes, include Clearing and Cooling Powder (see sunburn in Chapter 12), or Talcum and Indigo Powder.

❦ Talcum and Indigo Powder
滑黛粉
huá dài fěn

Talcum *(hua shi)*
Indigo Pulverata Levis *(qing dai)*

PREPARATION & DOSAGE: Mix five parts Talcum *(hua shi)* with one part Indigo Pulverata Levis *(qing dai)* and grind together into a fine powder. Store in an amber glass jar with an airtight lid.

Traditional vs. Biomedical Treatment

Traditional treatment is perhaps no more and no less effective than biomedical methods. The disadvantage of traditional remedies is their lengthy preparation time. Despite this, they may be appreciated for their non-pharmaceutical approach to resolving this condition, especially as an alternative to corticosteroids.

Prevention

In addition to treatment with the above remedies, frequent and immediate diaper changes will usually clear up diaper dermatitis quickly. Rubber or plastic pants should not be worn since they prevent the evaporation of contactant and facilitate its penetration into the skin. During diaper changes, warm water rather than soap should be used to clean the area, since soap may irritate the skin. To aid in healing, the child should be permitted to go diaper-less for short periods throughout the day.

CHAPTER NOTES

1. Dai, Y.F. and Liu, C.J. *Medicinal Uses of Fruits (Yao yong guo pin)*. Nanning: Guangxi People's Publishing House, 1982.

2. Yang, G.X., "Myrrha and Lonicera Decoction in the Treatment of Skin Diseases," *Chinese Journal of Integrated Traditional and Western Medicine,* 10(8): 492; 1990.

3. Zhang, S.H., Guo, Y.L., Huang, T.J., and Zhang J.L., "External Application of Asarum, Dahurica, Schizonepeta, Ledebouriella Powder in the Treatment of Localized Eczema," *Henan Traditional Chinese Medicine,* 10(4): 24; 1990.

4. He, T.A., "External Application of Indigo, Alumen, and Zanthoxylum Powder in the Treatment of Eczema, *Yunnan Journal of Traditional Chinese Medicine,* 11(2): 28; 1990.

5. Liu, Q.W., "Mirabilitum Used for the Treatment of Acute Eczema," *New Journal of Traditional Chinese Medicine,* 22(9): 40; 1990.

6. Dai and Liu, *Medicinal Uses of Fruits (Yao yong guo pin)*.

7. Ye, J.Q. *Traditional Chinese Food Medicinals and Folk Prescriptions (Shi wu zhong yao yu pian fang)*. Jiangsu: Jiangsu Science and Technology Press, 1980.

8. Ibid.

9. Wang, L.Y., "Eliminate Wind and Transform Stasis Decoction Used for the Treatment of Neurodermatitis," *Jiangsu Journal of Traditional Chinese Medicine,* 11(3): 10; 1990.

10. Guo, Y.B., "External Application of Table Vinegar Paste in the Treatment of Neurodermatitis," *Shaanxi Journal of Chinese Traditional Medicine,* 12(11): 510; 1991.

11. Ma, X.P., "Discussion of Acupuncture in the Treatment of Skin Diseases," *Jiangsu Journal of Traditional Chinese Medicine,* 13(6): 24-25; 1992.

CHAPTER 14

Inflammatory Reactions

Drug Eruptions
中药毒
zhòng yào dú, "medicine poisoning"

Drug eruptions are inflammatory reactions of the skin that occur subsequent to taking medication. In Chinese medicine, the term "medicine poisoning" encompasses adverse reactions of both the skin and the vital organs. Records of materia medica poisoning and their antidotes are found as early as the 4th century work *Emergency Formulas to Keep Up One's Sleeve* (341). A medico-legal text, *Collection of Records on Redressing Wrongs* (1247), contains the following passage: "Arsenic [and] *gou wen* [Gelsemium] toxin, [which after ingesting], a short time [later] the entire body develops small vesicles, [and becomes cyanotic] . . ." And for early stage arsenic poisoning, there is this note in *True Lineage of External Medicine* (1617): "[P]our the juice from crushed leaves of *dà lán gēn* [Folium Isatis] down the person's throat; light cases will be relieved."

Signs & Symptoms

Drug eruptions are among the most common side effects of therapeutic drug use. These reactions are important because they may be the first sign of a generalized hypersensitivity, or of a toxic reaction involving other structures and organs.

Changes in the skin range from a slight rash to the potentially life-threatening condition known as toxic epidermal necrolysis (peeling of the epidermis). The lesions themselves may be localized, or, as with many such eruptions, generalized. The reaction may be immediate, or delayed for hours, days, or even years.

Whereas Chinese medicine considers drug eruptions (medicine poisoning) to be caused by various materia medica, and modern biomedicine considers these conditions to be due to pharmaceuticals, the types of reactions are the same. The commonly seen eruption patterns are classified morphologically as follows: urticarial reactions, morbilliform eruptions, erythema multiforme, fixed drug eruptions, purpuric eruptions, exfoliative erythroderma, and toxic epidermal necrolysis. Urticarial and morbilliform eruptions are the most frequently occuring types.

Urticarial reactions. Urticaria (hives) is characterized by local, itchy wheals surrounded by redness. It is an immediate hypersensitivity reaction that is typically produced within 36 hours after drug administration, but can occur within minutes. The lesions vary in size from a small point to a large area. The epidermis is usually not involved, although the dermis and subcutaneous tissues may become so swollen that respiration is impaired, which may lead to life-threatening anaphylaxis. Urticarial lesions rarely last more than 24 hours.

Pharmaceuticals that can cause urticaria include penicillin and aspirin, among others. Chinese herbs known to induce urticaria include Radix Ginseng *(ren shen)*, Radix Isatidis seu Baphicacanthi *(ban lan gen)*, Herba Andrographitis Paniculatae *(chuan xin lian)*, Radix Salviae Miltiorrhizae *(dan shen)*, Radix Notoginseng *(san qi)*, Radix Astragali Membranacei *(huang qi)* and Fructus Schisandrae Chinensis *(wu wei zi)*. Among Chinese prepared medicines, Six-Miracle Pill *(liu shen wan)* and Yunnan White Medicine *(yun nan bai yao)* have been implicated.

Morbilliform eruptions. These are also known as maculopapular exanthems, and are the most frequently occuring of drug-induced eruptions. They are usually symmetric, starting as small red macules and papules that become confluent and form erythematous plaques. Morbilliform eruptions often start on the trunk. Mild fever is sometimes present, and itching is common. As opposed to urticaria, the dermis and epidermis are involved. The latency period for morbilliform eruptions is usually longer than for urticarial eruptions, but most occur within one week after a drug's introduction. Ordinarily, morbilliform eruptions disappear within two weeks after the drug is withdrawn.

Penicillins, barbiturates, sulfonamides and antibiotics are common drugs known to cause morbilliform eruptions, as are herbs such as Radix Trichosanthis Kirilowii *(tian hua fen)* as well as the Western herb, foxglove.

Erythema multiforme. This is an inflammatory eruption characterized by symmetric erythematous, edematous or bullous lesions. Onset is usually sudden, with eruptions appearing primarily on the distal portions of the extremities (palms and soles), and on the face; sore throat and malaise are common systemic symptoms. Bleeding lesions of the lips and oral mucosa can also occur. The skin lesions, also known as iris or "target" lesions, are symmetric, with concentric rings and central grayish discoloration of the epidermis. Itching may be present.

Drugs most often implicated in erythema multiforme are penicillin, sulfonamides, phenothiazines, thiazides and phenytoin.

Fixed drug eruptions. These are sharply defined, often single red or purple lesions of the skin or mucous membranes. The hallmark of these lesions is that they recur in the same spot each time the drug is administered. The face and genitalia are commonly involved. Although the redness resolves in days or weeks after drug withdrawal, the skin can remain hyperpigmented for long periods.

Penicillins, tetracyclines, phenolphthalein, benzodiazepines, as well as nonsteroidal anti-inflammatory drugs are common causes of fixed drug eruptions. The Chinese prepared medicine, Six-Miracle Pill *(liu shen wan)*, is also known to induce such eruptions.

Purpuric eruptions. These are purple macules and plaques that do not fade upon pressure; they may be of different sizes, but are usually small. They are most common on the legs, although they can occur anywhere. Often these lesions are a sign of a more serious drug-induced vasculitis of internal organs, the central nervous system, or the joints. Thus, the patient should be examined more carefully for involvement of these systems.

Drugs known to cause purpuric eruptions include anticoagulants, chlorothiazide and meprobamate, among others. Materia medica that have been found to induce this reaction include Cinnabaris *(zhu sha)*, Fructus Tribuli Terrestris *(bai ji li)*, Arillus Euphoriae Longanae *(long yan rou)*, Semen Nelumbinis Nuciferae *(lian zi)* and Bulbus Fritillariae Cirrhosae *(chuan bei mu)*. The Chinese prepared medicines, Six-Miracle Pill *(liu shen wan)*, Emperor of Heaven's Special Pill to Tonify the Heart *(tian wang bu xin dan)* and Red Ointment *(hong you gao)*, have also been implicated in purpuric eruptions.

Exfoliative erythroderma. This is a generalized severe redness and scaling of the skin. The onset may be rapid or insidious. The entire skin becomes red, scaly, thickened and sometimes crusted. Itching may be severe or absent. Fever may be present, or the patient may feel cold from excessive heat loss due to the increased blood flow to the skin and exfoliation (falling off of scales in layers). The condition may be life-threatening if signs of weight loss, lowered blood protein, iron deficiency or even congestive heart failure appear as the condition worsens.

Drugs that can cause exfoliative erythroderma include streptomycin, penicillin, sulfonamides, isoniazid and phenytoin.

Toxic epidermal necrolysis. This is an exceedingly serious and potentially life-threatening reaction. At first the skin is red and tender, followed by blistering. Perhaps most alarming is that the skin may peel off in large sheets with just gentle pressure. Extensive erosion, including the mucous membranes (eyes, mouth, and genitalia), takes place within one to three days of onset, and causes fluid and electrolyte imbalance and increases the risk of infection. Such cases require hospitalization.

Drugs that can cause toxic epidermal necrolysis include barbiturates, penicillins, sulfonomides, tetracyclines, nonsteroidal anti-inflammatory agents and phenytoin.

Differential Diagnosis

In addition to ascertaining whether a drug is responsible for a skin eruption, other causative factors should be investigated. The possibility of foods and beverages should be considered since there is an almost endless variety of chemical compounds used in the processing of such products. Also, other diseases, such as viral infections, may cause eruptions resembling those caused by drugs. In some instances it may be difficult to determine whether an illness or its treatment is the cause of an eruption. For example, erythema multiforme may follow an infection, or it may be due to drugs used to treat the infection.

Patients should be asked about all medications including nonprescription drugs, and prior experience with them. Some drug reactions occur after the medication has been discontinued (e.g., ampicillin), and other reactions can continue for weeks and months after use of the medication is discontinued. Individuals who take more than one drug at the same time may require rechallenge with the drug(s) in order to pinpoint the causative agent.

Identifying the causative agent of drug eruptions caused by materia medica may be more vexing, since they are contained in formulas that are usually made up of several substances. Just as any pharmaceutical is capable of causing an adverse reaction, so it is with any materia medica. However, as with pharmaceuticals like penicillin and tetracycline, certain materia medica have been implicated more often in causing adverse reactions, including skin eruptions. In many cases, these materia medica are ones that are toxic at low doses. Practitioners should thus familiarize themselves with these so that safe doses are prescribed.

Traditional Chinese Etiology

Constitutional insufficiency causes intolerance to medicinal toxin, which combines with pre-existing dampness and/or heat to accumulate in the skin. Severe cases are the result of accumulated toxic heat from the offending medicinal searing the nutritive and blood levels.

Treatment

All medications should be stopped immediately and the causative agent identified. Traditional treatment is based on the presenting patterns that are categorized below.

INTERNAL

Toxic heat combined with wind. This pattern is characterized by papules, red macules and/or wheals on the skin. Onset is rapid, and the upper body is more often affected. Warm temperatures will induce itching. Generalized symptoms may include fever and aversion to cold, headache, stuffy nose, coughing, a thin yellow tongue coating, and a floating, rapid pulse. This pattern corresponds with urticarial, morbilliform and purpuric eruptions. The strategy is to clear heat from the qi level and relieve toxicity, and cool the blood and reduce purple macules. The formula recommended for this pattern is Honeysuckle and Forsythia Powder Combined with White Tiger Decoction.

Honeysuckle and Forsythia Powder Combined with White Tiger Decoction
银翘散白虎汤化裁
yín qiáo sǎn bái hǔ tāng huà cái

Flos Lonicerae Japonicae *(jin yin hua)*	12g
Fructus Forsythiae Suspensae *(lian qiao)*	10g
Radix Paeoniae Rubrae *(chi shao)*	10g
Radix Rehmanniae Glutinosae *(sheng di huang)*	10g
Radix Scutellariae Baicalensis *(huang qin)*	10g
Gypsum *(shi gao)*	30g
Dry-fried Rhizoma Anemarrhenae Asphodeloidis *(chao zhi mu)*	6g
Dry-fried Fructus Arctii Lappae *(chao niu bang zi)*	6g
Radix Glycyrrhizae Uralensis *(gan cao)*	6g
Radix Dioscoreae Oppositae *(shan yao)*	15g

PREPARATION & DOSAGE: First decoct the Gypsum *(shi gao)* for 15-20 minutes before cooking the other ingredients. Administer in three doses daily.

Blood heat combined with dampness. This pattern is characterized by red macules, bullas, erosion and/or weeping skin lesions. The mucosa of the mouth and perineum may be affected. Generalized symptoms may include dryness of the mouth, dry stools, a red tongue with little coating, and a wiry, thin pulse. Erythema multiforme and fixed drug eruptions correspond to this pattern. The strategy is to clear and transform damp-heat, and cool the blood and relieve toxicity. The formula recommended for this pattern is Modified Rhinoceros Horn and Rehmannia Decoction [A].

Modified Rhinoceros Horn and Rehmannia Decoction [A]
犀角地黄汤加减
xī jiǎo dì huáng tāng jiā jiǎn

Cornu Rhinoceri *(xi jiao)*	1.3g
Testa Phaseoli Radiati *(lu dou yi)*	30g
Charred Radix Rehmanniae Glutinosae *(di huang tan)*	30g
Charred Flos Lonicerae Japonicae *(jin yin hua tan)*	30g
Semen Coicis Lachryma-jobi *(yi yi ren)*	30g
Radix Salviae Miltiorrhizae *(dan shen)*	12g
Dry-fried Cortex Moutan Radicis *(chao mu dan pi)*	12g
Radix Arnebiae seu Lithospermi *(zi cao)*	12g
Cortex Poriae Cocos *(fu ling pi)*	12g
Semen Phaseoli Calcarati *(chi xiao dou)*	15g
Herba Taraxaci Mongolici cum Radice *(pu gong ying)*	15g

PREPARATION & DOSAGE: Grind the Cornu Rhinoceri *(xi jiao)* into a powder and administer as a draft followed by the strained decoction. If Cornu

Bubali *(shui niu jiao)* is substituted, as is strongly recommended, 15g of the total 30g of this medicinal should be powdered or shaved and cooked separately for 15-20 minutes before adding the other ingredients. Administer in three doses daily.

Fire toxin sinking. This pattern is characterized by blisters with clear exudate or blood, swelling of the skin, and moist skin; the mucosa is usually involved. Generalized symptoms may include chills and high fever, extreme thirst, a purple tongue with a yellow sticky coating, and a wiry, slippery and flooding pulse. As the condition worsens, the skin may separate from the tissue below, and the accompanying symptoms of impaired consciousness and raving, jaundice and bloody urine may ensue. This pattern corresponds to the early stage of toxic epidermal necrolysis. The strategy is to clear the nutritive level and relieve toxicity, and enrich yin and drain heat. The formula recommended for this pattern is Defeat Toxin Decoction.

❧ Defeat Toxin Decoction
败毒饮
bài dú yǐn

Gypsum *(shi gao)*	60g
Rhizoma Coptidis *(huang lian)*	10g
Radix Scutellariae Baicalensis *(huang qin)*	15g
Fructus Gardeniae Jasminoidis *(zhi zi)*	15g
Radix Rehmanniae Glutinosae *(sheng di huang)*	30g
Radix Scrophulariae Ningpoensis *(xuan shen)*	15g
Cortex Moutan Radicis *(mu dan pi)*	10g
Radix Paeoniae Rubrae *(chi shao)*	10g
Fructus Forsythiae Suspensae *(lian qiao)*	15g
Radix Platycodi Grandiflori *(jie geng)*	10g
Herba Lophatheri Gracilis *(dan zhu ye)*	10g
Radix Glycyrrhizae Uralensis *(gan cao)*	10g
Mirabilitum *(mang xiao)*	15g

PREPARATION & DOSAGE: Decoct all of the ingredients except the Mirabilitum *(mang xiao)*. After cooking, dissolve it in the strained decoction. Administer in three doses daily.

Injury of both the qi and blood. This pattern is exhibited during the late stages of drug eruptions, when the qi and yin are exhausted. It is characterized by widespread exfoliation. Generalized symptoms may include malaise, loss of appetite, unformed stools, dryness of the mouth and lips with the desire to drink, a red tongue with denuded coating, and a thin, rapid pulse. This pattern corresponds to exfoliative erythroderma. The strategy is to benefit qi and enrich yin, and support normal qi to relieve toxicity. The formula recommended for this pattern is Modified Increase the Fluids Decoction.

❧ Modified Increase the Fluids Decoction
增液汤加减
zēng yè tāng jiā jiǎn

Radix Rehmanniae Glutinosae *(sheng di huang)*	30-60g
Flos Lonicerae Japonicae *(jin yin hua)*	12g
Radix Adenophorae seu Glehniae *(sha shen)*	12g
Radix Scrophulariae Ningpoensis *(xuan shen)*	12g
Radix Astragali Membranacei *(huang qi)*	12g
Testa Phaseoli Radiati *(lu dou yi)*	30g
Herba Dendrobii *(shi hu)*	30g
Radix Dioscoreae Oppositae *(shan yao)*	30g
Tuber Asparagi Cochinchinensis *(tian men dong)*	15g
Tuber Ophiopogonis Japonici *(mai men dong)*	15g
Rhizoma Polygonati Odorati *(yu zhu)*	15g
Semen Phaseoli Calcarati *(chi xiao dou)*	15g

PREPARATION & DOSAGE: Decoct and administer in 2-3 doses daily.

MODIFICATIONS: For dry stools, add Radix et Rhizoma Rhei *(da huang)* and Radix Platycodi Grandiflori *(jie geng)*; for severe itching, add Ramulus cum Uncis Uncariae *(gou teng)*, Cortex Dictamni Dasycarpi Radicis *(bai xian pi)* and Radix Sophorae Flavescentis *(ku shen)*. For impaired consciousness with raving, administer one-half or one Calm the Palace Pill with Cattle Gallstone, 2-3 times daily, until the patient regains consciousness, and then administer Modified Increase the Fluids Decoction.

EXTERNAL

For redness, macules and/or wheals, apply Three-Yellow Wash (see furuncles in Chapter 7), 3-5 times daily. For blisters, erosion and/or weeping lesions, apply Portulaca Wash (see herpes simplex in Chapter 8) as a wet compress for 15 minutes, 3-5 times daily. For dryness, scaling and/or itching of the skin, apply Indigo Ointment (see tinea in Chapter 9), Coptis Ointment (see herpes zoster in Chapter 8) or Black Ointment (see atopic dermatitis in Chapter 13), 2-3 times daily. For ulcers and/or erosion of the genitalia, apply Magarita Powder.

❧ Magarita Powder
珍珠散
zhēn zhū sǎn

Indigo Pulverata Levis *(qing dai)*	1.5g
Magarita *(zhen zhu)*	3g
Calomelas *(qing fen)*	30g

PREPARATION & DOSAGE: Grind the three ingredients together into a fine powder and store in an airtight glass container. Before application, wash the affected area with warm water only, and pat dry. Apply the powder directly to the lesions, 2-3 times daily.

ACUPUNCTURE

Acupoints that should be needled include PC-6 *(nei guan),* LI-11 *(qu chi),* SP-10 *(xue hai),* ST-36 *(zu san li),* BL-40 *(wei zhong)* and SP-6 *(san yin jiao).* First drain and then tonify ST-36 *(zu san li)* and SP-6 *(san yin jiao).* For all other points use draining manipulation. Treat once daily until the eruption has subsided.

CLINICAL NOTE: Acupoints affected by lesions should not be needled.

Traditional vs. Biomedical Treatment

Drug eruptions often require no further therapy once the causative agent is stopped. Traditional treatment will probably accelerate recovery because of its ability to address the root cause, while biomedical intervention is palliative through use of corticosteroids, antihistamines and antipruritic medications. Severe cases such as toxic epidermal necrolysis may benefit from a combined traditional and biomedical approach, the former to neutralize the medicinal toxin, and the latter to prevent infection and to monitor fluid and electrolyte imbalance.

Prevention

After the offending agent has been identified, patients should avoid using it. They should also inform their physician or practitioner of their allergy.

Severe cases of drug eruption, such as toxic epidermal necrolysis, may require a combined traditional and Western treatment approach, since it generally takes longer for herbs to render their effects. Thus, patients may need to be put on antibiotic therapy in order to prevent infection.

Erythema Multiforme
猫眼疮
māo yǎn chuāng, "cat eye sore"

Erythema multiforme is an inflammatory skin eruption characterized by nodular wheals and target-like plaques. The Chinese name of "cat eye sore" is found in several texts on external medicine, including *Golden Mirror of the Medical Tradition* (1742), which describes this disease as follows: "Cat eye sore is so named because of its appearance. [Often there is] no pain or itching; there is no bleeding or pus. [The sores] glimmer like cat eyes." Other names for this condition include "cold sore" *(hán chuāng),* because of its resemblance to chilblain lesions, and "wild goose sore" *(yàn chuāng),* because the condition often occurs during February and August, the times of the year when wild geese arrive in parts of China.

In over half of the cases no biomedical cause can be found. In the remainder, drugs, chemicals, physical agents, foods or various internal diseases are implicated.

Signs & Symptoms

Onset of erythema multiforme is typically sudden, with the appearance of red papules affecting any area of the body, but especially the arms, legs, palms and soles. Itching may be mild or absent. The lesions enlarge slowly and resolve centrally. A new crop of papules may develop later, often starting in the cleared center of a previous lesion, thus producing the distinctive iris "target" lesion.

In the bullous type of erythema multiforme, blisters appear in the center of plaques, and occasionally at the edges. When the blisters break, erosion and blood crusts occur. In the mouth and on other mucous membranes, crusts and ulcers take the place of blisters.

In Stevens-Johnson syndrome, the severe form of erythema multiforme, bullae develop on the oral mucosa, pharynx, anogenital region and conjunctiva. Typical lesions may or may not be present on the rest of the body. The patient may be unable to eat or drink because of the pain in the mouth and pharynx, thus resulting in fluid and electrolyte imbalance. When the trachea and bronchia are affected, there is a risk of death from asphyxiation. Involvement of the conjunctiva may cause blindness due to corneal scarring.

Differential Diagnosis

At the outset, the papules and wheals may resemble urticaria or insect bites. However, in most cases of urticaria the lesions disappear within a short time (minutes or hours). Erythema multiforme lesions usually appear in numbers, whereas insect bites typically do not. Tinea corporis may be confused with the annular lesions of erythema multiforme. Whereas tinea is a scaling disease, erythema multiforme is not. Usually upon appearance of the target lesions, erythema multiforme can be confirmed.

Traditional Chinese Etiology

The three primary causes of this condition are constitutional insufficiency, invasion of wind-heat and fire or heat toxin.

Constitutional insufficiency. This results in the invasion of external wind-cold, which lodges in the skin and tissues and causes disharmony between the protective and nutritive levels, thus giving rise to the lesions.

Invasion of wind-heat. The wind-heat, along with pre-existing damp-heat, accumulate and lodge in the skin and tissues, where they produce the lesions.

Fire or heat toxin. This is often the result of intolerance to certain foods or medicinal substances, or the result of other diseases. The fire or heat toxin penetrates and sears the blood, causing blood heat to be driven outward to the skin and tissues, such that the lesions arise.

Treatment

INTERNAL

Constitutional insufficiency. This pattern presents with lesions that are purple, swelling of the fingers and toes, and a sensation of coldness of the skin. Generalized symptoms may include an aversion to cold, coldness of the limbs, abdominal pain, unformed stools, a thin white tongue coating, and a soggy pulse. The condition either recurs or is exacerbated during exposure to cold temperatures. The strategy is to harmonize the nutritive level and dispel cold.

Formulas that are recommended for this pattern include Modified Tangkuei Decoction for Frigid Extremities [B], or Prepared Aconite Decoction.

❧ Modified Tangkuei Decoction for Frigid Extremities [B]
当归四逆汤加减
dāng guī sì nì tāng jiā jiǎn

Radix Angelicae Sinensis *(dang gui)*	9g
Ramulus Cinnamomi Cassiae *(gui zhi)*	9g
Radix Paeoniae Rubrae *(chi shao)*	9g
Herba cum Radice Asari *(xi xin)*	6g
Honey-toasted Radix Glycyrrhizae Uralensis *(zhi gan cao)*	6g
Fructus Zizyphi Jujubae *(da zao)*	4-5 pieces
Fructus Liquidambaris Taiwanianae *(lu lu tong)*	6g
Radix et Rhizoma Notopterygii *(qiang huo)*	6g
Radix Aristolochiae Fangchi *(fang ji)*	6g

PREPARATION & DOSAGE: Decoct and administer in three doses daily.

❧ Prepared Aconite Decoction
炙附汤
zhì fù tāng

Radix Lateralis Aconiti Carmichaeli Praeparata *(fu zi)*	4.5-9g
Radix Codonopsitis Pilosulae *(dang shen)*	9g
Rhizoma Zingiberis Officinalis *(gan jiang)*	3-4.5g
Rhizoma Atractylodis *(cang zhu)*	9g
Rhizoma Atractylodis Macrocephalae *(bai zhu)*	9g
Cortex Cinnamomi Cassiae *(rou gui)*	1.5-3g
Radix Ligustici Chuanxiong *(chuan xiong)*	9g
Radix Angelicae Sinensis *(dang gui)*	9g
Honey-toasted Radix Glycyrrhizae Uralensis *(zhi gan cao)*	3-9g

PREPARATION & DOSAGE: Decoct and administer in 2-3 doses daily.

CLINICAL NOTE: Boil the Radix Lateralis Aconiti Carmichaeli Praeparata *(fu zi)* for 30-60 minutes before adding the other ingredients, as this reduces its toxicity.

Invasion of wind heat with pre-existing dampness. This pattern presents with lesions that are red; blisters are not uncommon. Generalized symptoms may include fever, throat pain, dryness of the mouth, soreness of the joints, dry stools, a thin or sticky yellow tongue coating, and a slippery, rapid pulse. In general, there does not appear to be a seasonal occurrence to this pattern, although a number of cases do show up during the warm months. The strategy is to scatter wind, clear heat and drain dampness. The formula recommended for this pattern is Buchnera, Moutan, and Batryticatus Decoction.

Buchnera, Moutan, and Batryticatus Decoction
鬼丹僵蚕汤
guǐ dān jiāng cán tāng

Herba Buchnerae Cruciatae *(gui yu jian)*	10g
Cortex Moutan Radicis *(mu dan pi)*	10g
Radix Salviae Miltiorrhizae *(dan shen)*	10g
Radix Rehmanniae Glutinosae *(sheng di huang)*	10g
Radix Paeoniae Rubrae *(chi shao)*	10g
Radix Arnebiae seu Lithospermi *(zi cao)*	10g
Radix Angelicae Sinensis *(dang gui)*	10g
Bombyx Batryticatus *(jiang can)*	10g

PREPARATION & DOSAGE: Decoct and administer in a single dose daily.

Patterns that show marked damp-heat may be treated with Clear the Flesh and Leach Out Dampness Decoction.

Clear the Flesh and Leach Out Dampness Decoction
清肌渗湿汤
qīng jī shèn shī tāng

Rhizoma Atractylodis *(cang zhu)*	3g
Cortex Magnoliae Officinalis *(hou po)*	3g
Pericarpium Citri Reticulatae *(chen pi)*	3g
Radix Glycyrrhizae Uralensis *(gan cao)*	3g
Radix Bupleuri *(chai hu)*	3g
Caulis Mutong *(mu tong)*	3g
Rhizome Alismatis Orientalis *(ze xie)*	3g
Radix Angelicae Dahuricae *(bai zhi)*	3g
Rhizoma Cimicifugae *(sheng ma)*	3g
Rhizoma Atractylodis Macrocephalae *(bai zhu)*	3g
Fructus Gardeniae Jasminoidis *(zhi zi)*	3g
Rhizoma Coptidis *(huang lian)*	3g

PREPARATION & DOSAGE: Decoct in 400ml of water for 15 minutes. Then add 3 slices of Rhizoma Zingiberis Officinalis Recens *(sheng jiang)* and 20 strands of Medulla Junci Effusi *(deng xin cao)*, and continue decocting until about 320ml of fluid remain. Administer the decoction warm in one dose daily.

Fire or heat toxin. This pattern usually has a sudden onset, accompanied by an aversion to cold, high fever, headache, malaise, dryness and pain of the throat, chest pain and cough, and even nausea and vomiting, diarrhea and joint pain. Lesions may cover the entire body, including the mucous membranes of the mouth and genitalia. The lesions are often a mixture of red papules, blisters and erosions that bleed and crust over. The tongue is red with a yellow coating, and the pulse is slippery and rapid. The strategy is to enrich yin and clear heat, and cool the blood and relieve toxicity. The formula recommended for this pattern is Modified Universal Benefit Decoction to Eliminate Toxin.

❧ Modified Universal Benefit Decoction to Eliminate Toxin
普济消毒饮加减
pǔ jì xiāo dú yǐn jiā jiǎn

Fructus Arctii Lappae *(niu bang zi)*	3g
Radix Scutellariae Baicalensis *(huang qin)*	15g
Rhizoma Coptidis *(huang lian)*	15g
Flos Lonicerae Japonicae *(jin yin hua)*	3g
Fructus Forsythiae Suspensae *(lian qiao)*	3g
Radix Isatidis seu Baphicacanthi *(ban lan gen)*	3g
Radix Sophorae Tonkinensis *(shan dou gen)*	3g
Radix Rehmanniae Glutinosae *(sheng di huang)*	6g
Radix Paeoniae Rubrae *(chi shao)*	6g
Radix Arnebiae seu Lithospermi *(zi cao)*	3g
Rhizoma Smilacis Glabrae *(tu fu ling)*	3g
Radix Glycyrrhizae Uralensis *(gan cao)*	3g

PREPARATION & DOSAGE: Decoct and administer in two doses daily.

MODIFICATIONS: For nausea and vomiting, add Rhizoma Pinelliae Ternatae *(ban xia)*, Pericarpium Citri Reticulatae *(chen pi)* and Caulis Bambusae in Taeniis *(zhu ru)*; for watery stools, replace Flos Lonicerae Japonicae *(jin yin hua)* and Radix Scutellariae Baicalensis *(huang qin)* with their charred forms.

EXTERNAL
Wheals, papules and blisters may be treated with Jade Red Ointment.

❧ Jade Red Ointment
玉红膏
yù hóng gāo

Radix Angelicae Sinensis *(dang gui)*	60g
Radix Angelicae Dahuricae *(bai zhi)*	15g
Radix Glycyrrhizae Uralensis *(gan cao)*	36g
Radix Arnebiae seu Lithospermi *(zi cao)*	6g
Sanguis Draconis *(xue jie)*	12g
Calomelas *(qing fen)*	12g
White Beeswax	60g
Sesame Oil	500ml

PREPARATION & DOSAGE: Steep the first four ingredients in the sesame oil for three days. Then boil the oil over low heat until the herbs turn brown.

Filter and discard the dregs. Add the beeswax, Sanguis Draconis *(xue jie)* and Calomelas *(qing fen)* to the oil; reheat if necessary in order to dissolve the beeswax. Stir thoroughly and pour into an amber glass jar. Allow to congeal. Apply liberally to the affected areas, once daily, with a sterile cotton swab.

For erosion of the skin, either Three-Yellow Wash (see furuncles in Chapter 7) or Indigo Ointment (see tinea in Chapter 9) is recommended, with application 3-4 times daily.

For ulcers and erosion of the mouth, Terminalia Wash may be used, followed by application of Enrich the Yin and Generate Flesh Powder.

❧ Terminalia Wash
青果水洗剂
qīng guǒ shuǐ xǐ jì

Fructus Terminaliae Chebulae Immaturus *(zang qing guo)*	9-15g
Herba Equiseti Hiemalis *(mu zei)*	9g
Flos Trollii *(jin lian hua)*	6g

PREPARATION & DOSAGE: Decoct in 1 liter of water until 250ml remains. Filter and discard the dregs. Rinse the mouth for 1-2 minutes with the decoction, 3-5 times daily.

❧ Enrich the Yin and Generate the Flesh Powder
养阴生肌散
yǎng yīn shēng jī sǎn

Cornu Rhinoceri *(xi jiao)*	0.3g
Secretio Moschus *(she xiang)*	0.3g
Indigo Pulverata Levis *(qing dai)*	6g
Calcined Gypsum *(duan shi gao)*	6g
Pasta Acaciae seu Uncariae *(er cha)*	6g
Borax *(peng sha)*	6g
Cortex Phellodendri *(huang bai)*	6g
Radix Gentianae Longdancao *(long dan cao)*	6g
Herba Menthae Haplocalycis *(bo he)*	3g

PREPARATION & DOSAGE: Grind the ingredients together into a fine powder. Use a sterile cotton swab to apply the powder to lesions after rinsing the mouth with Terminalia Wash.

CLINICAL NOTE: Ten times the amount of Cornu Bubali *(shui niu jiao)* is usually substituted for Cornu Rhinoceri *(xi jiao)*, both due to expense and the fact that all species of rhinoceros are endangered.

Traditional vs. Biomedical Treatment

Traditional measures are more effective in promoting quicker healing than biomedical treatment, which often consists of corticosteroids to relieve inflammation. In severe cases, combining traditional formulas with antibiotics that prevent infection can be considered. In cases where oral lesions makes feeding difficult, intravenous fluids and electrolyte replacement may be necessary, perhaps combined with Terminalia Wash and Enrich the Yin and Generate the Flesh Powder, as described above.

Prevention

When the cause can be found, it should be eliminated or avoided. During treatment with herbal formulas the patient should abstain from foods and beverages that may produce dampness and heat, such as spicy and greasy foods, shrimp, lamb, sweets and coffee. Even after the lesions have healed, patients should either avoid or moderate their intake of such foods and beverages.

Urticaria
风瘾疹
fēng yǐn zhěn, "wind-type concealed rash"

Urticaria, or hives, is an inflammatory reaction of the skin characterized by local wheals and redness. The term "concealed rash" was first recorded in *Basic Questions,* Chapter 64: "Excess in the lesser yin [causes] skin painful obstruction and concealed rash." Additional names for this condition include "wind rash" *(fēng zhěn),* "wind itch concealed rash" *(fēng sāo yǐn zhěn)* and "wind rash lumps" *(fēng zhěn kuài),* among others. Through the ages, as Chinese physicians gained experience in treating urticaria, they learned that it has many causes, as described below under traditional etiology.

Biomedically, urticaria is an allergic reaction limited to the skin. It often results from: an allergy to certain foods; medications; insect stings or bites; heat, cold, or sunshine; pollen, molds, or animal danders. Hives may appear as a symptom of some viral infections such as hepatitis, measles, and mononucleosis. Parasitic infections are common causes of urticaria in tropical climates. Non-infectious diseases are sometimes associated with urticaria, including lupus erythematosus, and hyper- and hypothyroidism. Some women develop urticaria during menstruation. Psychological factors may play a role in the etiology of chronic urticaria.

Signs & Symptoms

The first symptom is itching, soon followed by the development of large or small pink wheals caused by vascular dilatation and edema. The lesions vary from a few millimeters to several centimeters in diameter. Large lesions may appear as circles of redness and swelling that resolve centrally. Individual lesions usually last less than 24 hours. Acute hives generally has a course between one and seven days. With chronic conditions, unexplained remissions may recur up to years later.

Differential Diagnosis

Other skin conditions sometimes confused with urticaria include allergic contact dermatitis, erythema multiforme, multiple insect bites, pityriasis rosea and scabies. The specific differentiation can often be made by history and physical examination, or biopsy if the diagnosis is in doubt. In chronic urticaria, an underlying chronic disease should be ruled out through a careful history and physical examination, and routine screening tests.

Traditional Chinese Etiology

The traditional causes of urticaria are numerous. Typically, individuals prone to urticaria have an intolerant constitution to begin with. Then, when confronted with external excesses such as wind, cold, heat or other harmful factors that cannot be tolerated (such as certain foods, medicinals and the like), their skin and tissues develop the lesions. The more common types of urticaria and their causes are discussed below.

Wind-cold. The initial onset occurs during attack by wind-cold, when the protective and nutritive levels are in disharmony. As time passes, deficiency of the exterior and instability of the protective level result. Thus, when again attacked by wind and/or cold, urticaria recurs.

Wind-heat. The initial onset occurs when wind-heat attacks and lodges in the skin and injures the nutritive and blood levels, causing disharmony between the protective and nutritive levels. As the condition becomes protracted, the wind-heat stagnates in the tissues and interstices. Thus, when again attacked by wind-heat, the urticaria is provoked.

Wind-dampness. This is often due to improper diet, such as overindulgence in spicy or greasy foods, which causes disharmony of the Spleen/Stomach such that dampness is produced. Protracted dampness transforms into heat, which in turn provokes wind that combines with the dampness. Thus, when the wind-dampness cannot be expressed externally or drained internally, it stagnates in the skin and interstices and produces urticaria.

Spleen/Stomach dysfunction. Pre-existing Spleen/Stomach dysfunction is the source of this pattern. Disturbance of the Spleen/Stomach's transportive and transformative mechanisms results in qi stagnation, intestinal accumulation of parasites, or deficiency cold of the Spleen/Stomach, all of which leave the body susceptible to ensuing attack by wind, thus leading to urticaria.

Blood heat. This pattern is caused by emotional provocation such that heat stagnates in the Heart channel and transforms into fire, which then enters the blood. Blood heat in turn transforms into wind, thus producing urticaria.

Blood stasis. Urticaria of this type occurs when there is pre-existing blood stasis, and the qi of the protective and nutritive levels is not disseminated, such that when either wind and cold or wind and heat mutually contend, lesions break out.

Blood deficiency. This pattern occurs in individuals who are blood deficient. When the Liver does not have enough blood to nourish itself, one of the results is the provocation of wind, which in this case causes urticaria.

Disharmony between the conception vessel and penetrating channel. This type of urticaria occurs in women, usually those who, after giving birth, do not regain harmony between the conception and penetrating vessels, and who also have insufficiency of qi of the protective and nutritive levels, such that the skin is not sufficiently nourished. Thus, when attacked by external wind, or when internal wind is provoked, the lesions arise.

Treatment

Successful treatment of urticaria requires careful pattern differentiation.

INTERNAL

Wind-cold. Wheals are itchy and pale or slightly red. Upon exposure to cold, the condition is either produced or exacerbated. Often, mere washing of hands with cold water, or exposure to cool or cold wind, will bring on urticaria. Warmth relieves the condition. Typically, it worsens during cold weather and improves during the warmer months. Generalized symptoms may include an aversion to cold, an elevated temperature, absence of perspiration and thirst, generalized pain, a pale tongue with a thin white coating, and a pulse that is floating and tight, or slow and moderate. The treatment strategy for the initial attack is to dispel wind and scatter cold, and regulate and harmonize the protective and nutritive levels. The formula recommended for this pattern is Modified Schizonepeta and Ledebouriella Powder to Overcome Toxin.

❧ Modified Schizonepeta and Ledebouriella Powder to Overcome Toxin
荆防败毒散加减
jīng fáng bài dú sǎn jiā jiǎn

Herba seu Flos Schizonepetae Tenuifoliae *(jing jie)*	4.5g
Radix Ledebouriellae Divaricatae *(fang feng)*	4.5g
Ramulus Cinnamomi Cassiae *(gui zhi)*	4.5g
Herba Ephedrae *(ma huang)*	4.5g
Radix Paeoniae Lactiflorae *(bai shao)*	4.5g
Radix Gentianae Qinjiao *(qin jiao)*	4.5g
Cortex Dictamni Dasycarpi Radicis *(bai xian pi)*	4.5g
Rhizoma Zingiberis Officinalis Recens *(sheng jiang)*	3 pieces
Herba Lemnae seu Spirodelae *(fu ping)*	4.5g
Radix Glycyrrhizae Uralensis *(gan cao)*	1.5g

PREPARATION & DOSAGE: Decoct and administer in a single dose daily. The decoction should be sipped slowly after a meal.

For recurrent conditions of this pattern, the strategy is to stabilize the protective level so that cold will be resisted. The recommended formula is Jade Windscreen Powder plus Modified Cinnamon Twig Decoction [A].

🌸 Jade Windscreen Powder
玉屏风散
yù píng fēng sǎn

Radix Astragali Membranacei *(huang qi)*	30g
Rhizoma Atractylodis Macrocephalae *(bai zhu)*	60g
Radix Ledebouriellae Divaricatae *(fang feng)*	60g

PREPARATION & DOSAGE: Grind the ingredients into a fine powder. Administer 9g daily as a draft. Then administer Modified Cinnamon Twig Decoction [A]. (This is Modified Schizonepeta and Ledebouriella Powder to Overcome Toxin, as described above, minus Herba Ephedrae *[ma huang]*).

Wind-heat. Wheals are red and extremely itchy, and are markedly raised above the skin. The lesions are warm to the touch. Warmth or heat either bring on or exacerbate the condition, and cool or cold environments relieve it. Generalized symptoms may include headache, slight fever, sore throat, restlessness, thirst, dry stools, a red tongue with a white or yellow coating, and a floating, slippery and rapid pulse. The treatment strategy is to dispel wind and clear heat. Initial attacks may be treated with Modified Honeysuckle and Forsythia Powder [B].

🌸 Modified Honeysuckle and Forsythia Powder [B]
银翘散加减
yín qiáo sǎn jiā jiǎn

Flos Lonicerae Japonicae *(jin yin hua)*	12g
Fructus Forsythiae Suspensae *(lian qiao)*	12g
Dry-fried Fructus Arctii Lappae *(chao niu bang zi)*	10g
Folium Daqingye *(da qing ye)*	10g
Radix Rehmanniae Glutinosae *(sheng di huang)*	10g
Herba seu Flos Schizonepetae Tenuifoliae *(jing jie)*	6g
Radix Ledebouriellae Divaricatae *(fang feng)*	6g
Dry-fried Cortex Moutan Radicis *(chao mu dan pi)*	6g
Radix Glycyrrhizae Uralensis *(gan cao)*	6g

PREPARATION & DOSAGE: Decoct and administer in two doses daily.

MODIFICATIONS: For protracted cases, modify as follows: for dry stools, increase the dosage of Radix Rehmanniae Glutinosae *(sheng di huang)*; for pain and swelling of the throat, add Radix Isatidis seu Baphicacanthi *(ban lan gen)* and Radix Sophorae Tonkinensis *(shan dou gen)*; for restlessness, add Cortex Lycii Radicis *(di gu pi)*, Concha Margaritaferae *(zhen zhu mu)* and Concha Ostreae *(mu li)*; for recalcitrant cases, administer powdered Lumbricus *(di long)* separately.

Wind-dampness. Wheals are pale and often edematous; bullas may occur in severe cases. Onset is precipitated by damp and humid conditions. The tongue is pale and covered by a thin, white, sticky coating. The pulse is wiry and slippery. The treatment strategy is to strengthen the Spleen and overcome dampness, and dispel wind and stop the itching. The formula recommended for this pattern is Modified Calm the Stomach Powder.

❧ Modified Calm the Stomach Powder
平胃散加减
píng wèi sǎn jiā jiǎn

Rhizoma Atractylodis *(cang zhu)*	12-15g
Rhizoma Atractylodis Macrocephalae *(bai zhu)*	12-15g
Cortex Magnoliae Officinalis *(hou po)*	9-12g
Pericarpium Citri Reticulatae *(chen pi)*	9-12g
Sclerotium Poriae Cocos Rubrae *(chi fu ling)*	6-9g
Rhizome Alismatis Orientalis *(ze xie)*	6-9g
Radix Ledebouriellae Divaricatae *(fang feng)*	6-9g
Fructus Xanthii Sibirici *(cang er zi)*	6-9g
Radix Sophorae Flavescentis *(ku shen)*	6-9g
Radix Glycyrrhizae Uralensis *(gan cao)*	3-6g

PREPARATION & DOSAGE: Decoct and administer in a single dose daily.

Spleen/Stomach dysfunction. Wheals are pale red and large, resembling clouds. Individuals with Spleen/Stomach qi stagnation often suffer nausea and vomiting, and abdominal pain and distention during urticaria outbreaks; the tongue is pale with a white coating. Individuals with intestinal parasitosis have tongues with white spots. Cases presenting with accumulated cold of the Spleen/Stomach suffer recurrent urticaria and generalized symptoms of aversion to cold, cold limbs, discomfort in the stomach region, disturbed appetite, weariness, abdominal pain and daybreak diarrhea, absence of thirst, a pale tongue with white coating, and a submerged, slow and thin pulse. The strategy is to strengthen the Spleen and harmonize the Stomach, and dispel wind and stop the itching. The recommended formula for this pattern is Modified Immature Bitter Orange and Atractylodes Macrocephala Powder.

❧ Modified Immature Bitter Orange and Atractylodes Macrocephala Powder
枳术散加减
zhǐ zhú sǎn jiā jiǎn

Dry-fried Fructus Citri seu Ponciri Immaturus *(chao zhi shi)*	6g
Fructus Amomi *(sha ren)* (add last)	6g
Pericarpium Citri Reticulatae *(chen pi)*	6g

Herba seu Flos Schizonepetae Tenuifoliae *(jing jie)* 6g
Radix Ledebouriellae Divaricatae *(fang feng)* 6g
Dry-fried Rhizoma Atractylodis Macrocephalae *(chao bai zhu)* 10g
Rhizoma Cyperi Rotundi *(xiang fu)* 10g
Radix Linderae Strychnifoliae *(wu yao)* 10g
Radix Aucklandiae Lappae *(mu xiang)* 10g

PREPARATION & DOSAGE: Decoct and administer in two doses daily.

For cases with intestinal parasites, the strategy is to reduce parasite accumulation and support the Spleen. The formula recommended for this pattern is Modified Six-Gentleman Decoction with Aucklandia and Amomum.

❦ Modified Six-Gentleman Decoction with Aucklandia and Amomum
香砂六君子汤加减
xiāng shā liū jūn zǐ tāng jiā jiǎn

Rhizoma Cyperi Rotundi *(xiang fu)* 6g
Fructus Amomi *(sha ren)* (add last) 6g
Ginger-prepared Rhizoma Pinelliae Ternatae *(jiang ban xia)* 6g
Fructus Pruni Mume *(wu mei)* 6g
Radix Codonopsitis Pilosulae *(dang shen)* 10g
Rhizoma Atractylodis Macrocephalae *(bai zhu)* 10g
Pericarpium Citri Reticulatae *(chen pi)* 10g
Sclerotium Poriae Cocos *(fu ling)* 10g
Massa Fermentata *(shen qu)* 10g
Fructus Crataegi *(shan zha)* 10g
Radix Glycyrrhizae Uralensis *(gan cao)* 4.5g

PREPARATION & DOSAGE: Decoct and administer in two doses daily.

For cases with deficiency cold patterns, the strategy is to warm the middle and strengthen the Spleen, and regulate and harmonize the protective and nutritive levels. The formula recommended for this pattern is Modified Prepared Aconite Decoction to Regulate the Middle Plus Modified Cinnamon Twig Decoction.

❦ Modified Prepared Aconite Decoction to Regulate the Middle Plus Modified Cinnamon Twig Decoction
附子理中汤加桂枝汤加减
fù zǐ lǐ zhōng tāng jiā guì zhī tāng jiā jiǎn

Radix Lateralis Aconiti Carmichaeli Praeparata *(fu zi)* 9g
Rhizoma Zingiberis Officinalis *(gan jiang)* 9g
Radix Codonopsitis Pilosulae *(dang shen)* 9g

Charred Rhizoma Atractylodis Macrocephalae *(bai zhu tan)* 9g
Honey-toasted Radix Glycyrrhizae Uralensis *(zhi gan cao)* 9g
Ramulus Cinnamomi Cassiae *(gui zhi)* 9g
Dry-fried Radix Paeoniae Lactiflorae *(chao bai shao)* 9g
Sclerotium Poriae Cocos *(fu ling)* 9g
Fructus Pruni Mume *(wu mei)* 6g
Radix Ledebouriellae Divaricatae *(fang feng)* 9g

PREPARATION & DOSAGE: Decoct and administer in two doses daily.

CLINICAL NOTE: To reduce its toxicity, Radix Lateralis Aconiti Carmichaeli Praeparata *(fu zi)* should be boiled for 30-60 minutes before adding the other ingredients.

Blood heat. At onset the patient has a sensation of burning and prickly itching. Lesions are bright red, and scratching results in linear wheal and flare reactions (also known as dermographism or "write-on-skin"). The condition is worse at night. Generalized symptoms include restlessness, dry mouth and thirst with a desire to drink, canker sores, a red tongue without coating, and a wiry, slippery and rapid pulse. The strategy is to cool the blood and clear heat, and eliminate wind and stop the itching. The formula recommended for this pattern is Modified Eliminate Wind Powder [B].

❦ Modified Eliminate Wind Powder [B]
消风散加减
xiāo fēng săn jiā jiăn

Radix Ledebouriellae Divaricatae *(fang feng)* 4.5g
Radix Rehmanniae Glutinosae *(sheng di huang)* 9g
Radix Angelicae Sinensis *(dang gui)* 6g
Radix Sophorae Flavescentis *(ku shen)* 3g
Rhizoma Atractylodis *(cang zhu)* 3g
Periostracum Cicadae *(chan tui)* 3g
Radix Salviae Miltiorrhizae *(dan shen)* 3g
Fructus Arctii Lappae *(niu bang zi)* 3g
Rhizoma Anemarrhenae Asphodeloidis *(zhi mu)* 3g
Gypsum *(shi gao)* 6g
Semen Sesami Indici *(hei zhi ma)* 3g
Radix Glycyrrhizae Uralensis *(gan cao)* 3g

PREPARATION & DOSAGE: Decoct and administer in two doses daily.

Blood deficiency. This type of urticaria is often seen in the elderly and in individuals recovering from long illnesses. The wheals are pale red, and the condition is worse during the night and when the individual is tired. Generalized symptoms include a pale tongue with a very thin or nonexistent coating, and a wiry, thin pulse. The strategy is to extinguish wind and anchor the yang. The formula recommended for this pattern is Augmented Four-Substance Decoction.

❧ Augmented Four-Substance Decoction
四物汤加味
sì wù tāng jiā wèi

Radix Angelicae Sinensis *(dang gui)*	9g
Radix Rehmanniae Glutinosae *(sheng di huang)*	9g
Radix Paeoniae Lactiflorae *(bai shao)*	9g
Radix Ligustici Chuanxiong *(chuan xiong)*	3g
Radix Polygoni Multiflori *(he shou wu)*	6g
Herba seu Flos Schizonepetae Tenuifoliae *(jing jie)*	6g
Radix Ledebouriellae Divaricatae *(fang feng)*	6g
Fructus Tribuli Terrestris *(bai ji li)*	9g
Radix Astragali Membranacei *(huang qi)*	6g
Radix Glycyrrhizae Uralensis *(gan cao)*	3g
Os Draconis *(long gu)*	3g
Concha Ostreae *(mu li)*	3g

PREPARATION & DOSAGE: Decoct and administer in two doses daily.

Disharmony between the penetrating and conception vessels. The lesions appear about 2-3 days prior to menstruation and disappear after the flow stops. The lower abdomen, lower back and yin aspects of the thighs are primarily affected. Women with this pattern often suffer menstrual cramps, irregular periods, a purple tongue with no coating, and a wiry, thin pulse. The strategy is to adjust the penetrating and conception channels. The formula recommended for this pattern is Modified Two-Immortal Decoction [A].

❧ Modified Two-Immortal Decoction [A]
二仙汤加减
èr xiān tāng jiā jiǎn

Rhizoma Curculiginis Orchioidis *(xian mao)*	6g
Radix Angelicae Sinensis *(dang gui)*	6g
Radix Ligustici Chuanxiong *(chuan xiong)*	6g
Herba Epimedii *(yin yang huo)*	12g
Radix Rehmanniae Glutinosae *(sheng di huang)*	12g
Radix Rehmanniae Glutinosae Conquitae *(shu di huang)*	12g
Semen Cuscutae Chinensis *(tu si zi)*	12g
Fructus Lycii *(gou qi zi)*	12g
Fructus Ligustri Lucidi *(nu zhen zi)*	12g
Herba Ecliptae Prostratae *(han lian cao)*	12g
Dry-fried Cortex Moutan Radicis *(chao mu dan pi)*	10g

Herba Leonuri Heterophylli *(yi mu cao)* 10g

PREPARATION & DOSAGE: Decoct and administer in 1-2 doses daily.

EXTERNAL

For all patterns, itching may be relieved by decocting together 2-3 of any of the following herbs in equal amounts, and then using the warm decoction as a wash: Herba Artemisiae Yinchenhao *(yin chen hao)*, Radix Sophorae Flavescentis *(ku shen)*, Lignum Sappan *(su mu)*, Fructus Xanthii Sibirici *(cang er zi)*, Herba Lemnae seu Spirodelae *(fu ping)* and Radix Clematidis *(wei ling xian)*. Apply 3-5 times daily until the wheals resolve.

ACUPUNCTURE

Filiform needling . The primary acupoints are LI-11 *(qu chi)*, LI-4 *(he gu)*, SP-10 *(xue hai)*, BL-40 *(wei zhong)*, BL-17 *(ge shu)* and TB-10 *(tian jing)*. For nausea and vomiting, add PC-6 *(nei guan)*; for abdominal pain, add ST-25 *(tian shu)*; for menstrual cramps and irregularity, add SP-6 *(san yin jiao)*. Use draining manipulation, and retain the needles for 15 minutes. Treat once daily during acute attacks, and 1-2 times per week thereafter in order to control and eventually resolve the condition.

Ear acupuncture. Recommended acupoints include Lung, Spleen, Shenmen, Stop Wheezing and Occiput. Needle 2-3 points during each session, and retain needles for 20-30 minutes. Treatment regimen is the same as above.

Bloodletting. Bloodletting may be performed on the following points: Ear Apex, M-UE-1 *(shi xuan)* or M-LE-12 *(qi duan)*. Treat once daily during an acute outbreak, until the lesions resolve. At each session, bloodlet only one pair of points, squeezing 2-3 drops from each point.

MOXIBUSTION

Moxa roll, direct or warming needle moxibustion may be applied to the same acupoints as indicated under filiform needling above. Treat for 15 minutes, once daily, until the lesions disappear.

CUPPING

Cupping may be performed on two sets of points: [A] GV-14 *(da zhui)*, BL-12 *(feng men)* and BL-18 *(gan shu)*; [B] GV-12 *(shen zhu)*, BL-13 *(fei shu)* and BL-20 *(pi shu)*. Treat once daily or every other day, alternating the point sets. Cupping may be applied alone or in combination with acupuncture.

EMPIRICAL REMEDIES

[A] For urticaria due to wind-heat, combine 3g Herba Menthae Haplocalycis *(bo he)* and 3g Periostracum Cicadae *(chan tui)* with 350ml of water and 150ml of rice wine, and decoct for 5 minutes. Administer 2-3 times daily, or until the wheals resolve.[1]

[B] Large areas of urticarial wheals due to heat may be washed with a decoction of 250g of fresh wintermelon skin. Administer 4-5 times daily, or until the wheals resolve.[2]

[C] Decoct 500g of mashed fresh Japanese star fruit (Fructus Averrhoae Carambolae, *yáng táo)*. Wash the affected areas for 5-10 minutes with the decoction, three times daily, until the hives resolve.[3]

[D] Mash one whole grapefruit (with skin), the more sour the better, and then decoct for 10 minutes. Wash the affected areas for 10 minutes with the decoction, three times daily. While using this external remedy, the patient should eat 60g of fresh grapefruit, three times daily, until the lesions disappear.[4]

Traditional vs. Biomedical Treatment

Acute urticaria is generally self-limiting, and treatment is chiefly palliative. With chronic urticaria, treatment may be more complicated and requires close practitioner-patient cooperation in order to successfully manage the condition. In all cases of urticaria, when the cause is known, it should be avoided or treated.

Traditional treatment may be more effective in resolving the root of the condition, especially for chronic urticaria. Biomedical intervention usually involves administration of antihistamines and corticosteroids, which ordinarily address the immediate reaction, but they may not resolve the root problem.

Prevention

Elimination or avoidance of the causative agent is the best prevention. A correct pattern differentiation and appropriate traditional therapy can help prevent future attacks. Individuals prone to damp-heat accumulation should either moderate their intake or abstain from certain foods and beverages, such as spicy and greasy foods, sweets, lamb, capon, shrimp, alcohol and coffee.

CHAPTER NOTES

1. Ye, J.Q. *Traditional Chinese Food Medicinals and Folk Prescriptions (Shi wu zhong yao yu pian fang)*. Jiangsu: Jiangsu Science and Technology Press, 1980.
2. Dou, G.X. *Guide to Food Therapy (Yin shi zhi liao zhi nan)*. Jiangsu: Jiangsu Science and Technology Press, 1981.
3. Dai, Y.F. and Liu, C.J. *Medicinal Uses of Fruits (Yao yong guo pin)*. Nanning: Guangxi People's Publishing House, 1982.
4. Ibid.

CHAPTER 15

Scaling Disorders

Psoriasis
银屑病
yín xiè bìng, "silver scale disease"

Psoriasis is a chronic, recurrent disease marked by thickened patches of inflamed, red skin, frequently covered by silvery scales. Through the ages the Chinese have referred to this condition by many names: "white dagger sore" *(bái bǐ),* "pine skin tinea" *(sōng pí xuǎn)* and "snake lice" *(shé shī),* among others. *Golden Mirror of the Medical Tradition* (1742) provides the following description of one of the causes of psoriasis: "White dagger sore . . . is caused by pathogenic wind lodging in the tissue and skin, and also by blood dryness [making it] difficult to nourish the exterior."

The biomedical cause of psoriasis is unknown. There appears to be a genetic predisposition that may be related to a defect in the production of the epidermal layer of the skin. New skin cells are formed about ten times faster than normal, but the rate at which old cells are shed remains the same. Thus, live cells accumulate and form the characteristic thickened patches covered with dead, flaking cells. Caucasions seem to be more affected than other races. The condition typically recurs in flare-ups which may be precipitated by such factors as illness, emotional stress, and skin damage.

Signs & Symptoms

Onset of psoriasis is often slow. Sites typically affected include the scalp, elbows, knees, palms and soles, back, and buttocks. In about one-third of cases, the nails are involved. Lesions are characteristically round, well-demarcated, pink, scaling plaques of various sizes covered with large, adherent, silver scales. When the nails are affected, pitting of their surface is common.

Psoriatic arthritis affects about five percent of psoriasis patients, with the psoriasis preceding or following joint inflammation. Pustular psoriasis occurs following a sudden onset of high fever; the sterile pustules can be found on the palms and soles, or over the entire skin. Guttate psoriasis ordinarily affects children and may appear immediately after an upper respiratory tract infection or streptococcal pharyngitis; the lesions are characterized by small, red, drop-like papules covered by fine scales, spread over the entire body. Erythroderma psoriaticum is a rare form of psoriasis characterized by diffuse redness of the skin, covered by fine scales; intractable cases can be debilitating.

Differential Diagnosis

The diagnosis of psoriasis is usually obvious. However, the many different sizes and shapes of lesions may be misleading, and skin biopsy may be necessary to confirm the diagnosis. Skin diseases that may be confused with psoriasis include seborrheic dermatitis, secondary syphilis, fungal infections and eczema. But in psoriasis, traumatic removal of the superficial scales will typically reveal tiny bleeding points, known as Auspitz's sign.

Traditional Chinese Etiology

The causal basis of psoriasis is pre-existing deficiency at the nutritive and blood levels that provokes wind and dryness, such that the skin loses its nourishment. In early psoriasis, attack by wind-cold or wind-heat may also be involved, causing disharmony between the protective and nutritive levels, and disrupting the flow of qi and blood so that the pathogenic factors become lodged in the tissue and skin. Or, pre-existing damp-heat may smoulder and accumulate in the tissue and skin, thus causing the lesions. As the disease progresses, wind-cold, wind-heat or damp-heat transform into heat, consuming and injuring the qi and blood, such that blood deficiency and wind-dryness (blood dryness) result and exacerbate the condition.

Another possible result of deficiency at the nutritive and blood levels is impeded flow of qi and blood, which leads to stagnation in the tissue and skin, thus forming the lesions.

As the condition becomes more protracted, patterns of Organ dysfunction emerge. In psoriasis, the Liver and Kidney are particularly affected, such that insufficiency of these two Organs results in disharmony between the penetrating channel and conception vessel, leading to even more pronounced deficiency at the nutritive and blood levels.

The fire or heat toxin type of psoriasis results from the following causes: unresolved emotional disturbance transforming into fire; attack by heat toxin; or wind-cold or dampness transforming into heat, and then dryness, to form dry-heat, which then transforms into toxin. The heat toxin wanders about and enters the nutritive and blood levels, and into the Organs, such that the qi and blood, especially in the tissue and skin, contend, thus producing the lesions.

The blood heat pattern usually results from heat in the Heart and/or Liver channels, which may be caused by emotional disturbance. As the heat accumulates, it enters the blood level, and sears the tissue and skin, thus producing psoriatic lesions.

Treatment

Successful management of psoriasis entails meticulous pattern differentiation and patience during treatment, which may be lengthy for chronic cases.

INTERNAL

The major patterns of psoriasis and their treatments are described below.

Wind-cold. This type is usually seen in children, early cases, or in psoriatic arthritis. The lesions are pale red, and the scales are white and thick, and easily shed upon scratching; itching is minimal. The condition recurs or is exacerbated during winter, and improves or disappears altogether during summer. Generalized symptoms may include aversion to cold, joint soreness or pain, a pale tongue with a thin coating, and a soggy, slippery pulse. The strategy is to dispel wind and scatter cold, and nourish the blood and moisten dryness. The formula recommended for this pattern is Modified Cinnamon Twig Decoction [B].

❦ Modified Cinnamon Twig Decoction [B]
桂枝汤加减
guì zhī tāng jiā jiǎn

Ramulus Cinnamomi Cassiae *(gui zhi)*	3g
Radix Glycyrrhizae Uralensis *(gan cao)*	3g
Radix et Rhizoma Notopterygii *(qiang huo)*	3g
Radix Ledebouriellae Divaricatae *(fang feng)*	3g
Radix Paeoniae Rubrae *(chi shao)*	12g
Radix Angelicae Sinensis *(dang gui)*	12g
Cortex Dictamni Dasycarpi Radicis *(bai xian pi)*	12g
Radix Ligustici Chuanxiong *(chuan xiong)*	6g
Herba Ephedrae *(ma huang)*	6g
Semen Pruni Armeniacae *(xing ren)*	6g

PREPARATION & DOSAGE: Decoct and administer in three doses daily.

Blood heat. The lesions of this pattern are red macules or papules that increase and proliferate rapidly. The scales are heaped up, and are easily shed when scratched. Itching is sometimes intense. The condition is more severe during the summer. Generalized symptoms may include aversion to heat, restlessness, thirst, dry stools, yellow and scanty urine, a red tongue with a thin yellow or white coating, and a slippery, rapid pulse. The strategy is to clear the nutritive level and cool the blood, and relieve toxin and reduce spots.

Formulas recommended for this pattern include Cool the Blood and Eliminate Wind Powder (see seborrheic dermatitis in Chapter 13), or Modified Rhinoceros Horn and Rehmannia Decoction [B].

❦ Modified Rhinoceros Horn and Rehmannia Decoction [B]
犀角地黄汤加减
xī jiǎo dì huáng tāng jiā jiǎn

Cornu Rhinoceri *(xi jiao)*	1.5g
Radix Rehmanniae Glutinosae *(sheng di huang)*	30g
Dry-fried Cortex Moutan Radicis *(chao mu dan pi)*	10g
Radix Paeoniae Rubrae *(chi shao)*	10g
Radix Arnebiae seu Lithospermi *(zi cao)*	10g
Flos Carthami Tinctorii *(hong hua)*	10g
Charred Flos Lonicerae Japonicae *(jin yin hua tan)*	15g
Radix Sanguisorbae Officinalis *(di yu)*	15g
Gypsum *(shi gao)*	15g
Calcitum *(han shui shi)*	15g
Radix Adenophorae seu Glehniae *(sha shen)*	10g
Tuber Ophiopogonis Japonici *(mai men dong)*	10g
Radix Scrophulariae Ningpoensis *(xuan shen)*	10g

PREPARATION & DOSAGE: Decoct and administer in three doses daily.

CLINICAL NOTE: Ten times the amount of Cornu Bubali *(shui niu jiao)* is usually substituted for the Cornu Rhinoceri *(xi jiao)*, both due to expense and the fact that all species of rhinoceros are endangered.

Blood dryness. Psoriatic lesions of this pattern are usually pale red macules that are moist and covered by a thin layer of tightly adhering scales. The course of disease is slow, with new lesions appearing sporadically. Generalized symptoms may include light-headedness, pallor, a pale tongue with a thin white coating, and a soggy, thin pulse. The strategy is to nourish the blood and dispel wind, and moisten dryness. Formulas recommended for this pattern include Modified Nourish the Blood and Moisten the Skin Decoction, or Overcome Psoriasis Formula.

❦ Modified Nourish the Blood and Moisten the Skin Decoction
养血润肤饮加减
yǎng xuè rùn fū yǐn jiā jiǎn

Radix Rehmanniae Glutinosae *(sheng di huang)*	15g
Radix Rehmanniae Glutinosae Conquitae *(shu di huang)*	15g
Tuber Asparagi Cochinchinensis *(tian men dong)*	10g
Tuber Ophiopogonis Japonici *(mai men dong)*	10g
Radix Scrophulariae Ningpoensis *(xuan shen)*	10g
Radix Polygoni Multiflori *(he shou wu)*	10g
Ramulus cum Uncis Uncariae *(gou teng)*	10g
Radix Angelicae Sinensis *(dang gui)*	10g
Radix Adenophorae seu Glehniae *(sha shen)*	12g

Radix Trichosanthis Kirilowii *(tian hua fen)*	12g
Semen Phaseoli Calcarati *(chi xiao dou)*	12g
Dry-fried Radix Paeoniae Lactiflorae *(chao bai shao)*	12g

PREPARATION & DOSAGE: Decoct and administer in 2-3 doses daily.

❧ Overcome Psoriasis Formula
克银方
kè yín fāng

Radix Rehmanniae Glutinosae *(sheng di huang)*	30g
Radix Scrophulariae Ningpoensis *(xuan shen)*	30g
Semen Cannabis Sativae *(huo ma ren)*	10g
Rhizoma Menispermi Daurici *(bian fu ge gen)*	10g
Radix Sophorae Flavescentis *(ku shen)*	10g

PREPARATION & DOSAGE: Decoct and administer in 1-2 doses daily.

Blood stasis. Cases are usually chronic and recurrent. The lesions are dark or hyperpigmented and covered by thick, hard and adherent scales. Occasionally, lichenification has developed. Longstanding lesions may overlap, causing the skin to take on a map-like appearance. Sometimes these large lesions may be affected by pain and/or fissures. The tongue is often purple or has purple spots, and is covered by a thin coating, and the pulse is generally choppy or thin and slow. The strategy is to invigorate the blood and scatter stasis.

Formulas recommended for this pattern include Invigorate the Blood and Scatter Stasis Decoction, or White Dagger Sore Decoction.

❧ Invigorate the Blood and Scatter Stasis Decoction
活血散瘀汤
huó xuè sàn yū tāng

Lignum Sappan *(su mu)*	9-15g
Radix Paeoniae Rubrae *(chi shao)*	9-15g
Radix Paeoniae Lactiflorae *(bai shao)*	9-15g
Flos Carthami Tinctorii *(hong hua)*	9-15g
Semen Persicae *(tao ren)*	9-15g
Herba Buchnerae Cruciatae *(guǐ yǔ jiān)*	15-30g
Rhizoma Sparganii Stoloniferi *(san leng)*	9-15g
Rhizoma Curcumae Ezhu *(e zhu)*	9-15g
Radix Aucklandiae Lappae *(mu xiang)*	3-9g
Pericarpium Citri Reticulatae *(chen pi)*	9-15g

PREPARATION & DOSAGE: Decoct and administer in 1-2 doses daily.

❧ White Dagger Sore Decoction
白疕汤
bái bǐ tāng

Radix Rehmanniae Glutinosae *(sheng di huang)* 30g
Radix Angelicae Sinensis *(dang gui)* 15g
Rhizoma Smilacis Glabrae *(tu fu ling)* 25g
Radix Paeoniae Rubrae *(chi shao)* 15g
Radix Salviae Miltiorrhizae *(dan shen)* 20g
Herba cum Radice Violae Yedoensitis *(zi hua di ding)* 20g
Fructus Forsythiae Suspensae *(lian qiao)* 15g
Radix Scrophulariae Ningpoensis *(xuan shen)* 20g
Semen Cannabis Sativae *(huo ma ren)* 15g
Cortex Dictamni Dasycarpi Radicis *(bai xian pi)* 20g
Rhizoma Curcumae Ezhu *(e zhu)* 20g

PREPARATION & DOSAGE: Decoct and administer in 1-2 doses daily.

Damp-heat. Lesions of this type of psoriasis are typically dark red macules of uneven size, covered by greasy or thick, crust-like scales. The skin below the scales may be moist, or show weeping of exudate. Pustules may be present in some cases. The sites affected are the palms and soles, trunk, extremities and skin folds. The condition is worse in humid environments. Generalized symptoms may include an oppressive sensation in the chest, disturbed appetite, malaise, heaviness of the lower extremities, increased vaginal discharge, a thin, yellow, sticky tongue coating, and a soggy, slippery pulse. The strategy is to clear heat and drain dampness. The formula recommended for this pattern is Modified Dioscorea Decoction to Leach Out Dampness [A].

❧ Modified Dioscorea Decoction to Leach Out Dampness [A]
萆薢渗湿汤加减
bèi xiè shèn shī tāng jiā jiǎn

Rhizoma Atractylodis *(cang zhu)* 10g
Cortex Phellodendri *(huang bai)* 10g
Herba Lycopi Lucidi *(ze lan)* 10g
Sclerotium Polypori Umbellati *(zhu ling)* 10g
Rhizoma Dioscoreae Hypoglaucae *(bei xie)* 15g
Semen Coicis Lachryma-jobi *(yi yi ren)* 15g
Radix Salviae Miltiorrhizae *(dan shen)* 15g
Ramus Lonicerae Japonicae *(ren dong teng)* 30g
Rhizoma Smilacis Glabrae *(tu fu ling)* 30g
Herba Taraxaci Mongolici cum Radice *(pu gong ying)* 30g
Fructus Liquidambaris Taiwanianae *(lu lu tong)* 4.5g
Radix Cyathulae Officinalis *(chuan niu xi)* 4.5g
Pericarpium Citri Reticulatae Viride *(qing pi)* 4.5g

PREPARATION & DOSAGE: Decoct and administer in 2-3 doses daily.

Fire or heat toxin. The erythematous or pustular lesions of this pattern develop and spread swiftly, often coalescing together. They are covered by fine scales that shed easily. Itching, burning and pain are usually present. Generalized symptoms may include high fever, thirst, dry stools, yellow urine, a scarlet tongue with a thin coating, and a wiry, slippery and rapid pulse. The strategy is to cool the blood, clear heat, and relieve toxin.

Formulas recommended for this pattern include Combined Coptis Decoction to Relieve Toxin and Five-Ingredient Decoction to Eliminate Toxin, or Rehmannia and Scrophularia Decoction.

❧ Combined Coptis Decoction to Relieve Toxin and Five-Ingredient Decoction to Eliminate Toxin
黄连解毒汤五味消毒饮化裁
huáng lián jiě dú tāng wǔ wèi xiāo dú yǐn huà cái

Herba Taraxaci Mongolici cum Radice *(pu gong ying)*	15g
Flos Lonicerae Japonicae *(jin yin hua)*	15g
Herba cum Radice Violae Yedoensitis *(zi hua di ding)*	15g
Rhizoma Coptidis *(huang lian)*	6g
Radix Scutellariae Baicalensis *(huang qin)*	6g
Cortex Phellodendri *(huang bai)*	6g
Charred Fructus Gardeniae Jasminoidis *(zhi zi tan)*	6g
Radix Rehmanniae Glutinosae *(sheng di huang)*	10g
Radix Paeoniae Rubrae *(chi shao)*	10g

PREPARATION & DOSAGE: Decoct and administer in 1-2 doses daily.

❧ Rehmannia and Scrophularia Decoction
生玄饮
shēng xuán yǐn

Radix Rehmanniae Glutinosae *(sheng di huang)*	15g
Radix Scrophulariae Ningpoensis *(xuan shen)*	15g
Fructus Gardeniae Jasminoidis *(zhi zi)*	15g
Radix Isatidis seu Baphicacanthi *(ban lan gen)*	15g
Herba Taraxaci Mongolici cum Radice *(pu gong ying)*	10g
Flos Chrysanthemi Indici *(ye ju hua)*	10g
Radix Platycodi Grandiflori *(jie geng)*	10g
Radix Angelicae Sinensis *(dang gui)*	10g
Radix Paeoniae Rubrae *(chi shao)*	10g
Radix Trichosanthis Kirilowii *(tian hua fen)*	10g
Bulbus Fritillariae Cirrhosae *(chuan bei mu)*	12g
Rhizoma Smilacis Glabrae *(tu fu ling)*	12g
Herba cum Radice Violae Yedoensitis *(zi hua di ding)*	12g
Radix Glycyrrhizae Uralensis *(gan cao)*	6g

PREPARATION & DOSAGE: Decoct and administer in 1-2 doses daily.

For heat toxin patterns that produce pustular lesions, the strategy is to clear heat and relieve toxin, and support the interior and drain pus. Modified Gentiana Longdancao Decoction to Drain the Liver is recommended for this pattern.

🍃 Modified Gentiana Longdancao Decoction to Drain the Liver
龙胆泻肝汤加减
lóng dǎn xiè gān tāng jiā jiǎn

Flos Lonicerae Japonicae *(jin yin hua)*	30g
Testa Phaseoli Radiati *(lu dou yi)*	30g
Radix Rehmanniae Glutinosae *(sheng di huang)*	10g
Fructus Forsythiae Suspensae *(lian qiao)*	10g
Herba Taraxaci Mongolici cum Radice *(pu gong ying)*	10g
Flos Chrysanthemi Indici *(ye ju hua)*	10g
Radix Astragali Membranacei *(huang qi)*	10g
Semen Coicis Lachryma-jobi *(yi yi ren)*	12g
Cortex Dictamni Dasycarpi Radicis *(bai xian pi)*	12g
Radix Angelicae Sinensis *(dang gui)*	12g
Radix Paeoniae Rubrae *(chi shao)*	12g
Radix Scutellariae Baicalensis *(huang qin)*	6g
Rhizoma Coptidis *(huang lian)*	6g
Radix Glycyrrhizae Uralensis *(gan cao)*	6g

PREPARATION & DOSAGE: Decoct and administer in 1-2 doses daily.

Liver and Kidney insufficiency. The macular lesions of this pattern are pale red and covered by a thin layer of grayish white scales. Generalized symptoms may include soreness in the lower back, weakness of the extremities, joint pain, light-headedness, tinnitus, a fat, tooth-marked tongue with a thin coating, and a soggy, thin pulse. The strategy is to nourish the Liver and enrich the Kidney. The formula recommended for this pattern is Ophiopogon, Schisandra, and Rehmannia Decoction.

🍃 Ophiopogon, Schisandra, and Rehmannia Decoction
麦味地黄汤
mài wèi dì huáng tāng

Tuber Ophiopogonis Japonici *(mai men dong)*	10g
Radix Rehmanniae Glutinosae *(sheng di huang)*	10g
Radix Rehmanniae Glutinosae Conquitae *(shu di huang)*	10g
Fructus Corni Officinalis *(shan zhu yu)*	10g
Dry-fried Cortex Moutan Radicis *(chao mu dan pi)*	10g
Fructus Schisandrae Chinensis *(wu wei zi)*	4.5g
Rhizome Alismatis Orientalis *(ze xie)*	4.5g
Sclerotium Poriae Cocos *(fu ling)*	4.5g
Herba cum Radice Lycopodii Clavati *(shen jin cao)*	15g
Rhizoma Homalomenae Occultae *(qian nian jian)*	15g
Herba Buchnerae Cruciatae *(guǐ yǔ jiān)*	15g
Rhizoma Cibotii Barometz *(gou ji)*	15g

Ramulus cum Uncis Uncariae *(gou teng)* 15g
Radix Angelicae Sinensis *(dang gui)* 12g
Radix Salviae Miltiorrhizae *(dan shen)* 12g

PREPARATION & DOSAGE: Decoct and administer in 1-2 doses daily.

With the Liver and Kidney insufficiency pattern, individuals who present with a sub-pattern of disharmony between the penetrating and conception vessels will often suffer additional generalized symptoms such as impotence and spermatorrhea (in men), and irregular menstruation, infertility or improvement or even remission of psoriatic lesions during pregnancy followed by recurrence after giving birth (in women). The strategy is to regulate and tonify the penetrating and conception channels, and support the yang and harmonize the blood. The formula recommended for this pattern is Modified Two-Immortal Decoction [B].

Modified Two-Immortal Decoction [B]
二仙汤加减
èr xiān tāng jiā jiǎn

Rhizoma Curculiginis Orchioidis *(xian mao)* 6g
Dry-fried Rhizoma Anemarrhenae Asphodeloidis *(chao zhi mu)* 6g
Dry-fried Cortex Phellodendri *(chao huang bai)* 6g
Dry-fried Cortex Moutan Radicis *(chao mu dan pi)* 6g
Herba Epimedii *(yin yang huo)* 12g
Radix Angelicae Sinensis *(dang gui)* 12g
Radix Morindae Officinalis *(ba ji tian)* 12g
Herba Cistanches Deserticolae *(rou cong rong)* 12g
Sclerotium Poriae Cocos *(fu ling)* 10g
Semen Cuscutae Chinensis *(tu si zi)* 10g
Radix Polygoni Multiflori *(he shou wu)* 15g
Radix Salviae Miltiorrhizae *(dan shen)* 15g

PREPARATION & DOSAGE: Decoct and administer in 1-2 doses daily.

EXTERNAL

For early psoriasis or erythematous macular lesions with minimal scaling, formulas that are warming are preferred. These include Arnebia and Coptis Ointment (see diaper dermatitis in Chapter 13), or Universally Linked Ointment. The application dosage for both is 1-2 times daily.

Universally Linked Ointment
普连膏
pǔ lián gāo

Cortex Phellodendri *(huang bai)* 60g
Radix Scutellariae Baicalensis *(huang qin)* 60g
Petroleum Jelly 240g

PREPARATION & DOSAGE: Separately grind the herbal ingredients into fine powders and then sift together well. Combine with the petroleum jelly, heating slightly if necessary. Store in an airtight glass jar.

For chronic recurrent lesions with heaped up scales, use Xanthium and Kochia Wash (see folliculitis in Chapter 7), or Liquidambar Wash, 3-4 times per week.

❧ Liquidambar Wash
路路通水洗剂
lù lù tōng shuǐ xǐ jì

Fructus Liquidambaris Taiwanianae *(lu lu tong)*	60g
Rhizoma Atractylodis *(cang zhu)*	60g
Radix Stemonae *(bai bu)*	15g
Folium Artemisiae Argyi *(ai ye)*	15g
Alumen Praeparatum *(ku fan)*	15g

PREPARATION & DOSAGE: Decoct the ingredients in 1-1.5 liters of water for 20 minutes. Discard the dregs and wash the affected sites with the warm decoction 1-2 times daily.

ACUPUNCTURE

For all patterns of psoriasis needle BL-40 *(wei zhong)* bilaterally with a 28 gauge needle. Apply strong draining manipulation for 5-10 minutes, then retain the needles for an additional 5-10 minutes. Upon withdrawing the needles, squeeze 1-2 drops of blood from the opening. Treat once every other day. Ten treatments constitute one course. Improvement of symptoms should be evident after one course.

CUPPING

For all types of psoriasis the following two groups of acupoints may be used: [A] GV-14 *(da zhui)*, BL-12 *(feng men)*, BL-18 *(gan shu)*; [B] GV-12 *(shen zhu)*, BL-13 *(fei shu)*, BL-20 *(pi shu)*. Cupping may be applied alone or following acupuncture at these points. Treat once every other day. Seven treatments constitute one course. Improvement should be evident after 2-3 courses.

EMPIRICAL REMEDIES

Plum-blossom needling combined with medicinal fumigation may be utilized as described below.[1]

Combine together Folium Artemisiae Argyi *(ai ye)* floss in an amount sufficient to form a 15cm long by 2.5cm diameter roll, 10g of powdered Sulphur *(liu huang)*, 10g of powdered Radix Angelicae Dahuricae *(bai zhi)*, 10g of powdered Radix Aucklandiae Lappae *(mu xiang)*, 10g of powdered Radix Angelicae Pubescentis *(du huo)* and 1g of powdered Borneol *(bing pian)*. Form a moxa roll about 1cm long by 2.5cm in diameter.

First wash the psoriatic lesions with warm water, and disinfect with alcohol.

Gently tap the lesions with a plum-blossom needle until tiny beads of blood appear. Light the moxa roll and fumigate the lesions with the smoke by allowing the lesions to face downward while the moxa roll is held below; as the smoke rises, the lesions are fumigated. After fumigation, the ashes are sprinkled onto the lesions. Treat once daily at bedtime for 15-20 minutes. Seven days constitute one course of therapy. Improvement is usually seen within 2-3 courses.

Traditional vs. Biomedical Treatment

Successful treatment of psoriasis is difficult. Because the biomedical cause of this condition remains uncertain, the conventional view of psoriasis as an incurable disease still holds. However, traditional treatment may prove to be more effective in achieving remission as long as the correct pattern is differentiated and the suitable therapy is administered, and more importantly, if the patient complies with treatment, which is often protracted. Literature from China regarding traditional treatment of psoriasis claims a better success rate over biomedical therapy in achieving long-term remission. Biomedical therapy is still limited to topical corticosteroids, tars, anthralin, phototherapy, as well as more complex regimens. Furthermore, long-term use of some pharmaceuticals (e.g.,corticosteroids) present side effect and toxicity problems.

Prevention

Patients should avoid factors that precipitate exacerbation and recurrence of lesions. Sound nutrition should be maintained, and patients should abstain from food and beverages that can produce accumulation of heat and dampness. These include spicy and greasy foods, sweets, meats such as lamb and capon, shrimp, alcohol and coffee. Additionally, some nutritional supplements such as vitamins and minerals are warming, and should be taken in moderation, or discontinued altogether.

Pityriasis Rosea
风癣
fēng xuǎn, "wind tinea"

Pityriasis is a common self-limited skin disease characterized by scaly lesions. Other Chinese names for this disorder are "wind-heat sore" *(fēng rè chuāng)* and "mother-son tinea" *(mǔ zǐ xuǎn)*. The Chinese translation of the biomedical term, "rose-colored chaff rash" *(méi guì kāng zhěn),* is due to the rose-colored lesions and the shedding scales that resemble chaff.

The biomedical cause is unknown, although viral infection has been suspected. The condition develops abruptly, usually in the spring and autumn. Although it may occur at any age, it is seen most frequently in young adults.

Signs & Symptoms

Pityriasis rosea begins with a tinea-like "herald" or "mother" patch found most often on the trunk. This is followed several days later by multiple similar lesions that usually first appear on the trunk, later spreading to the proximal portions of the extremities. On the trunk, the long axis of the lesions follows the lines of cleavage of the skin, rendering a "Christmas tree" pattern. Generalized symptoms are usually nonexistent, although malaise and headache have been reported in rare cases. Itching of varying intensity is not uncommon. The lesions usually disappear spontaneously within six weeks. Recurrences are rare.

Differential Diagnosis

The differential includes tinea infection, drug eruptions, and psoriasis. Secondary syphilis must also be considered. Tinea infections may be ruled out by microscopic examination of material from the lesions. Drug eruptions are confirmed by a history of drug ingestion and clearing of lesions when the medication is withdrawn. In syphilis, papular lesions affect the hands and feet, whereas in pityriasis rosea these areas are usually spared. Also, *condyloma lata* and mucous patches are common in secondary syphilis. A serologic test will often confirm a diagnosis of syphilis.

Traditional Chinese Etiology

Pityriasis rosea is caused by the combination of pre-existing heat and attack by wind or wind-heat, all of which accumulate in the skin and interstices, thus producing the eruption.

Treatment

Since this disorder is self-limited, treatment is aimed at symptom amelioration and hastening involution of the eruption. The strategy is to cool the blood and disperse wind, and clear heat and relieve toxin.

INTERNAL

Several formulas may be used to relieve the symptoms of pityriasis rosea.

❦ Modified Cool the Blood and Eliminate Wind Powder
凉血消风散加减
liáng xuè xiāo fēng sǎn jiā jiǎn

Radix Rehmanniae Glutinosae *(sheng di huang)*	18g
Radix Arnebiae seu Lithospermi *(zi cao)*	12g
Dry-fired Cortex Moutan Radicis *(chao mu dan pi)*	9g
Radix Paeoniae Rubrae *(chi shao)*	9g
Radix Scutellariae Baicalensis *(huang qin)*	9g
Tuber Curcumae *(yu jin)*	9g
Charred Fructus Gardeniae Jasminoidis *(zhi zi tan)*	6g
Periostracum Cicadae *(chan tui)*	6g
Radix Glycyrrhizae Uralensis *(gan cao)*	6g
Herba seu Flos Schizonepetae Tenuifoliae *(jing jie)*	3g

PREPARATION & DOSAGE: Decoct and administer in three doses daily.

❧ Rehmannia, Gypsum, and Anemarrhena Formula
地石知方
dì shí zhī fāng

Radix Rehmanniae Glutinosae *(sheng di huang)*	15g
Gypsum *(shi gao)*	15g
Rhizoma Anemarrhenae Asphodeloidis *(zhi mu)*	9g
Radix Scrophulariae Ningpoensis *(xuan shen)*	9g
Fructus Gardeniae Jasminoidis *(zhi zi)*	9g
Radix Scutellariae Baicalensis *(huang qin)*	9g
Fructus Arctii Lappae *(niu bang zi)*	9g
Periostracum Cicadae *(chan tui)*	6g
Cortex Moutan Radicis *(mu dan pi)*	12g
Rhizome Alismatis Orientalis *(ze xie)*	9g

PREPARATION & DOSAGE: Decoct and administer in 1-2 doses daily.

❧ Arnebia and Isatis Decoction
紫板汤
zǐ bǎn tāng

Radix Arnebiae seu Lithospermi *(zi cao)*	15g
Radix Isatidis seu Baphicacanthi *(ban lan gen)*	30g

PREPARATION & DOSAGE: Decoct and administer in 1-2 doses daily.

For conditions that persist beyond six weeks, blood dryness patterns may emerge. The strategy for treating such cases is to nourish the yin and moisten dryness, and calm the Liver and extinguish wind. The formula recommended for this pattern is Modified Invigorate the Blood, Moisten Dryness, and Generate Fluids Decoction.

❧ Modified Invigorate the Blood, Moisten Dryness, and Generate Fluids Decoction
活血润燥生津汤加减
huó xuè rùn zào shēng jīn tāng jiā jiǎn

Radix Angelicae Sinensis *(dang gui)*	10g
Dry-fried Radix Paeoniae Lactiflorae *(chao bai shao)*	10g
Tuber Asparagi Cochinchinensis *(tian men dong)*	10g
Tuber Ophiopogonis Japonici *(mai men dong)*	10g
Radix Rehmanniae Glutinosae *(sheng di huang)*	15g
Radix Rehmanniae Glutinosae Conquitae *(shu di huang)*	15g
Radix Adenophorae seu Glehniae *(sha shen)*	15g
Herba Dendrobii *(shi hu)*	15g
Radix Polygoni Multiflori *(he shou wu)*	15g

Flos Carthami Tinctorii *(hong hua)* 6g
Flos Campsitis Grandiflora *(ling xiao hua)* 6g
Haematitum *(dai zhe shi)* 30g
Semen Cassiae *(jue ming zi)* 30g

PREPARATION & DOSAGE: Decoct and administer in three doses daily.

MODIFICATIONS: For severe itching, add Ramulus cum Uncis Uncariae *(gou teng)*, Radix Sophorae Flavescentis *(ku shen)*, Cortex Dictamni Dasycarpi Radicis *(bai xian pi)* and Fructus Kochiae Scopariae *(di fu zi)*; for dry stools, add dry-fried Fructus Citri Aurantii *(chao zhi ke)*, wine-fried Radix et Rhizoma Rhei *(jiu chao da huang)*, Semen Cannabis Sativae *(huo ma ren)* and Radix Platycodi Grandiflori *(jie geng)*; for lesions located primarily on the lower abdomen and inner thighs, add dry-fried Cortex Eucommiae Ulmoidis *(chao du zhong)*, Semen Coicis Lachryma-jobi *(yi yi ren)* and Ramulus Sanjisheng *(sang ji sheng)*; for lesions located primarily under the axillae and hypochondria, add Radix Bupleuri *(chai hu)* and Herba Artemisiae Annuae *(qing hao)*.

EXTERNAL

Either Three-Yellow Wash (see furuncles in Chapter 7) or Clearing and Cooling Powder (see sunburn in Chapter 12) may be applied, three times daily.

ACUPUNCTURE

The acupoints that may be needled include LI-4 *(he gu)*, LI-11 *(qu chi)*, GV-14 *(da zhui)*, LI-15 *(jian yu)*, GB-21 *(jian jing)* and ST-36 *(zu san li)*. Treat once every other day, using draining manipulation, with or without needle retention.

Traditional vs. Biomedical Treatment

Traditional treatment can be helpful in accelerating recovery. Biomedical therapy usually consists of palliative measures such as the use of antipruritic applications or systemic antihistamines.

Prevention

Pityriasis rosea is a self-limited disorder in most cases. To prevent prolonging the course of eruption, patients should abstain from foods and beverages that produce heat, such as chili pepper, garlic and onions, and alcohol.

CHAPTER NOTES

1. Song, F.R., "Plum-blossom Needling Combined with Medicinal Fumigation in the Treatment of Psoriasis," *Journal of New Chinese Medicine*, 20(1): 39; 1988.

CHAPTER 16

Autoimmune Rheumatologic Skin Diseases

Lupus erythematosus, scleroderma and dermatomyositis are systemic disorders of the skin that are associated with various autoantibodies. In the past these diseases were collectively known as collagen diseases, connective tissue diseases or collagen-vascular diseases. While each is a separate entity, combinations of the disorders can occur (as evidenced by their many shared clinical and laboratory characteristics), thus making differential diagnosis difficult. However, if followed long enough, most patients present with classic symptoms specific to one of the disorders.

Lupus Erythematosus
红斑狼疮
hóng bān láng chuāng

Lupus erythematosus is a chronic inflammatory condition of the connective tissues and appears in two forms: discoid lupus erythematosus, which affects primarily the skin, and systemic lupus erythematosus, which affects multiple organ systems (including the skin) and can be fatal. In Chinese medicine, discoid lupus erythematosus is considered a skin disease that "produces spots" *(fā bān)*. Descriptions of this condition have not been found in the classical Chinese texts. Modern names include "red butterfly" *(hóng hú dié)* and "ghost face sore" *(guǐ liǎn chuāng)*.

The biomedical cause of lupus is unknown. Exposure to sunlight often precedes the first appearance of lesions. Other factors that may play a role in etiology include genetic predisposition, certain drugs, autoimmunity, sex hormones and circulating antigen-antibody complexes. The disease is more common in females, usually affecting them in their thirties.

Signs & Symptoms

The onset of symptoms may be acute or insidious. Once the condition appears, the symptoms periodically subside and recur with varying severity. The rash begins as one or more red, circular, thickened areas of skin that may or may not later scar. The cheek bone areas and bridge of the nose ("butterfly" distribution), as well as the scalp, ear canals, and ears, are often affected, resulting in permanent loss of hair in the affected areas. As the disease progresses, the lesions exhibit follicular plugging, scarring, atrophy, hyperpigmentation, and hypopigmentation. Mild transitory systemic symptoms such as pain and reduced white cell counts are common. Individuals with widespread skin lesions often have internal manifestations, pointing to systemic lupus erythematosus. About ten percent of patients initially diagnosed with discoid lupus erythematosus develop varying degrees of systemic symptoms.

Differential Diagnosis

Clinical appearance combined with skin biopsy will determine diagnosis. Facial lesions of discoid lupus erythematosus may resemble rosacea and seborrheic dermatitis. Unlike lupus, rosacea lesions will not present with pustules. Seborrheic dermatitis frequently affects the nasolabial areas, whereas lupus rarely does. Older lesions that have left hyperpigmented scarring or areas of hair loss will also distinguish lupus from these diseases.

Traditional Chinese Etiology

Lupus erythematosus can be of two etiologies: yin deficiency and exuberant fire, in which constitutional insufficiency precipitates Kidney yin deficiency, which in turn leads to deficiency heat; and qi deficiency and blood stasis, in which stagnation of qi and blood transforms into heat. In both cases, heat then enters the blood and injures the collaterals. As the heat becomes protracted, it accumulates and smolders in the skin and tissues, thus producing the lesions.

Treatment

The biomedical treatment for discoid lupus erythematosus calls for application of local corticosteroids; in more severe cases, antimalarials are prescribed. Once traditional treatment is begun, Western medications should be slowly discontinued. Patients taking oral pharmaceuticals simultaneously with oral herbal formulas should be closely monitored, as side effects may occur from the long-term use of pharmaceuticals. If possible, the pharmaceuticals should be stopped once herbal therapy is begun.

INTERNAL

Yin deficiency and exuberant fire. This pattern is generally seen in early lupus erythematosus. The lesions are red and papular, and are usually limited in number and often scattered. Generalized symptoms may include restlessness, night sweats, insomnia, fatigue, a red tongue tip with little coating, and a thin, rapid pulse. The strategy is to nourish yin and direct fire downward, and cool the blood and clear heat.

Formulas recommended for this pattern are Nourish the Liver and Tonify the Kidney Formula, or Rehmannia Formula to Nourish the Yin and Clear Heat.

❧ Nourish the Liver and Tonify the Kidney Formula
滋肝补肾方
zī gān bǔ shèn fāng

Radix Rehmanniae Glutinosae *(sheng di huang)*	15g
Radix Rehmanniae Glutinosae Conquitae *(shu di huang)*	15g
Rhizoma Anemarrhenae Asphodeloidis *(zhi mu)*	12g
Fructus Corni Officinalis *(shan zhu yu)*	15g
Radix Scrophulariae Ningpoensis *(xuan shen)*	10g
Cortex Moutan Radicis *(mu dan pi)*	10g
Radix Paeoniae Rubrae *(chi shao)*	15g
Radix Paeoniae Lactiflorae *(bai shao)*	15g
Sclerotium Poriae Cocos *(fu ling)*	20g
Radix Achyranthis Bidentatae *(niu xi)*	10g
Herba Ecliptae Prostratae *(han lian cao)*	15g
Herba Hedyotidis Diffusae *(bai hua she she cao)*	30g
Radix Salviae Miltiorrhizae *(dan shen)*	30g

PREPARATION & DOSAGE: Decoct and administer in 2-3 doses daily.

MODIFICATIONS: For persistent low fever, add Herba Artemisiae Annuae *(qing hao)* and Cortex Lycii Radicis *(di gu pi)*; for night sweats, add Fructus Schisandrae Chinensis *(wu wei zi)* and Plumula Nelumbinis Nuciferae *(lian xin)*; for alopecia, add Radix Polygoni Multiflori *(he shou wu)*, Fructus Ligustri Lucidi *(nu zhen zi)* and Fructus Lycii *(gou qi zi)*; for lesions affecting the face and ulcers of the mouth, add Folium Hibisci Mutabilis *(mu fu rong ye)* and Flos Rosae Multiflorae (qiang wei hua); for joint pain, add Radix et Rhizoma Polygoni Cuspidati *(hu zhang)*, Radix et Caulis Jixueteng *(ji xue teng)*, Herba Leonuri Heterophylli *(yi mu cao)* and Lumbricus *(di long)*.

❧ Rehmannia Formula to Nourish the Yin and Clear Heat
生地养阴清热方
shēng dì yǎng yīn qīng rè fāng

Radix Rehmanniae Glutinosae *(sheng di huang)*	30g
Fructus Ligustri Lucidi *(nu zhen zi)*	9g
Rhizoma Polygonati *(huang jing)*	12g

Radix Dipsaci Asperi *(xu duan)*	9g
Radix Scrophulariae Ningpoensis *(xuan shen)*	30g
Cortex Phellodendri *(huang bai)*	9g
Radix Platycodi Grandiflori *(jie geng)*	4.5g
Semen Pruni Armeniacae *(xing ren)*	9g
Concha Ostreae *(mu li)*	30g
Fructus Forsythiae Suspensae *(lian qiao)*	3g
Semen Phaseoli Radiati *(lu dou)*	12g
Semen Glycine Max *(hei da dou)*	12g

PREPARATION & DOSAGE: Decoct and administer in 1-2 doses daily.

Qi deficiency and blood stasis. This pattern is usually seen in protracted cases of lupus erythematosus. The lesions are widespread, purple, and are often atrophied. Generalized symptoms may include joint pain, occasional low fever, a pale tongue with thin coating, and a thin, choppy pulse. The strategy is to augment the qi and stabilize the source (qi), and invigorate the blood and reduce spots. The formulas recommended for this pattern are either Modified Tonify the Spleen Stomach, Drain Yin Fire, and Raise the Yang Decoction, or Single-Ingredient Astragalus Formula.

❧ Modified Tonify the Spleen Stomach, Drain Yin Fire, and Raise the Yang Decoction
补脾胃泻阴火升阳汤加减
bǔ pí wèi xiè yīn huǒ shēng yáng tāng jiā jiǎn

Radix Astragali Membranacei *(huang qi)*	12g
Radix Codonopsitis Pilosulae *(dang shen)*	12g
Rhizoma Atractylodis *(cang zhu)*	10g
Radix et Rhizoma Notopterygii *(qiang huo)*	3g
Rhizoma Cimicifugae *(sheng ma)*	3g
Radix Bupleuri *(chai hu)*	3g
Dry-fried Rhizoma Coptidis *(chao huang lian)*	6g
Dry-fried Radix Scutellariae Baicalensis *(chao huang qin)*	6g
Dry-fried Cortex Moutan Radicis *(chao mu dan pi)*	6g
Flos Carthami Tinctorii *(hong hua)*	4.5g
Radix Paeoniae Rubrae *(chi shao)*	4.5g
Calcitum *(han shui shi)*	15g

PREPARATION & DOSAGE: Decoct the Calcitum *(han shui shi)* first for 30 minutes before adding the other ingredients. Administer in three doses daily.

❧ Single-Ingredient Astragalus Formula
独味黄芪方
dú wèi huáng qí fāng

Radix Astragali Membranacei *(huang qi)*	30g

PREPARATION & DOSAGE: Decoct and administer in 1-2 doses daily for the first 2-3 weeks. Then increase the dosage to 60g for the next four weeks, and thereafter to 90g.

CLINICAL NOTE: The source text indicates that large doses of Radix Astragali Membranacei *(huang qi)* usually do not cause side effects.

EXTERNAL

For all forms of lupus erythematosus, either Coptis Ointment (see shingles), or Clearing and Cooling Ointment (see impetigo in Chapter 7), or Artemisia Annua Ointment may be applied 1-2 times daily. These external formulas may be used in conjunction with internal formulas.

❦ Artemisia Annua Ointment
青蒿膏
qīng hāo gāo

Herba Artemisiae Annuae *(qing hao)*	20g
Petroleum Jelly	80g

PREPARATION & DOSAGE: Grind the Herba Artemisiae Annuae *(qing hao)* into a fine powder and mix thoroughly with the petroleum jelly. Store in an airtight glass jar.

ACUPUNCTURE

Filiform needling. Acupoints that may be needled are LI-4 *(he gu)*, LI-11 *(qu chi)*, PC-3 *(qu ze)*, LI-20 *(ying xiang)* and ST-2 *(si bai)*. Retain needles for one hour during which even manipulation should be applied for 2-3 minutes at 15 minute intervals. Treat once daily, with ten treatments constituting one course. At every fifth session, GV-10 *(ling tai)* may be bloodlet. Improvement of symptoms should be seen within 2-3 courses, after which sessions may be reduced to once every other day, or every three days.

Ear acupuncture. Acupoints that may be needled are Heart, Liver, Shenmen, Lung and Adrenal. Retain needles for 1-2 hours. Treat once every four days, with seven treatments constituting one course. Improvement should be evident within 2-3 courses.

Traditional vs. Biomedical Treatment

Treatment in general is aimed at controlling the progression of the disease. Because therapy is usually long-term, a traditional approach may be more desirable because of the lower risk of side effects. In addition, herbs or other measures to enhance the immune system can be used concomitantly. Biomedical treatment generally involves topical corticosteroids for early lesions, or intralesional injection of corticosteroids for refractory lesions. Progressive lupus may require antimalarials, salicylate or systemic corticosteroids, all of which can cause severe side effects.

Prevention

Early treatment is the best recourse against permanent atrophy of the lesions. Exposure to sunlight (or ultraviolet light) should be minimized, and sunscreen preparations applied when necessary.

Patients should be counseled about adhering to therapy, since control requires tenacious long-term treatment. Dietary habits should be evaluated, and foods that are spicy or greasy should be avoided, as should alcohol. During acute outbreaks, bedrest is advised.

Scleroderma
皮痹
pí bì, "skin painful obstruction"

Scleroderma is a chronic disease characterized by widespread formation of fibrous tissue (sclerosis), degenerative changes, and vascular abnormalities in the skin. Painful obstruction *(bì)* disorders, including those of the skin, are mentioned in early Chinese medical texts such as *Basic Questions*. However, not until such later works as *Pattern, Cause, Pulse, and Treatment* (1702) is there a description of a condition that can be considered to be scleroderma.

Scleroderma has two primary forms—localized cutaneous (described below) and systemic. The latter, called progressive systemic sclerosis, is a rather involved disease characterized by pathologic changes of the cutaneous, gastrointestinal, vascular, pulmonary, cardiac and renal systems. This form is not discussed in this text.

The biomedical cause of scleroderma is unknown. More women are affected than men, with some individuals developing the systemic form.

Signs & Symptoms

The localized cutaneous forms of scleroderma include morphea, generalized morphea, linear scleroderma, morphea profunda, eosinophilic fascitis and pansclerotic morphea. Morphea starts with indurated pink-red to blue-red patches that are smooth and shiny, but feel firm. The sclerosis is limited to the dermis. The lesions later change to hard, slightly yellow to white plaques surrounded by violet borders. The condition becomes generalized when the entire skin is involved. In morphea profunda, the sclerosis affects the subcutaneous fat. In eosinophilic fascitis, the fascia is the area of build-up of fibrous tissue, which eventually limits movement. In pansclerotic morphea, even the underlying muscle tissue may be inflamed and sclerosing. In linear scleroderma, the lesions usually follow the course of a nerve; involvement of underlying muscle and bone leads to atrophy of the skin and muscle and to skeletization. When the forehead is affected, the condition is called sabre-cut-like scleroderma *(en coup de sabre).*

As the disease progresses, cosmetic appearance is disturbed if the face and scalp are involved. If the extremities are affected, the disease is a major physical handicap as well.

Differential Diagnosis

Scleroderma should be differentiated from lichen sclerosis et atrophicus, lupus erythematosus, panniculitis (inflammation of the subcutaneous fat), and scleredema (a scleroderma-like infiltration of the skin). In lichen sclerosis, the elastic fibers in the tissue are destroyed (as determined by histology), whereas they are not in scleroderma. In lupus erythematosus, direct immunofluorescence studies of skin biopsies will confirm diagnosis. Panniculitis requires a biopsy of a full-thickness piece of skin for histologic examination in order to confirm diagnosis. Scleredema often follows infectious diseases and is typically associated with diabetes.

Traditional Chinese Etiology

Scleroderma is due to invasion of the skin by cold-dampness that accumulates in the interstices, causing the qi and blood to congeal, thus blocking the collaterals, and giving rise to the lesions.

Treatment

INTERNAL

The strategy is to dispel wind and transform dampness, harmonize the nutritive level and clear the collaterals. Three formulas are commonly used in the treatment of this disorder: Modified Angelica Pubescens and Sangjisheng Decoction; Persica, Leonuris, Salvia, and Carthamus Decoction; or Angelica and Ligusticum Formula.

❧ Modified Angelica Pubescens and Sangjisheng Decoction
独活寄生汤加减
dú huó jì shēng tāng jiā jiǎn

Radix Angelicae Pubescentis *(du huo)*	9g
Ramulus Sangjisheng *(sang ji sheng)*	6g
Radix Aristolochiae Fangchi *(fang ji)*	6g
Radix Angelicae Sinensis *(dang gui)*	6g
Radix Ligustici Chuanxiong *(chuan xiong)*	6g
Radix Paeoniae Rubrae *(chi shao)*	6g
Radix Salviae Miltiorrhizae *(dan shen)*	6g
Flos Carthami Tinctorii *(hong hua)*	6g
Radix et Caulis Jixueteng *(ji xue teng)*	6g
Herba cum Radice Lycopodii Clavati *(shen jin cao)*	6g
Radix Achyranthis Bidentatae *(niu xi)*	6g
Ramulus Mori Albae *(sang zhi)*	6g

PREPARATION & DOSAGE: Decoct and administer in 1-2 doses daily.

❧ Persica, Leonuris, Salvia, and Carthamus Decoction
桃益参红汤
táo yì shēn hóng tāng

Radix Salviae Miltiorrhizae *(dan shen)* 15g
Radix et Caulis Jixueteng *(ji xue teng)* 15g
Herba Lycopi Lucidi *(ze lan)* 9g
Tuber Curcumae *(yu jin)* 9g
Herba Leonuri Heterophylli *(yi mu cao)* 9g
Lignum Sappan *(su mu)* 9g
Radix Ligustici Chuanxiong *(chuan xiong)* 9g
Radix Rehmanniae Glutinosae Conquitae *(shu di huang)* 15g
Semen Persicae *(tao ren)* 9g
Flos Carthami Tinctorii *(hong hua)* 9g
Radix Paeoniae Rubrae *(chi shao)* 9g
Radix Angelicae Sinensis *(dang gui)* 9g

PREPARATION & DOSAGE: Decoct and administer in 1-2 doses daily. Save the dregs and decoct again, and use the fluid as a warm wash 2-3 times daily.

❧ Angelica and Ligusticum Formula
归芎方
guī xiōng fāng

Radix Angelicae Sinensis *(dang gui)*
Radix Ligustici Chuanxiong *(chuan xiong)*
Flos Carthami Tinctorii *(hong hua)*
Radix Puerariae *(ge gen)*

PREPARATION & DOSAGE: Grind equal amounts of the herbs together into a fine powder, and administer by mouth in 4-8g doses, three times daily. (Gelatin capsules may be filled with the herb powder, and then swallowed with warm water.)

CLINICAL NOTE: The source text suggests that this formula should not be administered as a decoction because a higher efficacy is achieved with the raw herbs.

EXTERNAL

The following external remedies may be applied in treating scleroderma.

❧ Jade Dragon Plaster to Restore Yang
回阳玉龙膏
huí yáng yù lóng gāo

Dry-fried Radix Aconiti Kusnezoffii Praeparata *(chao zhi cao wu)* 90g
Roasted Rhizoma Zingiberis Officinalis *(wei gan jiang)* 90g
Dry-fried Radix Paeoniae Rubrae *(chao chi shao)* 30g
Radix Angelicae Dahuricae *(bai zhi)* 30g
Roasted Rhizoma Arisaematis *(wei nan xing)* 30g
Cortex Cinnamomi Cassiae *(rou gui)* 15g

PREPARATION & DOSAGE: Grind the ingredients together into a fine powder. Put 90g of the powder together with 240g of beeswax into a glass jar with an airtight lid. Put the glass jar (uncovered) into a saucepan, add water to the saucepan to a level about one-third the height of the glass jar, and slowly heat until the beeswax dissolves; then remove the jar from the water. Thoroughly mix the herbal concoction.

Apply the plaster while warm by first spreading a thin layer onto sterile gauze. Then affix to the affected area with a bandage or skin tape. One application can be used continuously for up to two weeks (remove when bathing).

❦ Melia and Zanthoxylum Dry Compress
棟椒药熨
liàn jiāo yào yùn

Fructus Meliae Toosendan *(chuan lian zi)* 60g
Fructus Zanthoxyli Bungeani *(chuan jiao)* 30g

PREPARATION & DOSAGE: Break up the Fructus Meliae Toosendan *(chuan lian zi)* into small pieces. Stir-fry the two ingredients together with 30g of table salt for 8-10 minutes. Then wrap the hot herbs in several layers of sterile gauze. Apply as a dry compress to the affected area for about 10 minutes, 2-3 times daily.

Gently massage Effective Scarlet Wine (see chilblain in Chapter 12) into the affected area for about ten minutes, 1-2 times daily.

EAR ACUPUNCTURE

Points that may be needled include Lung, Occiput, Endocrine, Adrenal, Spleen and Liver. Treat 2-3 times weekly, retaining needles for 30-60 minutes. Ten treatments constitute one course of therapy; allow one week's rest between courses.

MOXIBUSTION

Apply moxibustion to the affected area with a moxa roll for 20 minutes. Treat 2-3 times weekly. Six treatments constitute one course of therapy; allow one week's rest between courses.

EMPIRICAL REMEDIES

Primary acupoints that may be needled include BL-23 *(shen shu)*, SP-10 *(xue hai)*, GB-31 *(feng shi)*, SP-9 *(yin ling quan)*, SP-6 *(san yin jiao)* and ST-36 *(zu san li)*, all bilaterally, and GV-14 *(ming men)*. Secondary points are those located on the border of lesions that are to be treated. After needles are inserted in the primary points and even manipulation applied, additional needles are inserted transversely at 15° every 4cm or so along the borders of lesions. Qi is obtained through even manipulation. Electric stimulation is applied to each needle at tolerance level for 30 minutes. The source text[1] suggests that for maximum effect, treatment should be given once daily, with thirty treatments constituting one course of therapy. Most patients experience improvement within one course, and some may even show remission of their lesions after two courses.

Traditional vs. Biomedical Therapy

Traditional treatment can be effective in controlling the progression of the disease. It should always be considered, as biomedical intervention is only supportive and directed toward the organ system involvement.

Prevention

The morphea type of scleroderma often resolves spontaneously or following treatment. Early and aggressive treatment is necessary to prevent progressive atrophy of underlying muscle and bone associated with linear scleroderma, as well as to prevent the development of systemic autoimmune disease.

Avoiding cold foods and beverages, and wearing protective clothing during cold weather, will help prevent exacerbation of the condition. Physiotherapy, whirlpool baths and massage may help prevent contractures by invigorating the blood and qi.

Dermatomyositis
肌痹
jī bì, "muscle painful obstruction"

Onset may be acute (particularly in children) or protracted. Classic skin involvement is a red rash that erupts on the face, neck, upper back, chest, and arms, and around the nail beds. A characteristic violaceous rash appears on the eyelids, with swelling around the eyes. Erythematous atrophic papules frequently affect the extensor surfaces of the finger joints. The skin lesions may disappear completely, but may be followed by brownish pigmentation, vitiligo, scarring, or atrophy. Soft tissue calcifications, which mostly affect children, occur in about 50 percent of patients as small nodules on the extremities, shoulder, and pelvic girdle; ulceration of the nodules is not uncommon.

The biomedical etiology of dermatomyositis is unknown. The disease may be caused by an autoimmune reaction. The association of cancer with dermatomyositis (reported incidence of 10-40 percent in adults with malignant tumors) suggests that neoplasms may incite myositis as the result of an autoimmune reaction directed against a common antigen in muscles and tumors. In some cases, dermatomyositis occurs before the malignancy is discovered. The disease commonly affects individuals between the ages of forty and sixty, and in children from ages five to fifteen. Females are twice as likely to be afflicted as males.

Signs & Symptoms

Onset may be acute (particularly in children) or insidious. An acute infection may precede or bring on the initial symptoms, which include proximal muscle (muscles closest to the trunk) weakness, muscle pain, rash, multi-joint pain, Raynaud's phenomenon (discoloration of the fingers caused by vascular spasms), difficulty swallowing, and constitutional complaints such as fever and weight loss.

The cutaneous eruption of dermatomyositis consists of erythema over the upper cheeks (similar to that of lupus erythematosus) and forehead, and a dusky red rash of the arms and upper back. Edema around the eyes with a reddish purple hue to the eyelids, the malar erythema, and red atrophic papules over the interphalangeal and metacarpophalangeal knuckles are telltale signs. The skin lesions may disappear completely, but may be followed by brownish pigmentation, vitiligo, scarring or atrophy. Soft tissue calcifications, which most commonly affect children, occur in about half of patients as small nodules on the extremities, shoulder and pelvic area; these nodules may ulcerate.

Muscular involvement may occur before or after the appearance of cutaneous lesions. Onset of muscle weakness may be sudden and progress over weeks or months. Typically, the proximal muscles of the extremities, the anterior neck flexors, and the abdominal muscles are affected, and as the disease progresses, additional muscles are involved as well. Some patients develop severe contracture of the muscles, or extensive calcifications.

Differential Diagnosis

Differential diagnosis includes other connective tissue diseases, especially scleroderma and lupus erythematosus. Early lesions of dermatomyositis may resemble dermatitis or other inflammatory skin diseases such as erysipelas.

Five major criteria are helpful in diagnosing dermatomyositis: proximal muscle weakness, a characteristic skin rash, elevated muscle enzymes in the blood, electromyographic abnormalities and muscle biopsy changes.

Traditional Chinese Etiology

Three primary causes are apparent for this condition: blazing heat toxin, invasion of the skin by cold-dampness, and deficiency of Spleen and Kidney yang.

Blazing heat toxin. The Spleen and Lung are invaded by toxic wind-warmth that accumulates and transforms into heat and then into toxin. The heat toxin enters the qi and blood causing contention between the two, resulting in extreme heat, which then lodges in the skin and muscles, inciting the skin lesions and muscular difficulties.

Invasion of the skin by cold-dampness. Invasion of the skin and interstices by cold-dampness causes inability of source qi to warm the external surface of the body. The cold-dampness also causes blockage and stagnation of qi and blood so that channel qi is unable to be spread, and stagnation of the superficial connecting channels occurs, thus giving rise to the skin lesions and muscular difficulties.

Deficiency of Spleen and Kidney yang. Insufficient Spleen yang causes inability of the protective level to secure the exterior. Concomitant invasion of wind, cold and dampness impedes the flow of qi and blood. As the condition becomes protracted, deficiency of qi and blood result, injuring the Kidney yang. Thus, deficiency of both the Spleen and Kidney yang gives rise to the skin lesions and muscular difficulties.

Treatment

INTERNAL

Blazing heat toxin. Onset is acute and the skin rash is purplish red. Generalized symptoms include high fever, bitter taste in the mouth, dry throat, and pain and weakness of the muscles and joints. Severe cases may present impaired consciousness and/or restlessness. The tongue is purple and the coating thin, slightly dry and yellow, and the pulse is rapid. The strategy is to cool the nutritive level and clear toxin, and enrich the yin and clear heat.

Formulas recommended for this pattern are Clear Epidemics and Overcome Toxin Decoction (see erysipelas), and Scolopendra Formula.

❧ Scolopendra Formula
蜈蚣方
wú gōng fāng

Scolopendra Subspinipes *(wu gong)*
Buthus Martensi *(quan xie)*

PREPARATION & DOSAGE: Grind together equal amounts of the two ingredients, and then sift the powder several times to ensure complete mixing. Administer 1.5g, 2-3 times daily.

CLINICAL NOTE: Because of the toxicity of this formula, patients should be closely monitored for side effects, especially those affecting respiration. The source text indicates that this formula is suitable for acute severe cases of heat toxin pattern, and that improvement of symptoms should be seen within ten days; if not, discontinue and consider other remedies.

Invasion of the skin by cold-dampness. The course of disease of this pattern is insidious. Skin lesions appear as dark red, edematous patches. Systemic pain and weakness of muscles are apparent. The tongue is pale red and the coating thin white, and the pulse is submerged and slow, or submerged and thin. The strategy is to augment the qi and warm yang, and scatter cold and unblock the channels.

Formulas recommended for this pattern include Modified Yang-Heartening Decoction, or Enrich the Blood, Dispel Wind, and Dry Dampness Formula.

❧ Modified Yang-Heartening Decoction
阳和汤加减
yáng hé tāng jiā jiǎn

Prepared Herba Ephedrae *(zhi ma huang)*	3g
Cortex Cinnamomi Cassiae *(rou gui)*	3g
Radix Rehmanniae Glutinosae Conquitae *(shu di huang)*	30g
Fructus Liquidambaris Taiwanianae *(lu lu tong)*	6g
Radix Astragali Membranacei *(huang qi)*	10g
Radix Codonopsitis Pilosulae *(dang shen)*	10g
Sclerotium Poriae Cocos *(fu ling)*	10g
Radix Gentianae Qinjiao *(qin jiao)*	10g
Radix Salviae Miltiorrhizae *(dan shen)*	15g
Herba Buchnerae Cruciatae *(gui yu jian)*	15g
Radix Dioscoreae Oppositae *(shan yao)*	15g
Radix Glycyrrhizae Uralensis *(gan cao)*	15g

PREPARATION & DOSAGE: Decoct and administer in three doses daily.

❧ Enrich the Blood, Dispel Wind, and Dry Dampness Formula
养血消风燥湿方
yǎng xuè xiāo fēng zào shī fāng

Radix Angelicae Sinensis *(dang gui)*	15g
Radix Ligustici Chuanxiong *(chuan xiong)*	10g
Radix Paeoniae Rubrae *(chi shao)*	15g
Radix Rehmanniae Glutinosae *(sheng di huang)*	25g
Bombyx Batryticatus *(jiang can)*	10g
Periostracum Cicadae *(chan tui)*	15g
Cortex Phellodendri *(huang bai)*	15g
Rhizoma Atractylodis *(cang zhu)*	15g
Fructus Tribuli Terrestris *(bai ji li)*	15g
Radix Polygoni Multiflori *(he shou wu)*	15g
Cortex Dictamni Dasycarpi Radicis *(bai xian pi)*	25g
Fructus Forsythiae Suspensae *(lian qiao)*	25g
Radix Glycyrrhizae Uralensis *(gan cao)*	10g

PREPARATION & DOSAGE: Decoct and administer in 2-3 doses daily.

Deficiency of Spleen and Kidney yang. Skin lesions are dark red or scarlet. Other symptoms include muscle atrophy, joint pain, cyanosis of the digits, weight loss and reduced food intake, generalized weakness, cold sensation of the stomach, watery stools, and abdominal fullness. The tongue is fat and pale with little coating, and the pulse is submerged, thin and forceless. The treatment strategy is to tonify the Kidney and bolster yang, and strengthen the Spleen and augment the qi.

Formulas recommended for treating this pattern include Modified Kidney Qi Pill from the Golden Cabinet, or Codonopsis and Sangjisheng Tonifying and Augmenting Formula.

❧ Modified Kidney Qi Pill from the Golden Cabinet
金匮肾气丸加减
jīn guì shèn qì wán jiā jiǎn

Radix Rehmanniae Glutinosae Conquitae *(shu di huang)*	12g
Fructus Corni Officinalis *(shan zhu yu)*	12g
Radix Dioscoreae Oppositae *(shan yao)*	12g
Radix Codonopsitis Pilosulae *(dang shen)*	12g
Rhizoma Atractylodis Macrocephalae *(bai zhu)*	12g
Dry-fried Cortex Moutan Radicis *(chao mu dan pi)*	6g
Rhizome Alismatis Orientalis *(ze xie)*	15g
Radix Morindae Officinalis *(ba ji tian)*	15g
Herba Epimedii *(yin yang huo)*	15g

Semen Trigonellae Foeni-graeci *(hu lu ba)* 15g
Radix Astragali Membranacei *(huang qi)* 10g
Radix Glycyrrhizae Uralensis *(gan cao)* 10g

PREPARATION & DOSAGE: Decoct and administer in three doses daily.

MODIFICATIONS: For persistent high fever, add Cornu Antelopis *(ling yang jiao)*, Cornu Bubali *(shui niu jiao)*, Gypsum *(shi gao)* and dry-fried Rhizoma Anemarrhenae Asphodeloidis *(chao zhi mu)*; for moist skin and edema of the lesions, add Flos Lonicerae Japonicae *(jin yin hua)*, Flos Carthami Tinctorii *(hong hua)* and Flos Campsitis Grandiflorae *(ling xiao hua)*; for palpitations and shortness of breath, add Radix Adenophorae seu Glehniae *(sha shen)*, Tuber Ophiopogonis Japonici *(mai men dong)*, Fructus Schisandrae Chinensis *(wu wei zi)* and Caulis Perillae Frutescentis *(zi su geng)*; for persistent low-grade fever, add Cortex Lycii Radicis *(di gu pi)* and Herba Artemisiae Annuae *(qing hao)*.

The following remedy actually consists of two formulas that are used alternately in order to tonify and augment the Spleen and Kidney, and to nourish the blood and unblock the channels.

❦ Codonopsis and Sangjisheng Tonifying and Augmenting Formula
党参寄生补益方
dǎng shēn jì shēng bǔ yì fāng

[A] Radix Codonopsitis Pilosulae *(dang shen)* 15g
Rhizoma Atractylodis *(cang zhu)* 15g
Rhizoma Atractylodis Macrocephalae *(bai zhu)* 15g
Semen Coicis Lachryma-jobi *(yi yi ren)* 15g
Radix Paeoniae Lactiflorae *(bai shao)* 15g
Semen Persicae *(tao ren)* 12g
Radix Salviae Miltiorrhizae *(dan shen)* 15g
Radix Rehmanniae Glutinosae Conquitae *(shu di huang)* 12g
Radix Angelicae Sinensis *(dang gui)* 12g
Lignum Sappan *(su mu)* 9g
Ramulus Cinnamomi Cassiae *(gui zhi)* 9g

[B] Ramulus Sangjisheng *(sang ji sheng)* 15g
Radix Rehmanniae Glutinosae Conquitae *(shu di huang)* 12g
Radix Angelicae Sinensis *(dang gui)* 12g
Fructus Schisandrae Chinensis *(wu wei zi)* 6g
Fasciculus Vascularis Luffae *(si gua luo)* 6g
Radix Achyranthis Bidentatae *(niu xi)* 12g
Cornu Cervi Degelatinatium *(lu jiao shuang)* 12g

PREPARATION & DOSAGE: Decoct and administer in a single daily dose, alternating the two formulas every other day.

EXTERNAL

For early lesions, Speranskia, Cinnamon, and Carthamus Wash may be applied.

❧ Speranskia, Cinnamon, and Carthamus Wash
透桂红洗剂
tòu guì hóng xǐ jì

Herba Speranskiae seu Impatientis *(tou gu cao)*	30g
Ramulus Cinnamomi Cassiae *(gui zhi)*	25g
Flos Carthami Tinctorii *(hong hua)*	10g

PREPARATION & DOSAGE: Decoct and wash the affected areas with the warm decoction once daily.

ACUPUNCTURE

Acupuncture may be used as an adjunct to internal remedies. To help improve muscle tone, the following acupoints are recommended for needling: ST-36 *(zu san li)*, SP-6 *(san yin jiao)*, LI-11 *(qu chi)*, SP-9 *(yin ling quan)* and LI-15 *(jian yu)*. Even manipulation should be used, and electrotherapy may be applied. Treat once daily, with ten treatments constituting one course. Allow three days' rest between courses.

Traditional vs. Biomedical Treatment

Traditional treatment is perhaps more desirable than the biomedical use of corticosteroids in controlling the progression of dermatomyositis. Corticosteroids must often be used for months and even years, thus leading to the problems associated with their use.

Prevention

Early diagnosis and treatment is essential to prevent complications associated with dermatomyositis. Long remissions and apparent recovery have been reported, especially in children.

Patients in the acute phase should limit their activities until the inflammation subsides. Because of the association of malignancy with dermatomyositis, studies should be performed to detect any underlying cancers in all adults with dermatomyositis.

CHAPTER NOTES

1. Chang, Y.B., "Acupuncture in the Treatment of Scleroderma," *New Journal of Traditional Chinese Medicine,* 22(6): 31; 1990.

CHAPTER 17

Disorders of the Sweat Glands

Miliaria
痱子
fèi zǐ, "boiling rash"

Miliaria, also known as heat rash or prickly heat, is an acute inflammatory, itchy eruption caused by retained extravasated sweat. A miliaria-type disease was first mentioned in Chapter 3 of *Basic Questions*. Later, in *Discussion of the Origins of Symptoms of Diseases* (610), Chao Yuan-Fang presented a more detailed description of this condition:

> During the height of summer, the skin and interstices are open, [so that the body is] easily injured by wind and heat. Wind and heat toxin struggle within the skin, thus giving rise to boiling sores which resemble the bubbles of soup.

Biomedically, miliaria is caused by sweat-duct obstruction that causes sweat to be trapped below the surface. Rupture of the duct occurs, followed by formation of a vesicle containing retained sweat.

Signs & Symptoms

The term "miliaria" denotes three disorders differentiated by the level at which obstruction takes place and the type of vesicle that results. In miliaria crystallina, obstruction occurs at the superficial level. The minute, clear crystalline vesicles commonly affect elderly, bedridden patients, especially in the axillae and the neck areas. These vesicles rupture easily and may go unnoticed.

In miliaria rubra, or prickly heat, obstruction occurs in the epidermis, causing inflammation that results in redness and pruritus. The individual lesions are red macules, ranging from 1-3mm in diameter, with a tiny summit vesicle. The eruption usually affects the trunk and neck. Pustules may develop in persons with extensive eruption.

In miliaria profunda, obstruction takes place at the dermal-epidermal junction. Individuals with widespread recurrent miliaria rubra are particularly susceptible to this type. The eruption is characterized by nonpruritic whitish papules, about 1-3mm in diameter. Because of the extensive sweat gland obstruction, patients with miliaria profunda are predisposed to develop thermoregulatory failure accompanied by high body temperature and cardiorespiratory symptoms after heat exposure or exercise.

Differential Diagnosis

A history of exposure to heat usually confirms diagnosis of miliaria.

Traditional Chinese Etiology

Exposure to summerheat or to high temperature causes sweating. The discharge of sweat is inhibited, resulting in accumulation and steaming of summerheat-dampness, thus causing the skin eruption.

Treatment

INTERNAL

In treating miliaria, the strategy is to clear summerheat, promote urination and relieve toxicity. The formulas recommended for this pattern include Clear Summerheat Decoction, or Taraxacum, Viola, and Lonicera Decoction.

❧ Clear Summerheat Decoction
清暑汤
qīng shǔ tāng

Fructus Forsythiae Suspensae *(lian qiao)*
Radix Trichosanthis Kirilowii *(tian hua fen)*
Radix Paeoniae Rubrae *(chi shao)*
Radix Glycyrrhizae Uralensis *(gan cao)*
Talcum *(hua shi)*
Semen Plantaginis *(che qian zi)*
Flos Lonicerae Japonicae *(jin yin hua)*
Rhizome Alismatis Orientalis *(ze xie)*
Herba Lophatheri Gracilis *(dan zhu ye)*

PREPARATION & DOSAGE: The source text does not specify amounts for the ingredients. Decoct and administer in two doses daily until the eruption subsides.

❧ Taraxacum, Viola, and Lonicera Decoction
蒲地忍汤
pú dì rěn tāng

Herba Taraxaci Mongolici cum Radice *(pu gong ying)* 30g
Herba cum Radice Violae Yedoensitis *(zi hua di ding)* 30g
Ramus Lonicerae Japonicae *(ren dong teng)* 30g

PREPARATION & DOSAGE: Decoct and administer in three doses daily until the eruption subsides.

EXTERNAL

For miliaria crystallina and miliaria rubra, any one of the following external remedies may be applied: Three-Yellow Wash (see furuncles in Chapter 7), Clearing and Cooling Powder (see sunburn in Chapter 12), or Miliaria Powder.

❦ Miliaria Powder
痱子粉
fèi zǐ fěn

Semen Phaseoli Radiati *(lu dou)* (powdered)	10g
Borneol *(bing pian)* (powdered)	2.5g
Talcum *(hua shi)* (powdered)	87.5g

PREPARATION & DOSAGE: Mix the powdered ingredients together well. Sprinkle on the affected areas 2-3 times daily.

For miliaria profunda, mix either Light-Yellow Powder (see atopic dermatitis in Chapter 13) or Jade Dew Powder (see sunburn in Chapter 12) with vegetable oil to form an ointment, and apply 2-3 times daily.

EAR ACUPUNCTURE

To relieve the intense itching associated with miliaria rubra, the following points may be needled: Lung, Adrenal, Occiput and Shenmen. Retain needles for 30 minutes. Treat once daily until the itching subsides.

EMPIRICAL REMEDIES

[A] Mung bean and mint soup: Cook one cup of mung beans in 1.0 liter of water for 20 minutes. Just before turning off the heat, add 2-3 sprigs of fresh mint. Administer one cup five times daily until the miliaria is resolved.[1]

[B] Another remedy is to rub fresh watermelon or wintermelon rind on the affected areas 2-3 times daily.

Traditional vs. Biomedical Treatment

Treatment in general is to provide symptomatic relief. Traditional therapy may be more effective in accelerating recovery through use of both internal and external remedies that clear summerheat toxicity. Biomedical treatment is mainly palliative through application of a drying lotion such as calamine or 1% hydrocortisone in a hydrophilic lotion base.

Prevention

Miliaria resolves within a few days once the patient is removed from exposure to heat. For patients with severe conditions, a cool environment is essential. Gentle cleansing and application of one of the above herbal powders hastens recovery, as does administration of internal formulas.

Individuals prone to miliaria may try using the internal and/or external remedies as prophylaxis if they are aware of impending heat exposure, e.g., travel to warm, humid areas, or the arrival of hot weather.

Bromhidrosis
狐臭
hú chòu, "fox stench"

Bromhidrosis, or foul perspiration, is characterized by abnormal or excessive body odor resulting from degraded axillary sweat. Other Chinese names given to this condition include "body smell" *(tǐ qì),* "axillary smell" *(yè qì)* and "axillary stench" *(yè chòu),* among others. *Discussion of the Origins of Symptoms of Diseases* (610) provides the following description:

> [There are] persons who have axillary stench that resembles the smell of onion fermented beans, or it is said, persons [whose smell] resembles fox droppings, thus it is called fox stench. This is all [due to] blood and qi not being in harmony, [which then] accumulate [and cause] the foul smell.

Biomedically, bromhidrosis is caused by the decomposition of sweat and cellular debris by yeast and bacteria. Only sweat from the apocrine glands located in the axillae contains the substrate that gives rise to the offensive odor after interaction with bacteria.

Signs & Symptoms

Although the odor emanates specifically from the underarms, it results in an unpleasant general body odor. Some persons have unusual axillary odors ranging from musty to sweet to sour to rancid, reflecting variations in sweat composition. Because of preferential anosmia, some patients are unaware of their axillary odor unless informed of it.

Traditional Chinese Etiology

Accumulation of damp-heat produces turbidity that is discharged with sweat, thus giving rise to the foul-smelling perspiration.

Treatment

In Chinese medicine, treatment for bromhidrosis is generally by external means. However, if the condition is severe, internal formulas may be administered.

INTERNAL

The strategy is to clear heat and drain dampness, and transform turbidity with aromatic herbs. The formula recommended for this pattern is Sweet Dew Special Pill to Eliminate Toxin.

Sweet Dew Special Pill to Eliminate Toxin
甘露消毒丹
gān lù xiāo dú dān

		Decoction
Talcum (hua shi)	450g	(18-21g)
Radix Scutellariae Baicalensis (huang qin)	300g	(12-15g)
Herba Artemisiae Yinchenhao (yin chen hao)	330g	(24-30g)
Secretio Moschus (she xiang)	120g	(9-12g)
Fructus Forsythiae Suspensae (lian qiao)	120g	(12-15g)
Rhizoma Acori Graminei (shi chang pu)	180g	(4-6g)
Fructus Amomi Kravanh (bai dou kou)	120g	(10-12g)
Herba Menthae Haplocalycis (bo he)	120g	(6-9g)
Caulis Mutong (mu tong)	150g	(9-12g)
Rhizoma Belamcandae Chinensis (she gan)	120g	(9-12g)
Bulbus Fritillariae Cirrhosae (chuan bei mu)	150g	(6-9g)

PREPARATION & DOSAGE: Grind the ingredients together into a fine powder and administer 9g daily with warm water. Or form into small boluses using Massa Fermentata (shen qu), administering a total of 9g of the powder daily. A decoction may be made by using the amounts indicated in parentheses; administer 1-2 doses daily.

EXTERNAL

Several remedies may be applied locally after bathing, or after thoroughly cleansing the axillae with soap and water.

❦ Five-Fragrance Powder
五香散
wǔ xiāng sǎn

Lignum Aquilariae (chen xiang)	9g
Lignum Santali Albi (tan xiang)	9g
Radix Aucklandiae Lappae (mu xiang)	9g
Herba cum Radice Lysimachiae Foeni-Graci (ling ling xiang)	9g
Secretio Moschus (she xiang)	1g

PREPARATION & DOSAGE: Grind the ingredients together into a fine powder and store in an airtight amber glass jar. Apply three times daily by mixing, at each application, 0.15g powder with 25ml water, and then using a washcloth or several cotton balls dipped in the herbal remedy to wash the axillae.

❦ Aristilochia Powder
清木香散
qīng mù xiāng sǎn

Radix Aristolochiae (qing mu xiang)	60g
Radix Lateralis Aconiti Carmichaeli Praeparata (fu zi)	30g
Calcite (shi hui)	30g
Alumen (ming fan)	15g

PREPARATION & DOSAGE: Grind the ingredients together into a fine powder and store in an airtight amber glass jar. Apply to the axillae 1-2 times daily.

Fox Stench Powder
狐臭粉
hú chòu fěn

Calcitum *(han shui shi)*
Lithargyrum *(mi tuo seng)*

PREPARATION & DOSAGE: Grind equal amounts of the ingredients together into a fine powder and store in an airtight glass jar. Apply to the axillae 1-2 times daily.

Clove and Borneol Powder
丁香冰片散
dīng xiāng bīng piàn săn

Flos Caryophylli *(ding xiang)*	30g
Borneol *(bing pian)*	6g

PREPARATION & DOSAGE: Grind the ingredients together into a fine powder and store in an airtight amber glass jar. Apply to the axillae 1-2 times daily.

EMPIRICAL REMEDIES

[A] Grind 15g of Semen Euphoriae Longanae *(lóng yǎn hé)*, otherwise known as dragon eye fruit pits, and 9g of Fructus Piperis Nigri *(hu jiao)* together into a fine powder. Apply the powder to the axillae with a cotton ball 1-2 times daily.[2]

[B] 6g of Fructus Zanthoxyli Bungeani *(chuan jiao)*, 6g of Pericarpium Citri Reticulatae *(chen pi)*, 6g of Alumen Praeparatum *(ku fan)*, 6g of Radix Angelicae Dahuricae *(bai zhi)*, and 0.5g of Borneol *(bing pian)*. Grind the first four ingredients into a fine powder, then add the Borneol *(bing pian)* and continue grinding until an extra-fine powder is formed. Store in an airtight glass container.

Wash the axillae with soap and warm water, and towel dry. Sprinkle a small amount of the powder on a gauze pad and gently rub the powder into the axillae. Apply 2-3 times daily. Ten days is one course of treatment. The source text[3] indicates that most patients experience alleviation of odor after 2-3 courses.

Traditional vs. Biomedical Treatment

Many individuals respond to biomedical treatment involving application of deodorants containing aluminum chloride or other aluminum or zirconium salts. Topical antibiotics are also effective. Some patients with marked bromhidrosis who do not respond may be referred for surgical removal of the axillary apocrine sweat glands. However, such patients may wish to try traditional treatment before undergoing this procedure. Otherwise, traditional treatment remains desirable for those who prefer a non-chemical appraoch to management of this problem.

Prevention

Personal hygiene is important in controlling bromhidrosis. Careful bathing of the axillary skin with soap and water helps remove bacteria. Shaving of axillary hair reduces odor, as the hair serves to collect sweat and augments odor production. Clothing should be washed or dry-cleaned more frequently because their underarm sections may retain sweat and cause odor despite suppression of odor in the axillae.

Use of the above external remedies should be for a 1-2 week period followed by several remedy-free days to determine whether the odor has been resolved.

Diet may play a role in causing bromhidrosis, particularly foods that can give rise to heat and dampness, such as those that are spicy and greasy, as well as lamb, capon and shrimp. Patients should also abstain from alcohol and tobacco, as these can produce heat and dampness as well.

CHAPTER NOTES

1. Gu, B.H., ed. *Practical Textbook of Traditional Chinese External Diseases (Shi yong zhong yi wai ke xue)*. Shanghai: Shanghai Science & Technology Press, 1985.

2. Dai, Y.F. and Liu, C.J. *Medicinal Uses of Fruits (Yao yong guo pin)*. Nanning: Guangxi People's Publishing House, 1982.

3. Tian, Z.F., "An Empirical Formula for the Treatment of Axillary Stench," *Sichuan Journal of Traditional Chinese Medicine*, 8(3), 42; 1990.

CHAPTER 18

Acne and Rosacea

Acne
粉刺
fěn cì, "white thorns"

Acne is a chronic skin condition caused by inflammation of the hair follicles and sebaceous glands. In Chinese, the condition is called "white thorns" because of the resemblance of the lesion to thorns, and because of the white fluid that exudes when the lesion is squeezed. Other Chinese names for acne include "Lung wind white thorns" *(fèi fēng fěn cì),* "wine thorns" *(jiǔ cì)* and "early spring [pubescent] granules" *(qīng chūn lì).* Chen Shi-Duo, in *Profound Purpose from the Heavenly Abode* (1694), described the connection between acne and rosacea:

> Lung wind sores and red spot nose sores arise on the nose and face, [and] are diseases of the Lung channel. The Lung's orifice is the nose; [when] Lung qi is not clear, the nose therefore is injured. [Once] the nose is injured, [the disease] then spreads to the face.

Biomedically, the cause of acne is unknown, although the pathogenesis is fairly well-established. The lesions arise following sebaceous overactivity leading to plugging of the follicles by sebum. Bacteria, in particular *Propionibacterium acnes,* are trapped in the sebum plug, causing release of and irritation by accumulated fatty acids. This, along with foreign body reaction to the extrafollicular sebum, is the etiology of this disorder. Androgen hormones appear to activate sebaceous glands, thus onset of the condition occurs primarily during puberty, although acne can appear in neonates as well as for the first time in persons in their twenties and thirties, and may even persist into later life. In the latter circumstances, other factors such as medications, or contact with oil and grease, are often associated with increased tendency to acne.

Signs & Symptoms

Lesions of acne appear most frequently on the face, chest and back, where the sebaceous follicles are large. The first lesions are noninflammatory comedones (plugs of keratin and sebum in hair follicles). Open comedones are known as blackheads, closed ones as whiteheads. As time progresses, the dome-shaped comedones may develop into inflamed papules, superficial cysts and pustules. In severe cases, deep inflamed nodules and pus-filled cysts are present, with some having their openings on the skin surface where their contents are discharged. The scars that usually result from acne are pitted.

Differential Diagnosis

Diagnosis of acne is usually not difficult, since there are few other diseases that present with papules and pustules on the face. The lesions of rosacea appear commonly in the middle third of the face and are distinguished from those of acne by the absence of comedones, and the presence of flushing, telangiectasia, and rhinophyma. Folliculitis should also be considered, especially when lesions occur on the upper back; diagnosis in such cases may need to be confirmed through bacterial culture.

Traditional Chinese Etiology

The primary causes of acne are Lung heat, Stomach heat, blood heat, heat toxin, and damp toxin with blood stasis.

Lung heat. This is caused by the invasion of external wind, which causes pre-existing heat in the Lung channel to accumulate in the skin and tissues, thus giving rise to the lesions.

Stomach heat. This is typically caused by a high-fat diet or overeating of fried and/or spicy foods, which leads to accumulation of heat in the Spleen/Stomach. As the condition becomes protracted, the heat rises and lodges in the skin and tissues, thus producing the lesions.

Blood heat. This type of acne often has emotional disturbance as its source. The resulting qi stagnation, if unresolved, accumulates and transforms into heat that enters the blood level, and then lodges in the skin and tissues, thus causing the lesions.

Heat toxin. This is the result of the combination of Lung and/or Stomach heat with external toxin to form heat toxin that rises upward and lodges in the skin and interstices, thus producing the lesions.

Damp toxin with blood stasis. Acne of this type arises when pre-existing dampness accumulates in the skin and tissues followed by attack of external toxin, which then congeals with dampness to form damp toxin. Blockage of the channels and collaterals ensues, giving rise to disharmony between the qi and blood, and thus the lesions.

Treatment

Control of this often chronic disease requires careful pattern differentiation.

INTERNAL

Lung heat. Lesions of this pattern are characterized by whiteheads and blackheads that are papular and sometimes slightly itchy. The forehead, as well as the areas proximal to the nose, are most commonly affected. Generalized symptoms may include dryness of the nose and mouth, dry stools, a slightly red tongue with a thin white or yellow coating, and a floating, slippery pulse. The strategy is to clear and drain Lung heat.

Formulas recommended for treating this pattern include Eriobotrya Decoction to Clear the Lung, or Cool the Blood and Clear the Lung Decoction.

❧ Eriobotrya Decoction to Clear the Lung
枇杷清肺饮
pí pá qīng fèi yǐn

Folium Eriobotryae Japonicae *(pi pa ye)*	6g
Cortex Mori Albae Radicis *(sang bai pi)*	6g
Rhizoma Coptidis *(huang lian)*	3g
Cortex Phellodendri *(huang bai)*	3g
Radix Ginseng *(ren shen)*	1g
Radix Glycyrrhizae Uralensis *(gan cao)*	1g

PREPARATION & DOSAGE: Decoct and administer in three doses daily.

❧ Cool the Blood and Clear the Lung Decoction
凉血清肺饮
liáng xuè qīng fèi yǐn

Radix Rehmanniae Glutinosae *(sheng di huang)*	30g
Cortex Moutan Radicis *(mu dan pi)*	9g
Radix Paeoniae Rubrae *(chi shao)*	9g
Radix Scutellariae Baicalensis *(huang qin)*	9g
Rhizoma Anemarrhenae Asphodeloidis *(zhi mu)*	9g
Gypsum *(shi gao)*	30g
Cortex Mori Albae Radicis *(sang bai pi)*	9g
Folium Eriobotryae Japonicae *(pi pa ye)*	9g
Radix Glycyrrhizae Uralensis *(gan cao)*	6g

PREPARATION & DOSAGE: Decoct and administer in two doses daily.

MODIFICATIONS: For dry stools, add Radix et Rhizoma Rhei *(da huang)* and Folium Daqingye *(da qing ye)*.

Stomach heat. This pattern is characterized by whiteheads and blackheads that are papular. The areas around the mouth, chest and upper back are commonly affected. The face is prone to oiliness. Generalized symptoms may include a tendency to eat large amounts of food, halitosis, dry mouth and tongue, desire for cold beverages, dry stools, a red tongue with a sticky coating, and a submerged, slippery and forceful pulse. The strategy is to clear Stomach heat. The formula recommended for this pattern is Regulate the Stomach and Order the Qi Decoction.

꧁ Regulate the Stomach and Order the Qi Decoction
调胃承气汤
tiáo wèi chéng qì tāng

Radix et Rhizoma Rhei *(da huang)*	12g
Radix Glycyrrhizae Uralensis *(gan cao)*	6g
Mirabilitum *(mang xiao)*	9-12g

PREPARATION & DOSAGE: Cook the first two ingredients and strain the decoction before adding the Mirabilitum *(mang xiao)* to the resulting liquid. Administer in 1-2 doses daily.

Blood heat. Lesions of this pattern are papular, and primarily affect the areas near the nose and mouth as well as between the eyebrows. The capillaries of the face are often dilated so that exposure to heat or emotional stimulation brings on facial flush. Premenstrual women often experience an increase in skin lesions. Generalized symptoms may include dry stools, yellow urine, a tongue with a red tip and a thin coating, and a thin, slippery and rapid pulse. The treatment strategy is to cool the blood and clear heat.

Formulas recommended for this pattern include Four-Substance Decoction with Safflower and Peach Pit, or Cool the Blood Decoction with Five Flowers.

꧁ Four-Substance Decoction with Safflower and Peach Pit
桃红四物汤
táo hóng sì wù tāng

Radix Ligustici Chuanxiong *(chuan xiong)*	3g
Radix Angelicae Sinensis *(dang gui)*	6g
Radix Paeoniae Lactiflorae *(bai shao)*	6g
Radix Rehmanniae Glutinosae Conquitae *(shu di huang)*	6g
Semen Persicae *(tao ren)*	6g
Flos Carthami Tinctorii *(hong hua)*	3g

PREPARATION & DOSAGE: Decoct and administer in 1-2 doses daily.

꧁ Cool the Blood Decoction with Five Flowers
凉血五花汤
liáng xuè wǔ huā tāng

Flos Carthami Tinctorii *(hong hua)*	9-15g
Inflorescentia Celosiae Cristatae *(ji guan hua)*	9-15g
Flos Campsitis Grandiflorae *(ling xiao hua)*	9-15g
Flos Rosae Rugosae *(mei gui hua)*	9-15g
Flos Chrysanthemi Indici *(ye ju hua)*	9-15g

PREPARATION & DOSAGE: Decoct and administer in two doses daily.

Heat toxin. Lesions of this pattern are primarily pustules on an erythematous base. Pain may be present. Inflamed nodules are not uncommon. The upper back and chest are frequently involved. Residual scarring often occurs after healing. Generalized symptoms may include dry stools or constipation, scanty and yellow urine, a red tongue with yellow and dry coating, and a wiry and slippery, or a rapid pulse. The treatment strategy is to clear heat and relieve toxicity.

Formulas recommended for this pattern include Five-Ingredient Decoction to Eliminate Toxin (see folliculitis in Chapter 7), or Acne Decoction.

❧ Acne Decoction
痤疮煎剂
cuó chuāng jiān jì

Flos Lonicerae Japonicae *(jin yin hua)*	30g
Fructus Forsythiae Suspensae *(lian qiao)*	12g
Radix Scutellariae Baicalensis *(huang qin)*	12g
Radix Ligustici Chuanxiong *(chuan xiong)*	12g
Radix Angelicae Sinensis *(dang gui)*	12g
Radix Platycodi Grandiflori *(jie geng)*	9g
Radix Achyranthis Bidentatae *(niu xi)*	9g
Flos Chrysanthemi Indici *(ye ju hua)*	15g

PREPARATION & DOSAGE: Decoct and administer in 1-2 doses daily.

Damp toxin with blood stasis. Acne of this pattern is characterized by deep, painful inflamed nodules and pus-filled cysts on an erythematous base. The face, chest and back are generally involved, and the affected skin is oily. The residual scarring is usually pitted. Generalized symptoms may include headache and a sensation of heat throughout the body, a purple tongue with a yellow or white coating, and a slow or submerged and choppy pulse. The treatment strategy is to eliminate dampness and relieve toxicity, and invigorate the blood and dispel blood stasis. The formula recommended for this pattern is Eliminate Dampness and Relieve Toxicity Decoction.

❧ Eliminate Dampness and Relieve Toxicity Decoction
除湿解毒汤
chú shī jiě dú tāng

Cortex Dictamni Dasycarpi Radicis *(bai xian pi)*	15g
Semen Glycines Germinatum *(dou juan)*	12g
Semen Coicis Lachryma-jobi *(yi yi ren)*	12g
Rhizoma Smilacis Glabrae *(tu fu ling)*	12g
Fructus Gardeniae Jasminoidis *(zhi zi)*	6g
Cortex Moutan Radicis *(mu dan pi)*	9g
Flos Lonicerae Japonicae *(jin yin hua)*	15g

Fructus Forsythiae Suspensae *(lian qiao)* 12g
Herba cum Radice Violae Yedoensitis *(zi hua di ding)* 9g
Caulis Mutong *(mu tong)* 6g
Talcum *(hua shi)* 15g
Radix Glycyrrhizae Uralensis *(gan cao)* 6g

PREPARATION & DOSAGE: Decoct and administer in 1-2 doses daily.

EXTERNAL

For all patterns of acne, Upside Down Powder may be used.

❧ Upside Down Powder
颠倒散
diān dǎo sǎn

Radix et Rhizoma Rhei *(da huang)*
Sulphur *(liu huang)*

PREPARATION & DOSAGE: Separately grind equal amounts of the two ingredients into powder. Then combine the powders and grind again until extremely fine. Mix with cold water to form a liquid paste. After washing the affected area with soap and water, apply a thin layer of the herbal paste with a sterile cotton ball 1-2 times daily.

For heat toxin and damp toxin types of acne, Remove Spots Ointment is recommended.

❧ Remove Spots Ointment
去斑膏
qù bān gāo

Semen Hydnocarpi Anthelminticae *(da feng zi)* 30g
Semen Pruni Armeniacae *(xing ren)* 30g
Semen Persicae *(tao ren)* 30g
Hydrargyrioxydum rubrum *(hong fen)* 30g
Camphora *(zhang nao)* 30g

PREPARATION & DOSAGE: Grind the first three ingredients together into a fine powder, then add the remaining two ingredients and continue grinding until a paste forms. If the paste is dry, mix in a few drops of sesame oil. Store in an amber, airtight glass jar. After washing the affected areas with soap and water, apply the remedy by gently rubbing it into the skin with a sterile cotton ball. Apply once daily.

CLINICAL NOTE: Apply to a small inconspicuous area first in order to check for side effects. Due to the toxicity of this remedy, do not use long-term. Discontinue when inflammation is resolved, and continue treatment with other remedies.

EAR ACUPUNCTURE

Appropriate points for needling include Lung, Endocrine, Testicle and Cheek. Treat any two points during the first session, then alternate the points during subsequent sessions. Treat once daily or every other day, retaining the needles for 20-30 minutes. Ten treatments constitute one course. Improvement should be evident after 1-2 courses.

EMPIRICAL REMEDIES

The following associated points may be treated: BL-15 *(xin shu)*, BL-13 *(fei shu)*, BL-18 *(gan shu)*, BL- 20 *(pi shu)* and BL-23 *(shen shu)*. Select 2-3 points at the first session, then alternate points during subsequent sessions. Before treatment, massage or knead the skin surrounding the points. Then bloodlet the points, squeezing 2-3 drops of blood from each point. Treat once every other day, with six treatments constituting one course, and 2-3 days' rest between courses. Most patients experience improvement within 2-3 courses.

The source text[1] suggests that bloodletting these associated points of the back drains heat from their respective Organs—heat that has accumulated and given rise to the acne lesions.

Traditional vs. Biomedical Treatment

Treatment in general is aimed at controlling the symptoms, since in many cases acne is self-limiting. Traditional modalities may be more effective in eliminating the root of the condition through correct pattern differentiation and appropriate therapy. Biomedical means involve administration of pharmaceuticals such as vitamin A acid, salicylic acid, benzoyl peroxide and topical antibiotics, among others. Some individuals may be recommended for acne surgery or intralesional therapy.

Prevention

The course of acne varies greatly. Untreated acne can last for several years. Patients should be advised not to pick the lesions, particularly the crust covering an opened lesion; such manipulation may delay healing and produce a pitted scar. Women should avoid using comedogenic cosmetics, especially those that contain oils. Frequent washing of the face with soap and water is good practice for all acne patients.

Foods and beverages that can produce dampness and heat, such as spicy and greasy items, should be avoided. Alcohol and smoking can also give rise to acne.

Rosacea
酒渣鼻
jiǔ zhā bí, "wine dregs nose"

Rosacea is a chronic inflammation of the cheeks, nose, chin, and sometimes the entire face. Descriptions of this condition appear in early Chinese medical texts, such as Chapter 31 of *Basic Questions* where it is observed, "In a patient with Spleen heat, [the] nose [becomes] red first." In the *Compendium of Exter-*

nal Medicine (1665), Qi Kun provides a more detailed description of the cause and treatment of this disorder:

> A person with wine dregs nose, [the condition is caused by] blood heat steaming in the Lung channel first, and then by wind-cold attack, [resulting in] blood stasis which congeals so that [the skin] first [becomes] purple then dark. Treatment should ventilate the Lung, dispel blood stasis, so that the qi of the nutritive and protective levels flows freely to nourish new blood.

The biomedical cause of rosacea is unknown. The disease usually affects persons 20 to 50 years of age, and sometimes older. Women are affected more often than men, although in men the condition is more severe. Individuals with rosacea are more prone to blushing and flushing, and have ruddy complexions. Prolonged vasodilation can cause telangiectasis (permanent dilation of the blood vessels) and stimulation of the sebaceous glands, thus leading to acne-like papules and pustules.

Signs & Symptoms

Most patients indicate that their skin is sensitive and easily irritated, and that it feels hot to them, particularly during episodes of flushing. Redness affects the central areas of the face, although the forehead and chin are often involved as well. Upon pressure, the area blanches. Acne-like papules and pustules resemble acne, but comedones are not usually seen. When acneiform lesions are present, the condition is known as acne rosacea. In severe cases, pustules may evolve into cystic or granulomatous nodules. Enlargement of the nose due to sebaceous and fibrous hyperplasia is referred to as rhinophyma, or the "W. C. Fields" nose. Alcohol ingestion causes facial flushing, thus chronic alcoholism may predispose individuals with rosacea to rhinophyma. But by no means are all patients with rhinophyma alcoholics.

Differential Diagnosis

Rosacea is differentiated from acne by the presence of comedones in the latter. The butterfly erythema of lupus erythematosus may be confused with rosacea; however, laboratory findings will confirm a diagnosis of lupus.

Traditional Chinese Etiology

The four primary causes of rosacea are accumulated heat in the Lung and Stomach, clumped heat toxin, blood heat, and stagnation of qi and blood.

Accumulated heat in the Lung and Stomach. This is often due to overindulgence in alcohol or spicy foods, which causes heat to overpower the Stomach and then to steam the Lung. Heat then accumulates in the Lung and Stomach channels and rises to the nose area, thus causing the condition.

Clumped heat toxin. This is the result of pre-existing accumulated Lung and Stomach heat combining with attack by toxin. The heat toxin then rises through the Lung and Stomach channels to the face, causing the lesions.

Blood heat. This is often due to disharmonies of the penetrating and conception channels, such that blood heat stagnates in the skin and tissues of the nose area, giving rise to the lesions.

Stagnation of qi and blood. This can be caused by pre-existing disharmonies in the penetrating and conception channels or by pre-existing accumulated heat in the Lung and Stomach, after which attack by cold occurs. Heat is then unable to be ventilated and drained, and steams upward and clumps in the nose area, causing local stagnation of qi and blood, thus resulting in the condition.

Treatment

INTERNAL

Accumulated heat in the Lung and Stomach. This pattern is characterized by redness of the bulb of the nose. The redness blanches upon pressure. Generalized symptoms may include dryness of the nose and mouth, constipation, a red tongue with a thin yellow coating, and a wiry, slippery pulse. The treatment strategy is to clear heat and cool the blood. The formula Eriobotrya Decoction to Clear the Lung (see acne above) may be administered once daily.

Clumped heat toxin. In addition to redness, the bulb of the nose may also present with edema, pustules and pain, all of which, if severe, may affect the proximal areas of the nose. Generalized symptoms may include sensations of heat of the nose, thirst, dry stools, yellow urine, a red tongue with a yellow coating, and a floating and slippery, or a slippery and rapid pulse. The treatment strategy is to clear heat, cool the blood, and relieve toxicity. The formula Five-Ingredient Decoction to Eliminate Toxin (see folliculitis in Chapter 7) may be administered once daily.

Blood heat. In this pattern, the bulb of the nose is red, and scattered red papules surround the areas proximal to the nose and mouth; telangiectasis is evident on the cheeks. Generalized symptoms may include constipation, irregular menses in women, a red tongue with a thin yellow or white coating, and a wiry, slippery pulse. The treatment strategy is to cool the blood and clear heat, and regulate the penetrating and conception channels. The formula Cool the Blood Decoction with Five Flowers (see acne above) may be administered once or twice daily.

Stagnation of qi and blood. In this pattern, the bulb of the nose is dark red or purple, enlarged and moist, with telangiectasis, hypertrophy and enlarged openings of the sebaceous follicles; severe cases will show nodules or rhinophyma. Generalized symptoms may include a purple tongue with a sticky yellow coating, and a wiry, slow pulse. The treatment strategy is to invigorate the blood and dispel blood stasis, and soften masses and dissipate nodules. The formula Four-Substance Decoction with Safflower and Peach Pit (see acne above) may be administered once or twice daily for this pattern.

EXTERNAL

For papular or pustular lesions, apply Upside Down Powder (see acne above). For heat patterns, Rosacea Paste is recommended.

❧ Rosacea Paste
酒渣鼻膏
jiǔ zhā bí gāo

Lithargyrum *(mi tuo seng)* 60g
Radix Scrophulariae Ningpoensis *(xuan shen)* 30g
Sulphur *(liu huang)* 30g
Calomelas *(qing fen)* 24g

PREPARATION & DOSAGE: Grind the ingredients together into a fine powder. Mix with honey to form a paste. Store in an airtight glass jar. After washing the affected area with soap and water, rub with a small amount of the paste for 5 minutes, once in the morning and once before bedtime. Improvement is usually seen after 2-3 months of continuous application.

ACUPUNCTURE

Filiform needling. For all patterns of rosacea the primary acupoints for needling include M-HN-3 *(yin tang)*, GV-25 *(su liao)*, LI-20 *(ying xiang)*, ST-4 *(di cang)*, CV-24 *(cheng jiang)* and SI-18 *(quan liao)*. The secondary points are ST-5 *(da ying)*, LI-4 *(he gu)* and LI-11 *(qu chi)*. Needle any 3-4 points at the first session, then alternate points during subsequent sessions. Use draining manipulation, and retain needles for 20-30 minutes. Treat once every 2-3 days. Ten treatments constitute one course, with 4-5 days' rest between courses. Improvement should be seen within 2-3 courses.

Ear acupuncture. Points include External Nose, Lung, Endocrine and Adrenal. Treat once every other day, retaining needles for 20-30 minutes. Five treatments constitute one course, with 4-5 days' rest between courses. Improvement should be evident after 2-3 courses.

Traditional vs. Biomedical Treatment

Traditional treatment is perhaps more effective in resolving the root of the condition, which is typically caused by a pattern of heat as described above. Biomedical intervention relies primarily on topical or systemic antibiotics, or topical sulfurs, to address the acneiform component of the disease. In cases of excessive tissue of rhinophyma, surgical measures are often recommended.

Prevention

Early and persistent treatment is necessary to prevent telangiectasis and rhinophyma. In order to prevent vasodilation, patients should also be counseled about emotional factors that may trigger flushing and blushing. Potential irritants such as sunlight, heat and medications, if found to induce vasodilation, should also be avoided, as should alcohol and spicy foods, which produce heat. Frequent washing with soap and water is helpful in ridding the skin of oiliness.

CHAPTER NOTES

1. Jing, K., Wang, F.C. and Zhang, Y.X., "Bloodletting the Associated Points of the Five Yin Organs in the Treatment of Acne," *Beijing Journal of Traditional Chinese Medicine*, 8(3): 37; 1990.

CHAPTER 19

Disorders of Hair

Alopecia
油风
yóu fēng, "glossy wind"

Alopecia is the loss of hair in any area of the body that has hair. The Chinese name, "glossy wind" *(yóu fēng),* is derived from the suddenness of the condition (wind) and the shiny skin that remains (glossy) after the hair is gone. Other recorded names include "hair fall" *(fà luò)* and "ghost shaven head" *(guǐ tì tóu). Discussion of the Origins of Symptoms of Diseases* (610) describes this condition:

> A person who has wind excess of the head and sites [of the head] that are deficient, [will have] falling out of hair. . . . [The area] may be as large as a coin or as large as a finger. Hair does not grow, nor is there itching.

Biomedically, alopecia can result from genetic factors, aging or local or systemic disease.

Signs & Symptoms
Two general types of alopecia are distinguished: nonscarring and scarring. With nonscarring alopecia, hair loss occurs without scarring or scalp disease. With scarring alopecia, the skin after hair loss is characterized by the absence of hair follicles, and is hard and glistening and may show inflammation or atrophy. Such hair loss is usually due to mechanical trauma, burns, radiation, neoplasms and various skin diseases, such as lupus erythematosus. Since hair cannot regrow in the scarring type of alopecia, this chapter is devoted to nonscarring alopecia, which, through appropriate treatment, can often be resolved.

The major types of nonscarring alopecia are alopecia areata, telogen effluvium, drug-induced, and androgenic.

There are three forms of alopecia areata: localized, totalis, and universalis. Localized alopecia is characterized by complete hair loss in patches. The patch is typically circular, ranging in diameter from one to ten centimeters. Interestingly, the nails may also be involved, with ridging, pitting or splitting of the free edge. In alopecia totalis, the head hair is affected with sudden and generalized loss, leading to complete baldness; body hair is preserved. In alopecia areata universalis, all hair is lost from the body, including pubic, axillary, eyebrow and eyelid hair.

Telogen effluvium is characterized by shedding of hair rather than hair loss. This condition follows an acute illness, surgery or pregnancy. It may also be due to malnutrition, excessive dieting, blood loss or even severe psychologic stress.

Drug-induced alopecia occurs after taking cytotoxic drugs such as thallium compounds, or after overdoses of vitamin A.

The most common form of nonscarring hair loss is androgenetic alopecia, which includes male pattern baldness and diffuse female alopecia. In men, hair loss is familial and begins in the lateral frontal areas or over the vertex. In women, the condition results more in thinning of the hair than in hair loss, and affects the frontal and parietal regions, with complete baldness a rarity.

Differential Diagnosis

Nonscarring alopecia should be distinguished from scarring alopecia. Occasionally the patch of alopecia may appear scarred, in which case biopsy will help determine the type.

Traditional Chinese Etiology

Four primary causes of hair loss are identified: blood heat giving rise to wind, deficiency of yin and blood, deficiency of both qi and blood, and blood stasis.

Blood heat giving rise to wind. The source of this pattern is often emotional stimulation that leads to exuberant Heart fire. Heat then enters the blood, with blood heat giving rise to wind, and movement of wind causing hair loss.

Deficiency of yin and blood. This patterns is usually caused by a pre-existing deficiency of the Kidney. If Kidney yin is deficient, essence does not transform into blood. Since hair is the surplus of blood, if the blood is deficient, nourishment of the hair is compromised, and hair loss ensues. Deficiency of yin and blood can also result from general deficiency, which leads to loosening of the tissue interstices. When sweating occurs in the presence of wind in such a condition, wind easily enters the body. Overabundance of wind gives rise to blood dryness, and ultimately to deficient yin and blood, such that the hair loses its source of nourishment (blood); hair loss results.

Deficiency of both qi and blood. Hair loss after long-term illness or during the puerperium is caused by temporary deficiency of qi and blood, such that the hair loses nourishment, resulting in its loss.

Blood stasis. When long-term blood stasis exists under the skin and outside the tissues, the vessels and channels are blocked so that new blood is unable to reach and nourish the hair, resulting in hair loss.

Treatment

INTERNAL

Blood heat giving rise to wind. Hair loss is sudden and in circular patches. The underlying skin is glossy and accompanied by slight itching. Usually there are no generalized symptoms, or there may be restlessness, thirst, yellow urine and constipation. The tongue is often red with a thin yellow coating, and the pulse is wiry, slippery and rapid. The treatment strategy is to cool the blood and extinguish wind, and nourish the yin and protect the hair. The formula recommended for this pattern is Combined Four-Substance Decoction and Six-Ingredient Decoction with Rehmannia.

❧ Combined Four-Substance Decoction and Six-Ingredient Decoction with Rehmannia
四物汤六味地黄汤化裁
sì wù tāng, liù wèi dì huáng tāng huà cái

Radix Rehmanniae Glutinosae *(sheng di huang)*	15g
Fructus Ligustri Lucidi *(nu zhen zi)*	15g
Fructus Mori Albae *(sang shen)*	15g
Dry-fried Cortex Moutan Radicis *(chao mu dan pi)*	10g
Radix Paeoniae Rubrae *(chi shao)*	10g
Fructus Corni Officinalis *(shan zhu yu)*	10g
Radix Scrophulariae Ningpoensis *(xuan shen)*	12g
Semen Sesami Indici *(hei zhi ma)*	12g
Semen Cuscutae Chinensis *(tu si zi)*	12g
Haematitum *(dai zhe shi)*	30g
Sclerotium Poriae Cocos Pararadicis *(fu shen)*	12g
Radix Angelicae Sinensis *(dang gui)*	12g

PREPARATION & DOSAGE: Decoct and administer in three doses daily.

Deficiency of yin and blood. Hair loss in this pattern is insidious, and often affects persons in their twenties and thirties. The alopecia occurs over the vertex or at the lateral frontal areas. The scalp is frequently greasy or itchy with dandruff. Generalized symptoms may include light-headedness, tinnitus, soreness of the low back, tired limbs, a red tongue with little coating, and a thin, rapid pulse. The treatment strategy is to enrich and tonify the Liver and Kidney, and nourish the blood and dispel wind.

Formulas recommended for this pattern are Lu Family Decoction for Patchy Baldness, or Seven-Treasure Special Pill for Beautiful Whiskers.

❧ Lu Family Decoction for Patchy Baldness
陆氏斑秃汤
lù shì bān tū tāng

Radix Angelicae Sinensis *(dang gui)* 12g
Radix Paeoniae Rubrae *(chi shao)* 12g
Radix Paeoniae Lactiflorae *(bai shao)* 12g
Radix Ligustici Chuanxiong *(chuan xiong)* 10g
Radix Rehmanniae Glutinosae Conquitae *(shu di huang)* 12g
Radix Salviae Miltiorrhizae *(dan shen)* 15g
Radix Polygoni Multiflori *(he shou wu)* 12g
Radix Morindae Officinalis *(ba ji tian)* 12g
Herba Cistanches Deserticolae *(rou cong rong)* 12g
Fructus Ligustri Lucidi *(nu zhen zi)* 12g
Fructus Mori Albae *(sang shen)* 12g
Radix et Rhizoma Notopterygii *(qiang huo)* 10g
Herba seu Flos Schizonepetae Tenuifoliae *(jing jie)* 10g

PREPARATION & DOSAGE: Decoct and administer in 1-2 doses daily.

❦ Seven-Treasure Special Pill for Beautiful Whiskers
七宝美髯丹
qī bǎo měi rán dān

Radix Polygoni Multiflori *(he shou wu)*
  (steamed in black sesame seeds) 300g
Sclerotium Poriae Cocos *(fu ling)* 150g
Radix Achyranthis Bidentatae *(niu xi)* 150g
Radix Angelicae Sinensis *(dang gui)* 150g
Fructus Lycii *(gou qi zi)* 150g
Semen Cuscutae Chinensis *(tu si zi)* 150g
Fructus Psoraleae Corylifoliae *(bu gu zhi)*
  (deep-fried with black sesame seeds) 120g

PREPARATION & DOSAGE: Grind the ingredients into a powder and form with honey into 9g pills. Administer one pill in the morning and one in the evening with warm, salted water.

Deficiency of both qi and blood. This pattern presents with dry and brittle hair. Loss of hair is gradual and affects the entire scalp rather than specific areas. As opposed to the deficiency of yin and blood pattern, there is no itching of the scalp. Generalized symptoms may include weakness, a low and weak voice, pallor, palpitations, numbness of the limbs, a pale tongue with little coating, and a thin, weak pulse. The treatment strategy is to tonify both the qi and blood.

Formulas recommended for this pattern are Modified Eight-Treasure Decoction, or Ginseng Decoction to Nourish the Nutritive Qi.

❦ Modified Eight-Treasure Decoction
八珍汤加减
bā zhēn tāng jiā jiǎn

Radix Angelicae Sinensis *(dang gui)* 12g
Radix Rehmanniae Glutinosae Conquitae *(shu di huang)* 12g
Dry-fried Radix Paeoniae Lactiflorae *(chao bai shao)* 12g
Radix Codonopsitis Pilosulae *(dang shen)* 12g
Rhizoma Atractylodis Macrocephalae *(bai zhu)* 12g
Radix Astragali Membranacei *(huang qi)* 15g
Sclerotium Poriae Cocos *(fu ling)* 15g
Fructus Ligustri Lucidi *(nu zhen zi)* 15g
Radix Polygoni Multiflori *(he shou wu)* 15g
Semen Glycine Max *(hei da dou)* 15g
Radix Ligustici Chuanxiong *(chuan xiong)* 6g
Rhizoma Typhonii Gigantei *(bai fu zi)* 6g
Honey-toasted Radix Glycyrrhizae Uralensis *(zhi gan cao)* 6g

PREPARATION & DOSAGE: Decoct and administer in three doses daily.

❦ Ginseng Decoction to Nourish the Nutritive Qi
人参养营汤
rén shēn yǎng yíng tāng

Radix Paeoniae Lactiflorae *(bai shao)* 90g
Radix Angelicae Sinensis *(dang gui)* 30g
Pericarpium Citri Reticulatae *(chen pi)* 30g
Radix Astragali Membranacei *(huang qi)* 30g
Cortex Cinnamomi Cassiae *(rou gui)* 30g
Radix Ginseng *(ren shen)* 30g
Rhizoma Atractylodis Macrocephalae *(bai zhu)* 30g
Honey-toasted Radix Glycyrrhizae Uralensis *(zhi gan cao)* 30g
Radix Rehmanniae Glutinosae Conquitae *(shu di huang)* 22.5g
Fructus Schisandrae Chinensis *(wu wei zi)* 22.5g
Sclerotium Poriae Cocos *(fu ling)* 22.5g
Radix Polygalae Tenuifoliae *(yuan zhi)* 15g

PREPARATION & DOSAGE: Grind the ingredients into a powder and administer 12g once daily as a draft with three pieces of Rhizoma Zingiberis Officinalis Recens *(sheng jiang)* and two pieces of Fructus Zizyphi Jujubae *(da zao)*.

Blood stasis. Patients with this pattern often experience headache or a piercing pain of the scalp before hair loss begins. Actual hair loss occurs in patches; body hair may also be involved. In severe cases, complete loss of hair may result. Generalized symptoms may include thirst with the desire to drink, dream-disturbed sleep, nightmares, a cyanotic complexion, purple lips, a purple tongue with stasis spots, and a thin, choppy pulse. The treatment strategy is to invigorate the blood and dispel stasis. The formula recommended for this pattern is Unblock the Orifices and Invigorate the Blood Decoction.

Unblock the Orifices and Invigorate the Blood Decoction
通窍活血汤
tōng qiào huó xuè tāng

Radix Paeoniae Rubrae *(chi shao)*	3g
Radix Ligustici Chuanxiong *(chuan xiong)*	3g
Semen Persicae *(tao ren)*	9g
Flos Carthami Tinctorii *(hong hua)*	9g
Bulbus Allii Fistulosi *(cong bai)*	3g
Fructus Zizyphi Jujubae *(da zao)*	7 pieces
Rhizoma Zingiberis Officinalis Recens *(sheng jiang)*	9g
Secretio Moschus *(she xiang)*	0.15g

PREPARATION & DOSAGE: Decoct all the ingredients except Secretio Moschus *(she xiang)*. Add this ingredient and a small amount of rice wine to the strained decoction before administering once daily.

EXTERNAL

For all patterns of hair loss, Biota Ointment is recommended.

Biota Ointment
柏枝油
bǎi zhī yóu

Cacumen Biotae Orientalis *(ce bai ye)*	90g
Fructus Zanthoxyli Bungeani *(chuan jiao)*	90g
Rhizoma Pinelliae Ternatae *(ban xia)*	90g

PREPARATION & DOSAGE: Coarsely grind together all the ingredients. Decoct in 500ml of water until 250ml remains. Then add one teaspoon of honey, and boil for another 5 minutes. Strain and discard the dregs, and store the decoction in a glass container. Each time before applying, pour out the necessary amount and add one-half teaspoon of fresh ginger juice. Apply to hairless areas twice daily.

For deficiency of yin and blood, Artemisia Argyi Decoction is recommended.

Artemisia Argyi Decoction
海艾汤
hǎi ài tāng

Folium Artemisiae Argyi *(ai ye)*	6g
Flos Chrysanthemi Morifolii *(ju hua)*	6g
Herba Menthae Haplocalycis *(bo he)*	6g
Radix Ledebouriellae Divaricatae *(fang feng)*	6g
Rhizoma et Radix Ligustici *(gao ben)*	6g
Secretio Moschus *(she xiang)*	6g

Rhizoma et Radix Nardostachydis *(gan song)* 6g
Fructus Viticis *(man jing zi)* 6g
Herba seu Flos Schizonepetae Tenuifoliae *(jing jie)* 6g

PREPARATION & DOSAGE: Decoct the ingredients in 1.25 to 1.5 liters of water. Pour the decoction and its dregs into a large basin and allow the steam to envelop the face. When the fluid has suitably cooled, wash the head and massage the scalp with the decoction for 5 minutes. Then allow the remedy to settle into the scalp for another 5 minutes. Repeat the procedure. Rinse with warm water.

CLINICAL NOTE: Do not shampoo the hair immediately after using this remedy. If the hair needs washing, do so before applying the remedy.

For a pattern of deficiency of both qi and blood, Cordyceps Tincture is recommended.

❦ Cordyceps Tincture
冬虫夏草酊
dōng chóng xià cǎo dīng

Cordyceps Sinensis *(dong chong xia cao)* 60g
75% Alcohol 300ml

PREPARATION & DOSAGE: Soak the herb in the alcohol for seven days. Strain and discard the dregs, then use a cotton ball dipped in the remedy to rub the hairless areas 3-5 times daily.

CLINICAL NOTE: This treatment may be used for thin and slow-growing hair in children.

For baldness accompanied by severe itching in children, Brassica Powder is recommended.

❦ Brassica Powder
芜菁子散
wú jīng zǐ sǎn

Semen Brassicae Rapae (wu jing zi)

PREPARATION & DOSAGE: Grind any amount of the herb into a fine powder. Mix together with enough lard or oil to form an ointment. Apply to the head once daily.

ACUPUNCTURE

Filiform needling. The primary points for needling include GV-20 *(bai hui)*, ST-8 *(tou wei)* and Grow Hair point *(zhǎng fà diǎn),* an extra point located midway between GV-16 *(feng fu)* and GB-20 *(feng chi).* The secondary points are M-HN-13 *(yi ming)*, GV-23 *(shang xing)*, M-HN-9 *(tai yang)*, GB-20 *(feng chi)*, and M-HN-6 *(yu yao)* through to TB-23 *(si zhu kong)*. At the first session, in addition to needling the primary points, needle three secondary points. During ensuing sessions, needle the primary points and alternate the secondary points. Treatment should be once every other day. Use tonifying manipulation for deficiency patterns, and draining manipulation for symptoms of excess. Ten sessions constitute one course of therapy, with 4-5 days' rest between courses.

Encircling acupuncture may also be used, particularly for patchy areas of hair loss. Insert transversely four 32-34 gauge needles extending from the border of the patch toward the center. Retain the needles for 30 minutes, during which they should be manipulated every 10 minutes. Frequency of treatment should follow the schedule above.

Cutaneous acupuncture. Gently tap hairless patches with a plum-blossom needle until erythema or slight bleeding occurs. Tapping should be from the hair border toward the center of the patch. Frequency of treatment should follow the schedule above.

MOXIBUSTION

Use indirect moxibustion with ginger on BL-23 *(shen shu)*, BL-13 *(fei shu)*, ST-36 *(zu san li)*, TB-5 *(wai guan)*, GB-34 *(yang ling quan)* and on hairless patches (be careful not to singe the surrounding hair). Treatment should be once every 2-3 days. Five sessions constitute one course, with five days' rest between courses.

EMPIRICAL REMEDIES

[A] Apply warmed, mashed fresh ginger to areas of alopecia twice daily.[1]

[B] A combined internal-external method of treating alopecia is described below. The source text[2] states that the combined internal-external method treats both the branch and the root causes of alopecia. External formulas such as these are aimed at invigorating blood circulation, so that hair growth is promoted. Conditions of recent origin respond well to this method.

The internal formula is called Protect the Hair Decoction *(bǎo fà tāng)*, and is comprised of 15g Radix Polygoni Multiflori *(he shou wu)*, 15g Radix Angelicae Sinensis *(dang gui)*, 15g Herba Ecliptae Prostratae *(han lian cao)*, 15g Fructus Ligustri Lucidi *(nu zhen zi)*, 15g Fructus Mori Albae *(sang shen)*, 15g Fructus Schisandrae Chinensis *(wu wei zi)*, 15g Radix Rehmanniae Glutinosae *(sheng di huang)*, 10g Fructus Psoraleae Corylifoliae *(bu gu zhi)* and 10g Fructus Lycii *(gou qi zi)*.

MODIFICATIONS: For dizziness, soreness of the lower back and general weakness, add 15g Semen Cuscutae Chinensis *(tu si zi)*, 15g Fructus Rubi Chingii *(fu pen zi)*, and 15g Radix Dipsaci Asperi *(xu duan)*; for deficiency of blood, weariness, dream-disturbed sleep and palpitations, add 15g Semen Biotae Orientalis *(bai zi ren)*, 15g Fructus Alpiniae Oxyphyllae *(yi zhi ren)*, and 15g Caulis Polygoni Multiflori *(ye jiao teng)*; for dryness of the mouth, and symptoms of deficiency of fluids, add 10g Herba Dendrobii *(shi hu)* and 10g Tuber Ophiopogonis Japonici *(mai men dong)*.

PREPARATION & DOSAGE: Decoct and administer two doses daily.

The external formula is known as Generate Hair Treasure *(shēng fà bǎo)*, and is made up of 30g Mylabris *(ban mao)*, 70g Radix Ginseng *(ren shen)*, 100g Radix Ligustici Chuanxiong *(chuan xiong)*, 100g Semen Sinapis Albae *(bai jie zi)*, 100g Cortex Cinnamomi Cassiae *(rou gui)*, 200g Semen Persicae *(tao ren)*, 400g Radix Angelicae Sinensis *(dang gui)*, 400g Fructus Psoraleae Corylifoliae *(bu gu zhi)*, 800g Radix Salviae Miltiorrhizae *(dan shen)* and 800g Radix Astragali Membranacei *(huang qi)*.

PREPARATION & DOSAGE: Steep the ingredients in 40 liters of 75% alcohol for 7-10 days. Strain the dregs and pour the herbal fluid into smaller glass containers. With a cotton ball, rub the remedy onto areas of alopecia 2-8 times daily.

Traditional vs. Biomedical Treatment

Patients who have been balding for less than five years generally respond to treatment, whether traditional or biomedical. The term "respond" indicates new hair growth ranging anywhere from sparse to total coverage. Successful traditional treatment of alopecia requires careful differentiation of the presenting pattern. Practitioners should note that hair loss is not always due to Kidney deficiency. Indeed, the famous Qing dynasty physician Wang Qing-Ren (1768-1831) once observed that hair loss without apparent reason (such as that due to blood heat, yin and blood deficiency, or deficiency of both the qi and blood) is often caused by blood stasis, and should be treated as such. Traditional treatment also requires good patient-practitioner cooperation, as long-term therapy may be necessary before any results are seen.

Biomedical therapy of alopecia involves applying a topical solution of minoxidil. However, this medication can occasionally cause fluid retention, weight gain, hypotension or tachycardia. In addition, when treatment is discontinued, the newly regrown hair falls out. Hair transplantation is another biomedical means of addressing baldness.

Prevention

Recent cases of hair loss should be treated promptly to prevent further hair thinning and loss and to stimulate regrowth. Persons with blood heat patterns should avoid foods and beverages that produce heat, such as spicy items and alcohol.

CHAPTER NOTES

1. Dou, G.X. *Guide to Food Therapy (Yin shi zhi liao zhi nan)*. Jiangsu: Jiangsu Science and Technology Press, 1981.

2. Xiao, C.D., "Internal Administration and External Application of Chinese Herbs in the Treatment of Alopecia Areata," *Shaanxi Journal of Chinese Traditional Medicine,* 13(7): 301; 1992.

CHAPTER 20

Circulatory Disorders

Purpura
紫斑
zǐ bān, "purple spots"

A purpura is a small hemorrhage in the skin or mucous membrane that causes a purple macule or papule. There are many names for such lesions in Chinese. During the Sui-Tang dynasties (581-907) they were known as "spotted toxin" *(bān dú)*, and during the Ming-Qing (1368-1911) period as "purple spots" *(zǐ bān)*. The etiology determines whether purpuric lesions are categorized as yin or yang.

The biomedical causes of purpura are numerous, and range from trauma to blood disorders to vascular abnormalities. Western dermatologists have developed classification systems to aid diagnosis. One classification that helps in the recall of various types of purpura is based on whether the reason for the lesion is within the vessel, in the vessel wall itself, or in the supporting tissue. Other classifications are based on such factors as defects in the coagulation system, the presence or absence of inflammation, the palpability of the lesions, or the presence of an immunologic reaction. However, no one classification is adequate since more than one process may be taking place simultaneously.

Signs & Symptoms

Usually the first lesions are bluish or reddish-blue. With time and absorption the lesions turn shades of yellowish or reddish brown. Lesions a few millimeters in diameter are known as petechiae, and those larger than three centimeters are referred to as ecchymoses, "black-and-blue" discolorations, or bruises. Deeper accumulations of blood are called hematomas.

Differential Diagnosis

Diagnosis is based on the appearance of the lesions, which change in color over time. Also significant are the various laboratory tests that measure platelet count, prothrombin count, bleeding time and other factors involved in bleeding.

Traditional Chinese Etiology

This section will not describe purpura that are associated with febrile and infectious diseases such as typhus, sepsis, Rocky Mountain spotted fever, and the like.

There are five primary etiologies of purpura: reckless movement of blood, damp-heat sinking, Spleen does not govern blood, deficiency of Spleen and Kidney yang, and cold congealing blood.

Reckless movement of blood. This is seen in individuals who have pre-existing blood heat, such that when they eat foods that provoke wind (such as fish and shellfish), or when they are attacked by external wind, the blood heat contends with the wind excess. The result is reckless movement of blood that leads to the blood seeping through the collaterals and vessels, and congealing in the tissues and skin, thus forming the lesions.

Damp-heat sinking. This pattern comes about because of pre-existing damp-heat that blocks the collaterals and vessels such that qi and blood do not flow smoothly, and seep into the tissues and skin, giving rise to purpura. Dampness is a heavy excess and is sinking in nature; thus, lesions of this type affect the lower body.

Spleen does not govern blood. When Spleen qi is insufficient, the Spleen loses its ability to govern blood, such that blood escapes from the collaterals and vessels into the tissues and skin, producing purpura.

Deficiency of Spleen and Kidney yang. The source of this pattern is diminished life gate fire such that fire is unable to produce earth, resulting in deficiency of Spleen yang. The Spleen loses its ability to govern blood, and blood escapes into the tissues and skin, thus producing purpura.

Cold congealing blood. This pattern is usually seen in persons with pre-existing yang deficiency who are attacked by cold. Cold enters the collaterals and vessels causing blood to congeal, thus giving rise to purpura.

Treatment

Reckless movement of blood. This is a yang type of purpura that commonly affects young persons under 30 years of age. The onset is sudden with the lesions often appearing bilaterally on the extensor surfaces of the lower legs. Slight itching may be present. The lesions are usually the size of small coins and may coalesce; they do not fade upon pressure. Occasionally, the lesions may also present as minute raised papules. The purpura ordinarily resolves within 2-3 weeks, although reappearances are not uncommon. Generalized symptoms may include a sensation of heat in the body, restlessness, sore throat, thirst, malaise, a red tongue with a thin yellow coating, and a slippery and rapid, or a thin and rapid pulse. The treatment strategy is to clear heat and cool the blood, and invigorate the blood and eliminate spots.

The formulas recommended for this pattern are Cool the Blood Decoction with Five Roots, or Cool and Invigorate the Blood Formula.

❧ Cool the Blood Decoction with Five Roots
凉血五根汤
liáng xuè wǔ gēn tāng

Rhizoma Imperatae Cylindricae *(bai mao gen)*	30-60g
Radix Trichosanthis Kirilowii *(tian hua fen)*	15-30g
Radix Rubiae Cordifoliae *(qian cao gen)*	9-15g
Radix Arnebiae seu Lithospermi *(zi cao)*	9-15g
Radix Isatidis seu Baphicacanthi *(ban lan gen)*	9-15g

PREPARATION & DOSAGE: Decoct and administer in two doses daily.

❧ Cool and Invigorate the Blood Formula
凉血活血方
liáng xuè huó xuè fāng

Ramulus Sambuci Williamsii *(jie gu mu)*	9g
Radix Paeoniae Rubrae *(chi shao)*	9g
Radix Rubiae Cordifoliae *(qian cao)*	15g
Radix et Rhizoma Rhei Praeparata *(zhi da huang)*	9g
Herba Leonuri Heterophylli *(yi mu cao)*	15g
Radix Rehmanniae Glutinosae *(sheng di huang)*	15g
Herba Artemisiae Yinchenhao *(yin chen hao)*	12g
Radix Glycyrrhizae Uralensis *(gan cao)*	3g

PREPARATION & DOSAGE: Decoct and administer in 1-2 doses daily.

In severe cases of this pattern the purpura may be generalized and appear as dark purple patches. This is due to accumulated heat in the Stomach channel, which provokes reckless movement of blood such that heat injures the vessels and collaterals, resulting in blood seeping into the tissues. The legs may be swollen and appear cyanotic, and hemorrhaging and ulcers may affect the gums. The treatment strategy for this pattern is to clear Stomach heat and relieve toxicity, and cool the blood and transform spots. The recommended formula is Eliminate Spots with Indigo Decoction.

❧ Eliminate Spots with Indigo Decoction
消斑青黛饮
xiāo bān qīng dài yǐn

Indigo Pulverata Levis *(qing dai)*
Rhizoma Coptidis *(huang lian)*
Fructus Gardeniae Jasminoidis *(zhi zi)*
Radix Scrophulariae Ningpoensis *(xuan shen)*

Rhizoma Anemarrhenae Asphodeloidis *(zhi mu)*
Radix Rehmanniae Glutinosae *(sheng di huang)*
Cornu Rhinoceri *(xi jiao)*
Gypsum *(shi gao)*
Radix Bupleuri *(chai hu)*
Radix Ginseng *(ren shen)*
Radix Glycyrrhizae Uralensis *(gan cao)*
Rhizoma Zingiberis Officinalis Recens *(sheng jiang)*
Fructus Zizyphi Jujubae *(da zao)*

PREPARATION & DOSAGE: The source text does not indicate the amounts for the ingredients. Decoct and administer in 1-2 doses daily.

CLINICAL NOTE: It is strongly reccommended that Cornu Bubali *(shui niu jiao)* be substituted for Cornu Rhinoceri *(xi jiao)*, both because it is much less expensive, and because all species of rhinoceros are endangered.

Damp-heat sinking. This is a yang type of purpura, and often affects young females between the ages of 20 and 30. The lower legs and/or thighs are frequently involved. Initial lesions are flaming red and painful, and are often nodular (about 3-5cm in diameter). With time the lesions turn purple and the nodules dissipate without scarring. Generalized symptoms may include joint pain, heaviness and restricted movement of the limbs, a sticky sensation in the mouth, sticky stools causing a feeling of incomplete bowel evacuation, foul smelling vaginal discharge in women, a red tongue with a yellow sticky coating, and a slippery, rapid pulse. The treatment strategy is to invigorate the blood and unblock the channels. The formula recommended for this pattern is Unblock the Collaterals and Invigorate the Blood Formula.

❧ Unblock the Collaterals and Invigorate the Blood Formula
通络活血方
tōng luò huó xuè fāng

Radix Angelicae Sinensis *(dang gui)*
Radix Paeoniae Rubrae *(chi shao)*
Semen Persicae *(tao ren)*
Flos Carthami Tinctorii *(hong hua)*
Rhizoma Cyperi Rotundi *(xiang fu)*
Pericarpium Citri Reticulatae Viride *(qing pi)*
Semen Vaccariae Segetalis *(wang bu liu xing)*
Radix Rubiae Cordifoliae *(qian cao)*
Herba Lycopi Lucidi *(ze lan)*
Radix Achyranthis Bidentatae *(niu xi)*

PREPARATION & DOSAGE: The source text does not indicate the amounts for the ingredients. Decoct and administer in 1-2 doses daily.

Spleen does not govern blood. This is a yin type of purpura, with chronic recurrences. The lesions are dark purple and macular. Generalized symptoms may include a sallow or pale and lackluster complexion, lack of appetite, tiredness, shallow breathing, a low voice, a pale tongue, and a thin, weak pulse. As the condition becomes protracted, patients may suffer nosebleeds, bloody stools, or excessive uterine bleeding. The treatment strategy is to tonify the Spleen and benefit the qi, and guide the blood to return to the channels. The formula recommended for this pattern is Restore the Spleen Decoction.

❧ Restore the Spleen Decoction
归脾汤
guī pí tāng

Radix Ginseng *(ren shen)*	3-6g
Radix Astragali Membranacei *(huang qi)*	9-12g
Rhizoma Atractylodis Macrocephalae *(bai zhu)*	9-12g
Sclerotium Poriae Cocos *(fu ling)*	9-12g
Semen Zizyphi Spinosae *(suan zao ren)*	9-12g
Arillus Euphoriae Longanae *(long yan rou)*	6-9g
Radix Aucklandiae Lappae *(mu xiang)*	3-6g
Honey-toasted Radix Glycyrrhizae Uralensis *(zhi gan cao)*	3-6g
Radix Angelicae Sinensis *(dang gui)*	6-9g
Prepared Radix Polygalae Tenuifoliae *(zhi yuan zhi)*	3-6g

PREPARATION & DOSAGE: Decoct and administer in 1-2 doses daily.

Deficiency of Spleen and Kidney yang. This is a yin type of purpura that is chronic and recurs frequently. The lower extremities are primarily affected. The lesions are violet and range between 3-5cm; they do not coalesce. Generalized symptoms may include cold extremities, aversion to cold, loose stools, daybreak diarrhea, sallow complexion, low grade abdominal pain that is relieved upon warmth and pressure, and copious urine. All of these symptoms are exacerbated upon exposure to cold or when fatigued. The tongue is pale and the pulse is submerged and thin. The treatment strategy is to warm the yang and strengthen the Spleen, and tonify the gate of fire in order to produce earth.

Formulas recommended for this pattern are Fourteen-Ingredient Decoction to Strengthen the Middle, or Prepared Aconite Pill to Regulate the Middle.

❧ Fourteen-Ingredient Decoction to Strengthen the Middle
十四味建中汤
shí sì wèi jiàn zhōng tāng

Radix Angelicae Sinensis *(dang gui)* (shoots removed, then soaked in wine, and baked dry)
Radix Paeoniae Lactiflorae *(bai shao)* (filings)

Rhizoma Atractylodis Macrocephalae *(bai zhu)* (washed filings)
Honey-toasted Radix Glycyrrhizae Uralensis *(zhi gan cao)*
Radix Ginseng *(ren shen)* (shoots removed)
Tuber Ophiopogonis Japonici *(mai men dong)* (piths removed)
Radix Ligustici Chuanxiong *(chuan xiong)*
Cortex Cinnamomi Cassiae *(rou gui)* (coarse outer bark removed)
Radix Lateralis Aconiti Carmichaeli Praeparata *(fu zi)* (skin and nodes removed)
Herba Cistanches Deserticolae *(rou cong rong)* (soaked in wine overnight)
Rhizoma Pinelliae Ternatae *(ban xia)* (washed 7 times)
Honey-toasted Radix Astragali Membranacei *(zhi huang qi)*
Sclerotium Poriae Cocos *(fu ling)* (skin removed)
Radix Rehmanniae Glutinosae Conquitae *(shu di huang)*

PREPARATION & DOSAGE: Separately grind equal amounts of the ingredients into coarse powders, then mix together well. Decoct 9g in 220ml of water, adding three slices of Rhizoma Zingiberis Officinalis *(gan jiang)* and one piece of Fructus Ziziphi Jujubae *(da zao),* until 150ml remains. Discard the dregs and administer the warm decoction on an empty stomach. Administer in one dose daily.

❧ Prepared Aconite Pill to Regulate the Middle
附子理中丸
fù zǐ lǐ zhōng wán

Radix Lateralis Aconiti Carmichaeli Praeparata *(fu zi)*	90g
Rhizoma Zingiberis Officinalis *(gan jiang)*	90g
Radix Ginseng *(ren shen)*	90g
Rhizoma Atractylodis Macrocephalae *(bai zhu)*	90g
Honey-toasted Radix Glycyrrhizae Uralensis *(zhi gan cao)*	90g

PREPARATION & DOSAGE: Grind the ingredients together into a fine powder and form into 3g pills with honey. Make a draft of one pill and administer warm on an empty stomach. Administer in one dose daily.

Cold congealing blood. This is a yin type of purpura that primarily affects young women in their twenties. The lesions are purple and have a predilection for the face, nose, ears and dorsal surfaces of the hands and feet. The condition is relieved upon warmth and exacerbated when exposed to cold. Generalized symptoms may include a pale tongue with purple spots, and a submerged, thin and slow pulse. The treatment strategy is to warm the channels and scatter cold, and invigorate the blood and dispel stasis. The formula recommended for this pattern is Tangkuei Decoction for Frigid Extremities.

❧ Tangkuei Decoction for Frigid Extremities

当归四逆汤
dāng guī sì nì tāng

Radix Angelicae Sinensis *(dang gui)*	9g
Radix Paeoniae *(shao yao)*	9g
Ramulus Cinnamomi Cassiae *(gui zhi)*	9g
Herba cum Radice Asari *(xi xin)*	6g
Honey-toasted Radix Glycyrrhizae Uralensis *(zhi gan cao)*	6g
Fructus Zizyphi Jujubae *(da zao)*	25 pieces
Caulis Mutong *(mu tong)*	6g

PREPARATION & DOSAGE: Decoct and administer in three doses daily.

ACUPUNCTURE

The primary acupoints for needling include LI-11 *(qu chi)*, CV-6 *(qi hai)* and ST-36 *(zu san li)*. The secondary points are PC-6 *(nei guan)*, ST-25 *(tian shu)*, KI-9 *(zhu bin)* and BL-58 *(fei yang)*. Treat once daily or every other day. The primary points are needled during each treatment, along with two of the four secondary points; alternate pairs of secondary points at each session. Even manipulation should be utilized, and retain needles for 20 minutes.

For enhanced efficacy, acupuncture may be combined with the appropriate internal formula.

Traditional vs. Biomedical Treatment

In idiopathic cases, or those for which biomedical treatment is nonspecific (e.g., easy bruising, senile purpura, various immune and nonimmune purpuras), a traditional approach may lead to resolution of the root of the problem. Practitioners should be mindful that in Chinese medicine, purpura can be of different etiologies, and should not limit their differentiation solely to heat.

Prevention

Known causes, such as drugs that have produced the condition, should be discontinued. Traditional treatment of purpura may help prevent future episodes.

Leg Ulcers
臁疮
lián chuāng, "shin sores"

Leg ulcers are chronic open sores affecting the lower third of the legs. Several Chinese texts describe this condition. Among them is the following passage from *Complete Book of Ulcer Experience* (1695):

> Persons with medial or lateral shin sores [that are] next to *san li* [point] and to the side of *yin jiao* [point], develop [the sores] because of coldness in the Kidney channel attacking the lower burner; internally, because of attack by wind excess, and externally, because of struggle of cold; or [the sores] may be caused by bump injury. Developing this, [the lesion] slowly ulcerates, the pus fluid does not dry. Because of the chronic nature of these sores, the popular term for them is "old festering foot" *(laǒ làn tuǐ)*.

Biomedically, there are many causes of leg ulcers. The most common is venous disease and the second most common is arteriosclerosis. More than one pathologic process may be involved. Trauma, even slight ones, may trigger lesions in many of these diseases, and poses a particular problem in venous ulcers. Detailed descriptions of the various types of leg ulcers can be found in many Western dermatology textbooks.

Signs & Symptoms

Traditional Chinese dermatology divides the development of leg ulcers into two stages.

Initial stage. In most instances, itching precedes pain, with some cases experiencing alternating itching and pain. This is followed by erythema, edema, breakage of the skin, oozing, and then ulcer formation. Lesions that are not treated in a timely manner may then expand rapidly; the tissue inside the ulcer is inflamed with necrotic debris. The ulcer edges may be thick or thin. Often, a stench emanates from the wound. The tissue surrounding the ulcer may be either erythematous or deep purple, and affected by burning pain.

Advanced stage. As the ulcer progresses, the opening sinks and the edges become slightly smooth and round. The tissue within the ulcer may be grayish white or yellow, or deep purple. The exudate is often grayish black or green, and the odor is unbearable. The surrounding tissue is pigmented by hemosiderin (intracellular deposits of iron) and melanin, causing the skin to turn reddish brown. As the condition advances, the area becomes hardened with fibrosis, leading to chronic and disabling ulcers. Severe cases may present with deep ulcers revealing the bone. The size of the lesions may vary from small to those that involve much of the lower leg.

In modern biomedicine, the symptoms just described correspond to venous leg ulcers. Occupations and activities that require prolonged sitting and standing contribute to venous stasis, edema and venous insufficiency. Thus, the potential for developing leg ulcers is high in these individuals, particularly following trauma.

Traditional Chinese Etiology

There are four primary causes of leg ulcers: damp-heat lodged in the lower burner; Spleen deficiency leading to preponderance of dampness; blood stasis and qi stagnation; and yin deficiency of the Liver and Kidney.

Damp-heat lodged in the lower burner. This is primarily due to invasion of environmental dampness, which accumulates internally and transforms into heat. Damp-heat then invades the yang brightness channel, which is characterized by an abundance of qi and blood. Thus, qi and blood are "smoldered" by the damp-heat, causing ulceration of the skin and tissues.

Spleen deficiency leading to preponderance of dampness. Overwork and fatigue, or occupations that involve prolonged standing or lifting and carrying of heavy loads, can injure the middle qi and deplete Spleen qi. Dampness thus accumulates, blocking the channels and collaterals such that the skin and tissues lose their nourishment, causing ulcers to develop.

Blood stasis and qi stagnation. This is often initiated by trauma, either open or closed, causing qi and blood to stagnate, thus blocking the channels and collaterals. The skin and tissues then lose nourishment and ulcer formation ensues.

Yin deficiency of the Liver and Kidney. Ulcers of this type may arise following febrile illnesses or from overindulgence in sexual intercourse which depletes Kidney essence. The muscles and sinews of the lower extremities gradually lose nourishment, and along with downpouring of deficiency fire, ulcers form.

Treatment

Chinese medicine categorizes leg ulcers as either medial or lateral. Medial ulcers are associated with the three yin channels of the foot, and generally arise due to yin deficiency fire flourishing; such ulcers are often difficult to treat. The treatment strategy is aimed at enriching and tonifying yin. Lateral ulcers correspond to the three yang channels of the foot, and frequently develop because of damp-heat; such lesions are often easily resolved. The treatment strategy for the lateral pattern is to clear heat and leach out dampness.

INTERNAL

Damp-heat lodged in the lower burner. The lesion begins with pain, redness and swelling of the area, followed by breakage of the skin, oozing, severe itching and pus formation. As the lesion becomes chronic, the edges of the ulcer harden and become rounded. Serious cases may present with generalized symptoms such as aversion to cold, fever, dry mouth, yellow urine, a slippery and rapid pulse, and a thick, sticky tongue coating. The treatment strategy is to clear heat and relieve toxicity.

The formulas recommended for this pattern are Sublime Formula for Sustaining Life (see carbuncles), or Dioscorea Decoction to Leach Out Dampness [B].

❧ Dioscorea Decoction to Leach Out Dampness [B]
萆薢渗湿汤
bèi xiè shèn shī tāng

Rhizoma Dioscoreae Hypoglaucae *(bei xie)*
Semen Coicis Lachryma-jobi *(yi yi ren)*
Cortex Phellodendri *(huang bai)*
Sclerotium Poriae Cocos Rubrae *(chi fu ling)*
Cortex Moutan Radicis *(mu dan pi)*
Rhizome Alismatis Orientalis *(ze xie)*
Talcum *(hua shi)*
Medulla Tetrapanacis Papyriferi *(tong cao)*

PREPARATION & DOSAGE: The source text does not indicate amounts for the ingredients. Decoct and administer in 1-2 doses daily.

Spleen deficiency leading to preponderance of dampness. Lesions of this pattern are characterized by grayish white tissue inside the wound and weeping of copious and clear exudate. Generalized symptoms may include lack of appetite, tiredness of the limbs, dizziness, dry mouth, a slow pulse, and a pale tongue with a white coating. The treatment strategy is to strengthen the Spleen and transform dampness. The formula recommended for this pattern is Four-Gentleman Decoction Combined with Two-Marvel Powder.

❦ Four-Gentleman Decoction Combined with Two-Marvel Powder
四君子汤合二妙散
sì jūn zǐ tāng hé èr miào sǎn

Radix Ginseng *(ren shen)*	3g
Rhizoma Atractylodis Macrocephalae *(bai zhu)*	6g
Sclerotium Poriae Cocos *(fu ling)*	6g
Honey-toasted Radix Glycyrrhizae Uralensis *(zhi gan cao)*	3g
Cortex Phellodendri *(huang bai)*	9g
Rhizoma Atractylodis *(cang zhu)*	6g

PREPARATION & DOSAGE: Decoct and administer in 1-2 doses daily.

Blood stasis and qi stagnation. The lesion site is characterized by swelling and dark purple skin and tissue; varicosities may be evident. The ulcer itself is moist and the pain is sharp, the lower limb is heavy and numb, and walking is difficult. The pulse is choppy and the tongue is purple. The treatment strategy is to invigorate the blood and regulate the qi. The formula recommended for this pattern is Chaenomeles and Areca Powder.

❦ Chaenomeles and Areca Powder
木瓜槟榔散
mù guā bīng láng sǎn

Semen Arecae Catechu *(bing lang)*
Fructus Chaenomelis Lagenariae *(mu gua)*
Folium Perillae Frutescentis *(zi su ye)*
Pericarpium Citri Reticulatae *(chen pi)*
Radix Glycyrrhizae Uralensis *(gan cao)*
Radix Aucklandiae Lappae *(mu xiang)*
Radix Angelicae Sinensis *(dang gui)*
Radix Paeoniae Rubrae *(chi shao)*

PREPARATION & DOSAGE: The source text does not indicate the amounts for the ingredients. Decoct and administer in 1-2 doses daily.

Yin deficiency of the Liver and Kidney. The surrounding skin of the lesion is deep red, and there is either absence of pain or slight pain. Generalized symptoms may include low-grade or afternoon fever, loss of appetite, emaciation, dream-disturbed sleep, a rapid pulse, and a slightly red tongue with a thin coating. The treatment strategy is to enrich yin and direct fire downward. The formula recommended for this pattern is Six-Ingredient Pill with Rehmannia.

Six-Ingredient Pill with Rehmannia
六味地黄丸
liù wèi dì huáng wán

Radix Rehmanniae Glutinosae Conquitae *(shu di huang)*	240g
Fructus Corni Officinalis *(shan zhu yu)*	120g
Radix Dioscoreae Oppositae *(shan yao)*	120g
Sclerotium Poriae Cocos *(fu ling)*	90g
Cortex Moutan Radicis *(mu dan pi)*	90g
Rhizome Alismatis Orientalis *(ze xie)*	90g

PREPARATION & DOSAGE: Grind the ingredients together into a fine powder and form into small pills with honey. Administer in 9g doses three times daily.

EXTERNAL

For early lesions with symptoms of redness, swelling and pain (without ulceration), Golden-Yellow Powder According to One's Wishes (see folliculitis in Chapter 7) may be applied 2-3 times daily by mixing it with some honey to form a paste.

For early lesions that present with redness, swelling, itching and moist skin, Indigo Ointment (see tinea in Chapter 9) or Indigo Powder (see impetigo in Chapter 7) may be applied 2-3 times daily.

For lesions that have ulcerated and are exuding sticky pus, Five-Five Special Powder (described below) or Red Ointment (see lupus vulgaris in Chapter 7) may be applied twice daily, followed by Jade Red Ointment (see erythema multiforme in Chapter 14).

Five-Five Special Powder
五五丹
wǔ wǔ dān

calcined Gypsum *(duan shi gao)*	5g
Mimium *(qian dan)*	5g

PREPARATION & DOSAGE: Grind the ingredients together into a fine powder and store in an airtight amber glass jar.

For lesions that show necrotic debris or induration and have a foul odor, Seven-Three Special Powder or Eight-Two Special Powder (for both remedies, see carbuncles in Chapter 7) may be applied once daily, followed by Red Ointment (see lupus vulgaris in Chapter 7). Use this combined remedy for 3-5 consecutive days until necrotic material or induration is improved.

Lesions that have begun to heal, i.e., with exudate that is clearer and less pustular, with absence of necrosis and signs of new tissue growth, may be treated with Generate Flesh Powder (see carbuncles in Chapter 7).

Chronic lesions may be treated with Paper Sandwich Plaster.

❀ Paper Sandwich Plaster
夹纸膏
jiā zhǐ gāo

Mimium *(qian dan)*
Calomelas *(qing fen)*
Pasta Acaciae seu Uncariae *(er cha)*
Myrrha *(mo yao)*
Realgar *(xiong huang)*
Sanguis Draconis *(xue jie)*
Galla Rhois Chinensis *(wu bei zi)*
Vermilion *(yin zhu)*
Alumen Praeparatum *(ku fan)*

PREPARATION & DOSAGE: Grind equal amounts of the ingredients together into a fine powder. Cut two pieces of oil paper (wax paper may be substituted) slightly larger than the ulcer. Spread a layer of the medicinal powder between the two pieces of paper and affix the edges with an adhesive. Using a needle, prick several tiny holes in one of the papers and affix this side to the ulcer. This dressing should be changed once every three days.

Chronic lesions that are not healing because of insufficient nourishment due to patterns such as Spleen deficiency or blood stasis and qi stagnation may be treated with Remove Decay and Generate Flesh Formula, or Phoenix Mantle Formula.

❀ Remove Decay and Generate Flesh Formula
祛腐生肌方
qū fǔ shēng jī fāng

Hardboiled Eggs 10

PREPARATION & DOSAGE: Remove the egg yolks and crumble them into a sauce pan. Stir-fry over medium heat until oil from the yolks appears. Remove and discard the yolk residue, saving the oil only. Soak four or five pieces of 2" x 2" sterile gauze in the yolk oil, and then store in a sterile glass jar. Affix one or two pieces of the medicinal gauze to the ulcer. Change the gauze once daily.

❀ Phoenix Mantle Formula
凤凰衣方
fèng huáng yī fāng

Raw Egg 1

PREPARATION & DOSAGE: Sterilize the eggshell with alcohol. Make a small opening at one end of the shell and pour out the content of the egg. Then, using a sterile, smooth (non-serrated) surgical tweezer, gently remove the egg membrane through the opening, and immediately apply it to the ulcer. If there is much exudate, small openings may be poked into the membrane, and sterile dressing applied over it in order to absorb the exudate; the dressing should be removed after 24 hours. A new membrane can be applied every 2-3 days, although the source text indicates that most patients experience healing after 1-2 applications.

Other remedies that may be used for non-healing ulcers due to insufficient nourishment are cod liver oil or table sugar mixed in with Generate Flesh Powder (see carbuncles in Chapter 7), and applied in the same manner as Remove Decay and Generate Flesh Formula (see above).

ACUPUNCTURE

Treatment strategy and point prescriptions should be based on the principle that medial ulcers correspond to the three yin channels of the foot and generally develop due to flourishing of deficiency fire; and that lateral ulcers correspond to the three yang channels of the foot and are generally caused by conditions of damp-heat. Thus, in addition to local points proximal to the wound, point selection for medial ulcers should focus primarily along the three yin channels of the foot, and for lateral ulcers along the three yang channels of the foot.

MOXIBUSTION

Ulcer sites that are pale and cold to the touch may undergo indirect ginger or garlic moxibustion. Moxa cones, or any of the above medicinal powders (e.g., Seven-Three Special Powder, or the powder that comprises the Paper Sandwich Plaster) combined with moxa floss and formed into cones, can be burned atop a ginger or garlic wafer that is placed directly on the ulcer. Treatment is discontinued when the area feels warm. Therapy is once daily until the surrounding flesh regains its warmth. Other remedies may be used in conjunction with moxibustion.

EMPIRICAL REMEDIES

The first two remedies below may be applied to recalcitrant ulcers.

❦ Scolopendra Farewell Dinner[1]

蜈蚣饯

wú gōng jiàn

Tung Oil[2] 500ml
Radix Angelicae Pubescentis *(du huo)* 3g
Radix Angelicae Dahuricae *(bai zhi)* 3g
Radix Glycyrrhizae Uralensis *(gan cao)* 3g

Scolopendra Subspinipes *(wu gong)* 3g

PREPARATION & DOSAGE: Cook the herbal ingredients in the tung oil until a brown sediment results. Meanwhile, with the leg raised and supported, cleanse the ulcer site with hydrogen peroxide, and pat dry with sterile gauze. Make some flour dough and form into a strip, and surround the ulcer with the dough. Using a tablespoon, ladle the hot (not scalding) medicinal oil until the well formed by the dough is filled. Allow the oil to cool, and then spoon out. Remove the dough and apply Purple and Gold Plaster to Relieve Toxin (see below) to the ulcer, cover with oil or wax paper, and bandage loosely. Change the dressing every three days.

The source text indicates that this remedy is especially effective for long-standing ulcers that are unresponsive to other remedies—hence the name. In general, one application is sufficient, after which the diseased tissue will slough and healing will be initiated.

❦ Purple and Gold Plaster to Relieve Toxin[3]
解毒紫金膏
jiě dú zǐ jīn gāo

Calcined Melanteritum (duan lu fan) 500g
Gummi Pini (song xiang) 500g

PREPARATION & DOSAGE: Grind the ingredients together into a fine powder. Mix in sesame oil until a thick paste is formed. Apply a thin layer to the wound.

❦ Shin Sore Plaster[4]
臁疮膏
lián chuāng gāo

Radix et Rhizoma Notopterygii *(qiang huo)* 60g
Radix Angelicae Pubescentis *(du huo)* 60g
Radix Angelicae Sinensis *(dang gui)* 60g
Mimium *(qian dan)* 60g
Os Draconis *(long gu)* 60g
Calomelas *(qing fen)* 9g

PREPARATION & DOSAGE: Grind the ingredients together into a fine powder. Mix with sesame oil until a paste is formed. Spread a medium layer between two pieces of oil or wax paper and seal the edges with an adhesive. Punch fine holes on the side that is to be affixed to the ulcer site. Cleanse the ulcer with hydrogen peroxide and dab dry with sterile gauze. Affix the medicinal plaster over the ulcer for at least 3-4 days. Apply a fresh piece if healing has not begun.

[A] Mash one fresh fig into a pulp and apply to the previously cleansed ulcer site and bandage with sterile dressing. Or, grind one dried fig (completely desiccated) into a powder and sprinkle onto the ulcer, then bandage. Allow the remedy to remain in place for three days; apply afresh if healing has not begun.[5]

[B] Sprinkle a thick layer of powdered white sugar onto the previously cleansed ulcer. Cover with sterile gauze, then seal the entire ulcer site with adhesive tape. Avoid wetting the area while showering or bathing. Allow the remedy to remain in place for 5-7 days. Then remove the dressing and cleanse the ulcer site, and repeat the application if healing has not begun.

The source text[6] indicates that the amount of powdered sugar applied should be as thick as possible, and that the remedy should be left in place for at least five days before removing the dressing. Adjunct remedies, such as internal formulas or acupuncture, may be applied at the same time.

[C] For stubborn ulcers, stir-fry some soy bean residue (the dregs that remain after soy beans are milled to make tofu) until hot. Form a patty and apply to the previously cleansed ulcer. Affix a sterile dressing over the remedy. Apply a fresh patty once daily.[7]

[D] For ulcers of the Spleen deficiency or blood stasis and qi stagnation patterns, spread a thick layer of honey on sterile gauze and apply once or twice daily to the previously cleansed ulcer, and then bandage.[8]

Traditional vs. Biomedical Treatment

A traditional regimen may prove to be effective in cases that have failed to improve with biomedical treatment, which can include topical application of enzymes, benzoyl peroxide, gold leaf, hyperbaric oxygenation and antibiotics, among others. However, even traditional treatment may not be successful unless circulation is increased and venous stasis is reduced. This is accomplished through leg elevation and avoiding prolonged standing. A form-fitted elastic stocking may be used to maintain fluid dynamics.

Traditional external remedies should not be changed frequently. During the acute infection stage, or if weeping is severe, a once daily application suffices. After healing has begun, application can be once every 3-5 days.

Prevention

Individuals affected by venous incompetency ought to be told of the high risk of developing stasis dermatitis, which can lead to leg ulcers. Therefore, early treatment of venous stasis is critical to prevent dermatitis and leg ulcers. Since trauma to the lower leg in such patients can trigger lesions, the traumatized site should be attended to immediately. In addition, patients should be advised to elevate the leg for short periods throughout the day. Once the ulcer has healed, trauma again should be avoided and the ulcer site protected.

CHAPTER NOTES

1. Peng, H.R., ed. *Great Compendium of Famous Chinese Medical Formulas (Zhong hua ming yi fang ji da quan)*. Beijing: Gold Shield Press, 1990.

2. This is *tóng yóu,* a pale, yellow and pungent drying oil obtained from the seeds of tung trees and used chiefly in quick-drying varnishes and paints and as a waterproofing agent.

3. Peng, *Great Compendium of Famous Chinese Medical Formulas (Zhong hua ming yi fang ji da quan).*

4. Ibid.

5. Ye, J.Q. *Traditional Chinese Food Medicinals and Folk Prescriptions (Shi wu zhong yao yu pian fang).* Jiangsu: Jiangsu Science and Technology Press, 1980.

6. Ibid.

7. Ibid.

8. Ibid.

CHAPTER 21

Disorders of Pigmentation

Vitiligo
白癜风
bái diàn fēng, "white blotch wind"

Vitiligo is usually a progressive, chronic pigmentary anomaly of the skin characterized by depigmented white patches that are generally sharply demarcated. The earliest Chinese record of this condition is found in *Discussion of the Origins of Symptoms of Diseases* (610): "Persons with white blotch [disease], [the] skin of [their] face and neck, nape, body, turns white, and is different from [normal] flesh color, and does not itch or hurt." Another name given this disease is "white variegated wind" *(bái bó fēng).*

Biomedically, the white spots on the skin are understood to result from destruction of epidermal pigment cells. However, the causes and mechanisms of pigment cell destruction are unknown. Although various theories—including autocytotoxic, immunologic and neural—have been espoused, no compelling data proves which one (if any) is correct. Genetic factors probably predispose the pigment cells of some individuals to destruction.

Signs & Symptoms

The hallmark of vitiligo is the development of hypopigmented, and later, completely depigmented spots. Loss of pigment usually begins on the fingers, hands and wrists, but soon spreads to the face and feet. The individual lesions progress from hypopigmentation to depigmentation, with the spots growing increasingly larger, and new lesions appearing on the trunk and genitalia. The skin and mucous membranes are involved. Interestingly, patients with minimal skin depigmentation often have extensive depigmentation of the oral mucosa. Many patients spontaneously regain some or most of their pigment.

A more serious development of vitiligo is the destruction of pigment cells in the eyes. Seven percent of vitiligo patients have active but asymptomatic uveitis (inflammation of the posterior pigmented layer of the iris).

Vitiligo can develop at any age, although half of the patients acquire the condition before 19 years of age, and most are affected before the age of 50.

Differential Diagnosis

The paper-white spots and patches on the skin usually confirm diagnosis of vitiligo. However, thermal burns, radiation, deep lacerations or deep abrasions can also result in loss of pigment. Infections that leave deep scars, such as chickenpox or herpes zoster, often result in spots of depigmentation.

One type of depigmentation that is difficult to differentiate from vitiligo is chemically induced loss of pigmentation. Such lesions are confetti-like white macules or small, irregularly shaped white patches that appear on exposed surfaces such as the dorsum of the hand. Diagnosis is confirmed by history of exposure to chemicals, such as industrial cleaning solutions, germicidal agents, rubber products and the like.

Traditional Chinese Etiology

The three primary causes of vitiligo are invasion of external excesses, constrained Liver qi, and Kidney yin deficiency.

Invasion of external excesses. Wind, heat, cold and dampness can invade the exterior such that Lung qi is unable to disseminate. The excess accumulates in the channels and collaterals, causing disharmony between the blood and qi, or causing blood stasis and qi stagnation. The skin is thus unable to receive nourishment and the lesions result.

Constrained Liver qi. This is the result of anger and/or depression, which causes the Liver to lose its spreading and dispersing functions. Disharmony between the blood and qi ensues, causing blood stasis and qi stagnation such that the skin is unable to receive nourishment, thus giving rise to the lesions.

Kidney yin deficiency. Insufficient Kidney yin leads to flaring of Heart fire, which consumes yin blood, causing disharmony between qi and blood. The skin loses nourishment and the lesions develop.

Treatment

INTERNAL

Invasion of external excesses—wind-dryness pattern. This type of vitiligo is characterized by shiny lesions that mainly affect the head, although they may appear elsewhere. Onset and diffusion are rapid. Young individuals in their twenties are primarily affected. The strategy is to scatter wind and moisten dryness. The formula recommended for this pattern is Modified Two-Ultimate Pill.

❦ Modified Two-Ultimate Pill
二至丸加减
èr zhì wán jiā jiǎn

Fructus Ligustri Lucidi *(nu zhen zi)*	10g
Herba Ecliptae Prostratae *(han lian cao)*	10g
Fructus Mori Albae *(sang shen)*	15g
Fructus Tribuli Terrestris *(bai ji li)*	15g
Radix Salviae Miltiorrhizae *(dan shen)*	6g
Rhizoma Typhonii Gigantei *(bai fu zi)*	6g
Semen Sesami Indici *(hei zhi ma)*	6g
Radix Glycyrrhizae Uralensis *(gan cao)*	6g
Herba Lemnae seu Spirodelae *(fu ping)*	4.5g

PREPARATION & DOSAGE: Decoct and administer in three doses daily. Or, grind the ingredients together into a powder and mix with honey to form boluses; take 9g daily.

Invasion of external excesses—damp-heat. The lesions are usually pinkish, and often appear on the face about the seven orifices, or below the nape. The lesions increase in size during the summer and autumn. Itching is exacerbated after exposure to sunlight or heat. Usually persons in their late twenties and early thirties are affected. The strategy is to eliminate dampness and clear heat. The formula recommended for this pattern is Modified Linum Pill.

❧ Modified Linum Pill
胡麻丸加减
hú má wán jiā jiǎn

Semen Lini Usitatissimi (ya ma zi)	15g
Radix Sophorae Flavescentis *(ku shen)*	10g
Radix Ledebouriellae Divaricatae *(fang feng)*	10g
Rhizoma Acori Graminei *(shi chang pu)*	10g
Rhizoma Typhonii Gigantei *(bai fu zi)*	6g
Rhizoma Atractylodis *(cang zhu)*	6g
Radix Polygoni Bistortae *(quan shen)*	6g
Flos Carthami Tinctorii *(hong hua)*	6g
Periostracum Serpentis *(she yi)*	6g

PREPARATION & DOSAGE: Decoct and administer in three doses daily.

Invasion of external excesses—congealing of cold. Lesions of this type have a dark hue to them. The lower body is primarily affected, although the extremities may be as well. Lesions enlarge slowly and often never repigment. Usually the middle-aged and elderly are affected. The strategy is to scatter cold and clear the collaterals. The formula recommended for this pattern is Modified Miraculous Extinguish Wind Powder.

❧ Modified Miraculous Extinguish Wind Powder
神应消风散加减
shén yìng xiāo fēng sǎn jiā jiǎn

Radix Codonopsitis Pilosulae *(dang shen)*	10g
Radix Angelicae Dahuricae *(bai zhi)*	10g
Rhizoma Atractylodis *(cang zhu)*	10g
Radix Polygoni Multiflori *(he shou wu)*	15g
Radix et Caulis Jixueteng *(ji xue teng)*	15g
Caulis Polygoni Multiflori *(ye jiao teng)*	15g
Radix Salviae Miltiorrhizae *(dan shen)*	15g
Flos Carthami Tinctorii *(hong hua)*	6g
Fructus Liquidambaris Taiwanianae *(lu lu tong)*	6g
Buthus Martensi *(quan xie)*	1-2

PREPARATION & DOSAGE: Decoct and administer in three doses daily.

Constrained Liver qi. Lesions of this pattern appear pinkish, and are mainly localized, although they may be diffused throughout the body. Onset and spread are associated with emotional depression. Women are primarily affected, and often have accompanying menstrual irregularities. The strategy is to disperse Liver qi and relieve constraint. The formula recommended for this pattern is Modified Rambling Powder [B].

❧ Modified Rambling Powder [B]
逍遥散加减
xiāo yáo sǎn jiā jiǎn

Radix Angelicae Sinensis *(dang gui)*	10g
Dry-fried Radix Paeoniae Lactiflorae *(chao bai shao)*	10g
Sclerotium Poriae Cocos *(fu ling)*	10g
Radix Rehmanniae Glutinosae *(sheng di huang)*	10g
Tuber Curcumae *(yu jin)*	6g
Fructus Akebiae *(ba yue zha)*	15g
Herba Leonuri Heterophylli *(yi mu cao)*	15g
Fructus Xanthii Sibirici *(cang er zi)*	12g
Magnetitum *(ci shi)*	30g

PREPARATION & DOSAGE: Decoct and administer in three doses daily.

Kidney yin deficiency. Lesions of this pattern resemble porcelain and are spread throughout the body. Fatigue, overindulgence in sexual intercourse, or other activities that consume essence can cause the lesions to expand or increase in number. Men are primarily affected, with accompanying symptoms of impotence, dizziness and tiredness of the extremities. The strategy is to enrich and tonify the Liver and Kidney. The formula recommended for this pattern is White Spots Pitch-Black Decoction.

🌿 White Spots Pitch-Black Decoction
白斑乌黑汤
bái bān wū hēi tāng

Semen Astragali *(sha yuan ji li)*	15g
Fructus Ligustri Lucidi *(nu zhen zi)*	15g
Fructus Rubi Chingii *(fu pen zi)*	10g
Fructus Lycii *(gou qi zi)*	10g
Semen Sesami Indici *(hei zhi ma)*	15g
Fructus Tribuli Terrestris *(bai ji li)*	15g
Radix Paeoniae Rubrae *(chi shao)*	10g
Radix Paeoniae Lactiflorae *(bai shao)*	10g
Radix Ligustici Chuanxiong *(chuan xiong)*	10g
Radix Polygoni Multiflori *(he shou wu)*	10g
Radix Angelicae Sinensis *(dang gui)*	10g
Radix Rehmanniae Glutinosae *(sheng di huang)*	10g

PREPARATION & DOSAGE: Decoct and administer in two doses daily.

EXTERNAL

The following remedies may be applied externally to treat psoriasis.

🌿 Lithyargyrum Powder
密陀僧散
mì tuó sēng sǎn

Realgar *(xiong huang)*	6g
Sulphur *(liu huang)*	6g
Fructus Cnidii Monnieri *(she chuang zi)*	6g
Lithargyrum *(mi tuo seng)*	3g
Sulphur *(liu huang)*	3g
Calomelas *(qing fen)*	1.5g

PREPARATION & DOSAGE: Grind the ingredients together into a fine powder. Mix with vinegar to form a paste and apply on individual lesions; or sprinkle a thin layer of powder on the lesions. Bandage loosely with sterile gauze. Apply once daily.

CLINICAL NOTE: Due to its toxicity, this formula should not be used continuously for extended periods of time. After one week, alternate with other remedies and treatment methods.

🌿 White Blotch Wind Pill
白癜风丸
bái diàn fēng wán

Herba seu Flos Schizonepetae Tenuifoliae *(jing jie)*
Radix Ledebouriellae Divaricatae *(fang feng)*
Radix et Rhizoma Notopterygii *(qiang huo)*
Fructus Kochiae Scopariae *(di fu zi)*

Extremitas Radicis Angelicae Sinensis *(dang gui wei)*
Herba Speranskiae seu Impatientis *(tou gu cao)*
Realgar *(xiong huang)*
Alumen Praeparatum *(ku fan)*

PREPARATION & DOSAGE: Grind equal amounts of the ingredients into a fine powder. Mix with ground pig intestine to form a paste. Wrap a walnut-size wad of the medicinal paste in sterile gauze and gently rub the lesions for 5-10 minutes daily. Use fresh paste each day.

ACUPUNCTURE

Filiform needling. Recommended acupoints include LI-4 *(he gu)*, LI-11 *(qu chi)*, LR-2 *(xing jian)* and SP-6 *(san yin jiao)*. After obtaining needling sensation, electrostimulation (at tolerance level) may be applied for 20 minutes. Treatment should be once every other day, with ten sessions constituting one course.

Cutaneous needling. After sterilization, gently tap the lesion with a plum-blossom needle, starting at the lesion border and continuing inward in a concentric circle until the skin is flushed or a minute amount of blood is let. Treat once daily, with ten sessions constituting one course.

Ear acupuncture. Recommended points include Lung, Occiput, Hormone and Adrenal. Needle any two points on one ear, and the other two points on the other ear. Alternate points during subsequent sessions. Treat once every 2-3 days.

Acupuncture should be administered in conjunction with other treatment methods in order to obtain maximum therapeutic effect.

MOXIBUSTION

First bloodlet the miscellaneous point *jia xia* (located on the upper arm, on the lower third of the lateral aspect of the biceps); if blood does not appear, apply cupping to produce a few drops of blood. Then apply direct moxibustion to the miscellaneous point *jiu dian feng* (located on the palmar aspect of the hand, in the center of the transverse crease of the distal phalangeal joint) with moxa cones made up of the following powdered ingredients: 10g Galla Rhois Chinensis *(wu bei zi)*, 10g Folium Mori Albae *(sang ye)*, 10g Radix Clematidis *(wei ling xian)*, 10g Radix Angelicae Sinensis *(dang gui)*, 10g Radix Ligustici Chuanxiong *(chuan xiong)*, 10g Fructus Amomi Kravanh *(bai dou kou)*, 30g Rhizoma Acori Graminei *(shi chang pu)*, 30g Semen Sinapis Albae *(bai jie zi)* and 10g Buthus Martensi *(quan xie)*. Burn three small cones during each session, being careful not to produce blisters.

Treatment is once a week. At each session treat one aspect only, and alternate aspects during ensuing sessions.

EMPIRICAL REMEDIES

❧ Phytolacca Powder[1]
商陆散
shāng lù sǎn

Radix Phytolaccae *(shang lu)* 270g
Radix Ampelopsis Japonicae *(bai lian)* 90g
Radix Scutellariae Baicalensis *(huang qin)* 90g
Rhizoma Zingiberis Officinalis *(gan jiang)* 120g
Radix Lateralis Aconiti Carmichaeli Praeparata *(fu zi)* ... 30g
Inflorescentia Rhododendri Mollis *(nao yang hua)* 270g

PREPARATION & DOSAGE: Grind the ingredients into a fine powder. Administer 1.5g with wine, three times daily. The source text indicates that while taking this remedy neither pork nor cold water should be consumed.

Traditional vs. Biomedical Treatment

Traditional formulas are perhaps more effective than biomedical interventions in eliminating the root of this problem. Conventional biomedical treatment is of two types: repigmentation and depigmentation. The former is attempted with either topical or oral psoralens. When the latter is administered, the patient must undergo exposure to controlled doses of sunlight or ultraviolet lamp. Patients with extensive vitiligo who do not repigment with psoralens may undergo depigmentation with monobenzone to remove their remaining pigment; application of this drug permanently destroys the epidermal pigment cells. Surgical treatment may be tried when conventional therapies are unsuccessful.

Presently in China a combined traditional and biomedical approach is being researched. Herbs such as Radix Angelicae Dahuricae *(bai zhi)*, Radix Angelicae Pubescentis *(du huo)*, Radix et Rhizoma Polygoni Cuspidati *(hu zhang)*, Radix Rubiae Cordifoliae *(qian cao gen)*, Semen Cassiae *(jue ming zi)*, Radix Adenophorae seu Glehniae *(sha shen)*, Tuber Ophiopogonis Japonici *(mai dong)*, fresh Herba Portulacae Oleraceae *(ma chi xian)* and fig leaf have been found to contain furocoumarins, which on contact with the skin cause photosensitivity. Application of topicals containing extracts of these herbs, followed by exposure to sunlight or ultraviolet lamp, appears to induce repigmentation.

Prevention

Vitiligo is a condition that has great psychosocial impact on patients. Once diagnosed, immediate and persistent treatment should be undertaken to prevent lesions from increasing in size and number. Patients should also be advised to use sunscreens when outdoors, since areas of vitiligo are more susceptible to sunburn and such injury can extend the depigmentation response.

Individuals exhibiting patterns of disharmony that can be resolved through changes in lifestyle, diet and the like should be encouraged to make such changes, since in many cases relying solely on traditional remedies treats the symptoms and not always the root of the condition.

CHAPTER NOTES

1. Peng, H.R. *Great Compendium of Famous Chinese Medical Formulas (Zhong hua ming yi fang ji da quan)*. Beijing: Gold Shield Press, 1990.

CHAPTER 22

Disorders of Keratinization

Ichthyosis
蛇皮癬
shé pí xuǎn, "snake skin tinea"

Ichthyosis is the general term for a group of skin disorders characterized by excessive scaling. It was first recorded in *Discussion of the Origins of Symptoms of Diseases* (610):

> A person with snake body is called this [because] the skin resembles snake skin and has scales. . . . This [condition] is due to the aggregation of blood and qi which is thus unable to reach and moisten the skin.

Among other names for this condition are "fish scale wind" *(yú lín fēng)* and "fish scale disease" *(yú lín bìng)*.

Ichthyosis can be inherited or acquired; all types are characterized by excessive accumulation of scale on the skin surface. The inherited forms are classified biomedically according to clinical, genetic and histologic criteria. Scaling in some inherited forms is due to an increased rate of epidermal proliferation, similar to psoriasis, and in other forms to abnormal retention of stratum corneum (the most superficial layer of the epidermis, consisting of dead cells).

Acquired ichthyosis can be a symptom of several diseases. Internal malignant tumors, especially lymphoma, may first present as an ichthyotic scaling. Scaling can also appear as a result of chronic renal insufficiency and hypothyroidism, as well as from the use of certain drugs.

Signs & Symptoms

The several inherited forms of ichthyosis present differing symptomatologies, with the common feature being scaling. Onset is usually at birth and anytime during childhood. Symptoms of ichythosis vulgaris, the most common type of inherited ichthyosis, are limited to scaling and thickening of the palms and soles. Other types cause more serious symptoms ranging from abnormal serum values to dental and skeletal anomalies and developmental abnormalities. The different forms of ichthyosis have characteristic scales, from fine bran-like to large plate-like. These will be discussed in the treatment section.

Differential Diagnosis

With inherited forms of ichthyosis, usually the history will lead to a diagnosis, especially if the scaling has been present since childhood or birth. To confirm diagnosis of acquired ichthyosis, a thorough examination may be called for, since the distinction between overly dry skin due to environmental causes (harsh soaps, excessive bathing, low humidity) and ichthyosis as a feature of other diseases, is sometimes difficult.

Traditional Chinese Etiology

There are four common causes of this condition: blood deficiency/wind-dryness, blood heat/wind-dryness, damp-heat blocking the channels, and non-spreading of fluids.

Blood deficiency/wind-dryness. This is due to constitutional insufficiency that causes Kidney essence, and thus blood, to be deficient, such that the skin is not properly nourished. Protracted insufficient blood also leads to dryness, which then transforms into wind; wind then becomes lodged in the skin, giving rise to dryness and scaling of the skin.

Blood heat/wind-dryness. This is often caused by congenital blood heat or by protracted emotional disturbance that gives rise to fire. Fire then enters the blood and blood heat transforms into wind, all of which lodge in the skin and cause dryness and scaling.

Damp-heat blocking the channels. This may be due to congenital damp-heat, or in later life to a constant diet of sweet, spicy, greasy or broiled foods, which cause damp-heat to develop and accumulate, and then block the channels. The skin is thus unable to receive nourishment and becomes dry and scaly.

Non-spreading of fluids. Constitutional insufficient fluids can cause this type of ichthyosis, as can various factors in later life, such as lack of exercise, overindulgence in certain types of foods, or mental fatigue, which injures the Spleen such that fluids are not spread to the skin, thus giving rise to dryness and scaling.

Treatment

INTERNAL

Blood deficiency/wind-dryness. This pattern usually presents shortly after birth. It is characterized by fine bran-like scales that cover the trunk, and larger, more adherent scales over the extensor surfaces of the extremities. The face is often spared. Frequently, the palms and soles are thickened. The condition improves during summer and worsens during winter. There is occasional itching. Generalized symptoms may include a dry mouth and throat, little sweating, a pale dry tongue with a thin white coating, and a submerged, thin and weak pulse. The treatment strategy is to nourish the blood and moisten the skin, and enrich yin and produce fluids.

Formulas recommended for this pattern include Nourish the Blood and Moisten the Skin Decoction (see seborrheic dermatitis in Chapter 13), or Fish-Scale Formula.

❧ Fish-Scale Formula
鱼鳞方
yú lín fāng

Radix Astragali Membranacei *(huang qi)*	50g
Semen Sesami Indici *(hei zhi ma)*	40g
Radix Salviae Miltiorrhizae *(dan shen)*	25g
Fructus Kochiae Scopariae *(di fu zi)*	25g
Radix Angelicae Sinensis *(dang gui)*	20g
Radix Rehmanniae Glutinosae *(sheng di huang)*	20g
Radix Rehmanniae Glutinosae Conquitae *(shu di huang)*	20g
Fructus Lycii *(gou qi zi)*	20g
Radix Polygoni Multiflori *(he shou wu)*	20g
Cortex Dictamni Dasycarpi Radicis *(bai xian pi)*	20g
Radix Dioscoreae Oppositae *(shan yao)*	20g
Radix Sophorae Flavescentis *(ku shen)*	15g
Radix Ledebouriellae Divaricatae *(fang feng)*	15g
Radix Ligustici Chuanxiong *(chuan xiong)*	10g
Ramulus Cinnamomi Cassiae *(gui zhi)*	10g
Periostracum Cicadae *(chan tui)*	10g
Radix Glycyrrhizae Uralensis *(gan cao)*	10g

PREPARATION & DOSAGE: Decoct and administer in two doses daily.

MODIFICATIONS: For palpitations, sleeplessness and forgetfulness, add dry-fried Semen Zizyphi Spinosae *(chao suan zao ren)* and Cortex Albizziae Julibrissin *(he huan pi)*; for loss of appetite and abdominal fullness, eliminate Radix Rehmanniae Glutinosae *(sheng di huang)* and Radix Rehmanniae Glutinosae Conquitae *(shu di huang)*, and add Rhizoma Atractylodis Macrocephalae *(bai zhu)* and Endothelium Corneum Gigeriae Galli *(ji nei jin)*; for watery stools, eliminate Semen Sesami Indici *(hei zhi ma)*, Fructus Lycii *(gou qi zi)*, Radix Rehmanniae Glutinosae *(sheng di huang)* and Radix Rehmanniae Glutinosae Conquitae *(shu di huang)*, and add Rhizoma Atractylodis Macrocephalae *(bai zhu)* and Radix Dioscoreae Oppositae *(shan yao)*; for shortness of breath and spontaneous sweating, add Radix Codonopsitis Pilosulae *(dang shen)*.

Blood heat/wind-dryness. This pattern is characterized by small, dry, hard papules on an erythematous base. As the condition progresses, the papules develop into spiny ridges that later coalesce. The flexures are more affected than other areas of the body. Slight itching may be present. Often the tongue is red and the pulse is thin and rapid. The treatment strategy is to clear heat and cool the blood, and extinguish wind and moisten dryness. The formula recommended for this pattern is Cool the Blood and Moisten Dryness Decoction.

❦ Cool the Blood and Moisten Dryness Decoction
凉血润燥饮
liáng xuě rùn zào yǐn

Radix Rehmanniae Glutinosae *(sheng di huang)*
Cortex Moutan Radicis *(mu dan pi)*
Radix Arnebiae seu Lithospermi *(zi cao)*
Radix Rubiae Cordifoliae *(qian cao)*
Radix Scutellariae Baicalensis *(huang qin)*
Folium Daqingye *(da qing ye)*
Radix Scrophulariae Ningpoensis *(xuan shen)*
Tuber Ophiopogonis Japonici *(mai men dong)*
Herba Dendrobii *(shi hu)*
Radix Trichosanthis Kirilowii *(tian hua fen)*
Fructus Tribuli Terrestris *(bai ji li)*

PREPARATION & DOSAGE: The source text does not indicate amounts. Decoct and administer in 1-2 doses daily.

Damp-heat blocking the channels. This pattern is characterized by small, hard, spiny papules that later develop greasy, gray scales. As the condition progresses, the scales turn brown with a wart-like texture. A foul odor from macerated scales and secondary infection is common. Scaling is often bilateral, affecting the nape, back of the ears, face, trunk and extremities. The condition is worse in the summer and improves in the winter. Itching is often present. The tongue is red with blood-stasis spots and a yellow sticky coating, and the pulse is slippery and rapid. The treatment strategy is to clear heat and remove dampness, and invigorate the blood and clear the channels. The formula recommended for this pattern is Eliminate Dampness Decoction by Combining Calm the Stomach and Five-Ingredient Powder with Poria (see herpes zoster in Chapter 8).

Non-spreading of fluids. The features of this pattern are adherent, prickly brown scales on the trunk and extremities, with a characteristic tacked-on appearance. The condition worsens in the winter and improves in the summer. Generalized symptoms may include dryness of the eyes, accompanied by blurred vision (due to corneal opacities), a pale and dry tongue, and a submerged, thin and weak pulse. The treatment strategy is to assist the Spleen and nourish the Stomach, and nourish the blood and moisten dryness. The formula recommended for this pattern is Augmented Atractylodes Gelatin.

❦ Augmented Atractylodes Gelatin

加味苍术膏
jiā wèi cāng zhú gāo

Cortex Dictamni Dasycarpi Radicis *(bai xian pi)*	15g
Radix Angelicae Sinensis *(dang gui)*	30g
Rhizoma Atractylodis *(cang zhu)*	30g
Honey	1kg

PREPARATION & DOSAGE: Grind the herbs into a fine powder. Pour the honey into a non-metallic pot, and over low heat bring to a boil. Continue cooking until bubbles appear, then stir to break up the bubbles. Slowly mix in the herb powder, and stir thoroughly. Cook for another 5-10 minutes. Allow the concoction to congeal. Refrigerate to prevent spoilage. Administer 15g, 2-3 times daily.

EXTERNAL

For skin fissures and pain, either Moisten the Flesh Ointment (see seborrheic dermatitis in Chapter 13) or Prunus Ointment may be applied twice daily.

❦ Prunus Ointment
杏仁软膏
xìng rèn ruǎn gāo

Semen Pruni Armeniacae *(xing ren)*	30g
Lard	60g

PREPARATION & DOSAGE: Grind the Semen Pruni Armeniacae *(xing ren)* coarsely and mix thoroughly with the lard. Allow the concoction to steep for 3-4 days before applying twice daily.

Traditional vs. Biomedical Treatment

Before beginning treatment, determination should be made as to whether the dry skin is due to environmental causes (such as excessive bathing, harsh soaps, low humidity), or to acquired or inherited ichthyosis. Because acquired ichthyosis can be a manifestation of other diseases, patients should seek immediate medical attention to find the cause. The inherited forms of ichthyosis can benefit from traditional treatment, which addresses the root cause. Biomedical treatment is limited primarily to topical application of emollients, keratolitic agents, or alpha-hydroxy acid ointments to keep the skin moist.

Prevention

Inherited forms of ichthyosis may require long-term treatment before improvement in symptoms is seen. After the symptoms abate, patients may need follow-up treatment to prevent recurrence.

Corns
肉刺
ròu cì, "tissue thorns"

A corn is a horny induration and thickening of the stratum corneum (outermost layer of the skin) of the toes. Several Chinese medical classics describe this condition. Among them is the following passage from *Golden Mirror of the Medical Tradition* (1742):

> This condition arises on the toes, and resembles a chicken eye, thus the popular name [for this condition]. The root sinks into the tissue; [the corn] protrudes forth a hard crown, and is painful, [such that] walking is inconvenient. [Corns] can arise from either binding of feet, or from walking long distances in narrow shoes.

The biomedical cause of corns is recurrent pressure or friction over a bony prominence or abnormal bony growth (e.g., a spur).

Signs & Symptoms
Corns are pea-sized or slightly larger, and are almost always tender or painful. The plantar surface is the most commonly affected location. "Hard" corns occur over prominent protuberances, especially on the toes; "soft" corns occur between the toes (usually the 4th and 5th).

Differential Diagnosis
Diagnosis is confirmed by paring the stratum corneum with a sharp scalpel. A callus will reveal heaped up keratin and normal skin markings. A wart will appear sharply circumscribed, sometimes with soft macerated tissue or with central black dots resulting from thrombosed capillaries, and further paring will cause pinpoint bleeding. A corn, when pared, shows a sharply outlined translucent core that interrupts normal skin markings; continued paring will release the core, which can then be lifted out as a plug.

Traditional Chinese Etiology
Due to constant pressure and friction, the flow of qi and blood is disrupted, such that the skin and tissues are not properly nourished, thus giving rise to corns.

Treatment
Treatment consists of applying various external remedies. For recently-developed corns, Cibotium Wash is recommended.

❧ Cibotium Wash
狗脊水洗剂
gǒu jǐ shuǐ xǐ jì

Rhizoma Cibotii Barometz *(gou ji)*	30g
Pericarpium Citri Reticulatae *(chen pi)*	30g

Herba cum Radice Asari *(xi xin)* 15g
Rhizoma Cyperi Rotundi *(xiang fu)* 15g

PREPARATION & DOSAGE: Decoct the ingredients. First trim away the horny skin of the corn, then soak the affected foot in the warm decoction for 20 minutes, twice daily. Continue the treatment until the core is exposed and can be removed.

For chronic corns, Tissue Thorn Powder, or Hosta Ointment are the recommended remedies.

❧ Tissue Thorn Powder
肉刺散
ròu cì sǎn

Alumen *(ming fan)* 7g
Fructus Brucae Javanicae *(ya dan zi)* 15g
Copper Sulfate 3g

PREPARATION & DOSAGE: Stir-fry the Alumen *(ming fan)* and copper sulfate together in a cast iron saucepan until white clumps form. Grind the white clumps into a fine powder. Remove the hulls from the Fructus Brucae Javanicae *(ya dan zi)* and grind into a fine powder. Combine both powders thoroughly and store in an airtight amber glass jar. Before applying, mix a small amount of powder with cold water to form a paste. Pare away the horny skin of the corn and apply the remedy once daily. Affix with adhesive tape or a plastic bandage. Continue treatment until the core is exposed and can be removed.

❧ Hosta Ointment
紫玉赞膏
zǐ yù zān gāo

Folium Hostae Ventricosae *(zi yu zan ye)*
Galla Rhois Chinensis *(wu bei zi)*
Gummi Olibanum *(ru xiang)*
Myrrha *(mo yao)*
Globefish eye *(he tun mu)*
Sanguis Draconis *(xue jie)*
Pasta Acaciae seu Uncariae *(er cha)*
Mimium *(qian dan)*
Sesame Oil

PREPARATION & DOSAGE: The source text does not indicate the amounts. Globefish eye refers to the eye of the fish *Fugu ocellatus, F. vermicularis,* or *F. Obscuris (hé tún mù)*. Grind the ingredients together and mix with the sesame oil to form an ointment. Trim away the horny layer of the corn, and apply the remedy once daily. Bandage with adhesive tape or a plastic strip. Continue the treatment until the core is revealed and can be removed.

EMPIRICAL REMEDIES

[A] Bake gingko leaves in the oven until dried. Grind into a fine powder. Then form a paste with the powder and some rice that has been cooked into gruel. Apply the paste to the corn once daily. Bandage with a plastic strip.[1]

[B] Cook Fructus Pruni Mume *(wu mei)* into a thick paste. Apply once daily to the corn. Bandage with a plastic strip.[2]

[C] First soak the affected foot in hot water to soften the corn. Then trim away the horny layer. With the fingers, gently roll some spider web to form a small patty the size of the corn. Affix to the corn with adhesive tape. Remove the tape and spider web after 24 hours; the corn should be atrophied. In one week's time the corn should drop off spontaneously. The source text[3] indicates that a single treatment usually suffices, although another application may be necessary for deep-rooted corns.

Traditional vs. Biomedical Treatment

Traditional treatment may be desirable for patients who wish to avoid using biomedical keratolytic agents. However, no matter which treatment is chosen, if the cause is not eliminated, the corn will recur.

Prevention

Reduction, if not elimination, of the pressure or friction often produces relief and permanent cure, especially if the core of the corn is resolved. Soft, well-fitting shoes are important, and pads or rings of suitable sizes and shapes, as well as other special orthoses, may be helpful in preventing recurrence.

CHAPTER NOTES

1. Ye, J.Q. *Traditional Chinese Food Medicinals and Folk Prescriptions (Shi wu zhong yao yu pian fang)*. Jiangsu: Jiangsu Science and Technology Press, 1980.
2. Ibid.
3. Zhang, Z.X., "External Application of Spider Web to Treat Corns," *Shanxi Journal of Traditional Chinese Medicine*, 6(4): 12; 1990.

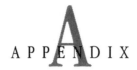

Supplemental Materia Medica

This appendix contains descriptions of materia medica mentioned in the text which are not among those included in *Chinese Herbal Medicine: Materia Medica (Revised Edition)* by Dan Bensky and Andrew Gamble. Since readers may be unfamiliar with these medicinal substances, we present basic information about them here in an abbreviated version of the format used in that book. The materia medica are arranged in alphabetical order by their *pīnyīn* names. Please note that for a very few of the substances listed below, little significant information was available to us beyond the most precise botanical or zoological name that we could find, together with its *pīnyīn* name.

白蔹
bái liǎn

Pharmaceutical name: Radix Ampelopsis Japonicae
Botanical name: *Ampelopsis japonicae* (Thunb.) Makino
Family: vitaceae
English: Japanese peppervine
Properties: bitter, sweet, acrid, cool
Channels entered: Heart, Liver, Spleen

ACTIONS & INDICATIONS:

♦ Clears heat, relieves toxicity: for deep-seated furuncles and swelling due to abscesses; treats malaria-like disorders.

♦ Dissipates clumps: for scrophula.

♦ Generates flesh and stops pain: for scalding of the skin, and bleeding hemorrhoids.

CAUTIONS & CONTRAINDICATIONS: Contraindicated in cases of deficiency cold of the Spleen/Stomach, and in cases of fire not due to excess.

DOSAGE: 3-9g

百药煎
bǎi yào jiān

Pharmaceutical name: Fermentatio Galla Rhois Chinensis
English: concoction made by fermenting together several herbs and tea leaves. The base herb is Galla Rhois Chinensis *(wu bei zi)*; other herbal constituents vary depending on the source text.
Literal English translation: "hundred medicine decoction"
Properties: sour, sweet, neutral
Channels entered: Lung, Stomach, Heart

ACTIONS & INDICATIONS:

♦ Moistens the Lung and transforms phlegm: for chronic cough with copious phlegm.

♦ Generates fluids and alleviates thirst: for sore throat; also treats dysenteric disorders, ulcers of the mouth and gum, abscesses and skin ulcers.

CAUTIONS & CONTRAINDICATIONS: Contraindicated in cases of cough due to externally-contracted excesses, damp-heat dysenteric disorders, and in cases of unresolved accumulation and stagnation.

DOSAGE: 3-9g

蓖麻子
bì má zǐ

Pharmaceutical name: Semen Ricini Communis
Botanical name: *Ricinus communis* L.
Family: euphorbiaceae
English: castor seed
Properties: neutral, bitter, acrid, toxic
Channels entered: Liver, Spleen, Lung, Large Intestine

ACTIONS & INDICATIONS:

♦ Reduces swelling and releases toxin: for swelling of carbuncles; scrofula.

♦ Drains downward and clears blockage: for abdominal swelling and floating edema, and dry stools.

CAUTIONS & CONTRAINDICATIONS: Contraindicated during pregnancy and in cases of loose stools. See **Toxicity** below.

DOSAGE: Sources do not indicate specific dosages. If administered orally, seeds should undergo processing with heat.

TOXICITY: Ingestion of raw castor seeds can be fatal. Reports indicate that death can occur in children after intake of 2-7 seeds, and in adults after intake of about 20 seeds. Toxic effects are rather slow and occur anywhere from three hours and three days, and can include burning pain in the throat and esophagus, nausea and vomiting, abdominal pain, diarrhea, and even bloody stools.

蝙蝠葛根
biān fú gé gēn

Pharmaceutical name: Rhizoma Menispermi Daurici
Botanical name: *Menispermum dauricum* DC.
Family: menispermaceae
English: Siberian moonseed root
Literal English translation: "bat kudzu"
Properties: bitter, cold
Channels entered: none noted

ACTIONS & INDICATIONS:
♦ Dispels wind and clears heat: for tonsillits, pharyngitis, and dysenteric disorders.
♦ Regulates qi and transforms dampness: for leg qi, edema, stomach pain with abdominal bloating, and wind-damp painful obstruction.

DOSAGE: 1.5-9g

楮叶
chǔ yè

Pharmaceutical name: Folium Broussonetiae Papyriferae
Botanical name: *Broussonetia papyrifera* (L.) Vent.
Family: mimosaceae
English: leaf of the paper mulberry
Properties: sweet, cool
Channels entered: none noted

ACTIONS & INDICATIONS:
♦ Cools the blood: for vomiting of blood, nosebleeds, excessive uterine bleeding, bleeding from trauma; also for tinea.
♦ Promotes urination: for edema.

DOSAGE: 3-6g

甘松
gān sōng

Pharmaceutical name: Rhizoma et Radix Nardostachydis
Botanical name: *Nardostachys chinensis* Batal., or *Nardostachys jatamanse* DC.
Family: valerianaceae

English: Chinese spikenard
Literal English translation: "sweet pine"
Properties: sweet, warm
Channels entered: Spleen, Stomach

ACTIONS & INDICATIONS:

♦ Regulates qi and arrests pain: for stomach pain and sensation of fullness in the abdomen.

♦ Awakens the Spleen and strengthens the Stomach: for hysteria or leg qi.

CAUTIONS & CONTRAINDICATIONS: Contraindicated in cases of qi deficiency and blood heat.

DOSAGE: 2-4.5g

蛤蜊粉
gé lí fěn

Pharmaceutical name: Conchae Pulvis Mactrae Quadrangularis
Zoological name: *Mactra quadrangularis* Deshayes
Family: veneridae
English: powdered clam shell
Properties: salty, cold
Channels entered: Lung, Kidney

ACTIONS & INDICATIONS:

♦ Clears heat, drains dampness, transforms phlegm, and softens masses: for coughing due to congested fluids, edema, goiter, and scalds and burns.

CAUTIONS & CONTRAINDICATIONS: Use with caution in cases that present Spleen/Stomach deficiency cold patterns, or in such cases add herbs that benefit the Spleen/Stomach.

DOSAGE: 3-9g

鬼羽箭
guǐ yǔ jiàn

Pharmaceutical name: Herba Buchnerae Cruciatae
Botanical name: *Buchnera cruciata* Buch.-Ham.
Family: scrophulariaceae
English: cruciate blueheart
Literal English translation: "ghost feather arrow"
Properties: bitter, cold
Channels entered: none noted

ACTIONS & INDICATIONS:

♦ Clears heat, cools the blood, and relieves toxicity: for measles-like rashes, seizures, swelling and pain due to wind toxin rashes.

CAUTIONS & CONTRAINDICATIONS: Contraindicated in cases of deficiency cold patterns and during pregnancy.

DOSAGE: 6-15g

鬼针草
guǐ zhēn cǎo

Pharmaceutical name: Herba Bidentis Bipinnatae
Botanical name: *Bidens bipinnata* L.
Family: asteraceae
English: Spanish needle, beggartick
Literal English translation: "ghost needle grass"
Properties: bitter, neutral, warm
Channels entered: none noted

ACTIONS & INDICATIONS:
♦ Clears heat and relieves toxicity: for malaria-like disorders, dysenteric disorders, hepatitis, insect bites and stings, and snakebite.
♦ Scatters blood stasis and eliminates swelling: for trauma and contusions.

CAUTIONS & CONTRAINDICATIONS: Contraindicated during pregnancy.

DOSAGE: 15-30g; if fresh herb is used, 30-60g

黑大豆
hēi dà dòu

Pharmaceutical name: Semen Glycine Max
Botanical name: *Glycine max* (L.) Merr.
Family: fabaceae
English: black bean
Literal English translation: "black big bean"
Properties: sweet, neutral
Channels entered: Spleen, Kidney

ACTIONS & INDICATIONS:
♦ Invigorates the blood and promotes urination: for floating edema.
♦ Dispels wind: for leg qi due to wind toxin, muscular tetany due to wind obstruction.
♦ Relieves toxicity: for abscesses and carbuncles; also relieves materia medica poisoning.

DOSAGE: 10-30g

红粉
hóng fěn

Pharmaceutical name: Hydrargyrioxydum rubrum

Chemical name: mercurous oxide
Properties: acrid, hot, extremely toxic
Channels entered: none noted

ACTIONS & INDICATIONS:

♦ Extracts toxin and draws out pus: for abscesses, carbuncles, and deep-seated furuncles, syphylitic lesions, and chronic exudation of pus.

♦ Removes decayed tissue and generates flesh: for fistulas and longstanding necrotic lesions.

CAUTIONS & CONTRAINDICATIONS: This is an extremely toxic substance and should not be administered orally. Long-term external use is not advised, as it may result in cumulative mercury poisoning. See **Toxicity** below.

DOSAGE: External use only in powders with other materia medica.

TOXICITY: Oral lethal dosage for humans is 0.1-0.7g.

鸡冠花
jī guān huā

Pharmaceutical name: Inflorescentia Celosiae Cristatae
Botanical name: *Celosia cristata* L.
Family: amaranthaceae
English: cock's comb
Properties: sweet, cool
Channels entered: Liver, Kidney

ACTIONS & INDICATIONS:

♦ Cools the blood and arrests bleeding: for bleeding hemorrhoids, bloody and pustular dysenteric disorder, vomiting of blood, coughing up of blood, bloody urine, and uterine hemorrhage.

DOSAGE: 4.5-9g

剪刀草
jiǎn dāo cǎo

Pharmaceutical name: Herba Clinopodii
Botanical name: *Clinopodium confine* (Hance.) O. Ktze., or *Clinopodium gracile* (Benth.) Matsum
Family: lamiaceae
English: clinopodium
Literal English translation: "scissors grass"
Properties: bitter, acrid, cool
Channels entered: none noted

ACTIONS & INDICATIONS:

♦ Dispels wind and clears heat: for headache due to attack by external excesses.

♦ Scatters blood stasis and eliminates swelling: for breast abscesses, deep-seated furuncles, hives, trauma, and contusions.

DOSAGE: 15-60g; 30-60g if fresh herb is used

接骨木
jiē gǔ mù

Pharmaceutical name: Ramulus Sambuci Williamsii
Botanical name: *Sambucus williamsii* Hance
Family: caprifoliaceae
English: twig of the red elderberry
Literal English translation: "connect bone wood"
Properties: sweet, bitter, neutral
Channels entered: none noted

ACTIONS & INDICATIONS:
♦ Dispels wind and drains dampness: sinew and bone pain due to wind-dampness; also for low back pain, edema, itching, and hives.
♦ Invigorates the blood and arrests pain: for postpartum dizziness due to blood stasis; also for bone fractures, and bleeding due to trauma and injury.

CAUTIONS & CONTRAINDICATIONS: Contraindicated during pregnancy. Some sources indicate that over-administration of this herb can result in vomiting.

DOSAGE: 9-15g

金莲花
jīn lián huā

Pharmaceutical name: Flos Trollii
Botanical name: *Trollius chinensis* Bge., or *Trollius asiaticus* L.
Family: ranunculaceae
English: globe flower
Literal English translation: "gold lotus flower"
Properties: bitter, cold
Channels entered: none noted

ACTIONS & INDICATIONS:
♦ Clears heat and relieves toxicity: for upper respiratory infections, tonsillitis, pharyngitis, acute otitis media, ulcers of the mouth, and deep-seated furuncles.

DOSAGE: 3-6g

韭菜
jiǔ cài

Pharmaceutical name: Folium Allii Tuberosi
Botanical name: *Allium tuberosum* Rottler

Family: liliaceae
English: Chinese chive
Properties: acrid, warm
Channels entered: Liver, Stomach, Kidney

ACTIONS & INDICATIONS:

♦ Warms the middle and promotes movement of qi: for blockage of the chest, difficulty in swallowing.

♦ Scatters blood: for nosebleeds, vomiting of blood, trauma, and contusions.

♦ Relieves toxicity: for insect bites and stings.

DOSAGE: 15-30g

狼毒
láng dú

Pharmaceutical name: Radix Stellerae seu Euphorbiae
Botanical name: *Stellera chamaejasme* L., *Euphorbia ebiacteolata* Hayata, or *E. fischeriana* Steud.
Family: thymelaeaceae
English: stellera?
Literal English translation: "wolf poison"
Properties: neutral, bitter, acrid, toxic
Channels entered: Lung, Liver, Spleen

ACTIONS & INDICATIONS:

♦ Guides water out and dispels phlegm: for abdominal edema, and accumulation due to phlegm, food, and parasites.

♦ Dissipates clumps: for scrofula and other tubercular conditions.

♦ Kills parasites: for scabies and tinea.

CAUTIONS & CONTRAINDICATIONS: Contraindicated during pregnancy and in cases with insufficient source qi. According to some sources, this herb is incompatible with Lythargyrum *(mi tuo seng)* and with vinegar. See **Toxicity** below.

DOSAGE: 1-2.5g.

TOXICITY: This is a highly toxic drug, although preparation usually removes much of its toxicity. Symptoms of toxicity include discomfort of the mouth and throat, nausea and vomiting, severe abdominal pain, diarrhea, headache and dizziness, malaise and weakness; severe cases may lead to respiratory arrest.

零陵香
líng líng xiāng

Pharmaceutical name: Herba Lysimachiae Foenum-Graci cum Radice
Botanical name: *Lysimachia foenum-graecum* Hance
Family: primulaceae
English: lysimachia

Literal English translation: "small hill fragrance"
Properties: acrid, sweet, warm
Channels entered: Lung

ACTIONS & INDICATIONS:

♦ Dispels wind-cold: for cold-induced disorders causing headache, stuffy nose, and stifling sensations in the chest.

♦ Cuts through turbidity: for foul body odor.

CAUTIONS & CONTRAINDICATIONS: Over-administration can lead to difficulty in breathing.

DOSAGE: 4.5-9g

凌霄花
líng xiāo huā

Pharmaceutical name: Flos Campsitis Grandiflorae
Botanical name: *Campsis grandiflora* (Thunb.) K.Schum
Family: bignoniaceae
English: flower of Chinese trumpet creeper
Literal English translation: "reach the clouds flower"
Properties: sour, cold
Channels entered: Liver

ACTIONS & INDICATIONS:

♦ Cools the blood and dispels stasis: for amenorrhea due to blood stasis, uterine masses; also for itching due to blood-heat, and for acne rosacea.

CAUTIONS & CONTRAINDICATIONS: Contraindicated in cases of qi and blood deficiency, and during pregnancy.

DOSAGE: 3-6g

龙葵
lóng kuí

Pharmaceutical name: Herba Solani Nigri
Botanical name: *Solanum nigrum* L.
Family: solanaceae
English: black solanum
Literal English translation: "dragon big-flowered plant"
Properties: bitter, cold
Channels entered: none noted

ACTIONS & INDICATIONS:

♦ Clears heat, resolves toxicity, invigorates blood, and reduces swelling: for sores, abscesses, erisypelas, trauma.

♦ Also used for chronic bronchitis and acute nephrites.

DOSAGE: 15-30g

龙眼核
lóng yǎn hé

Pharmaceutical name: Semen Euphoriae Longanae
Botanical name: *Euphoria longan* (Lour.) Steud.
Family: sapindaceae
English: pit of the longan fruit
Literal English translation: "dragon eye pit"
Properties: astringent
Channels entered: none noted

ACTIONS & INDICATIONS:

♦ Arrests bleeding and stops pain: for bleeding and pain due to trauma and injury.

♦ Regulates qi and transforms dampness: for hernia, scrophula, scabies and tinea, and sores due to dampness.

DOSAGE: 3-9g

绿矾
lǜ fán

Pharmaceutical name: Melanteritum
Chemical name: hydrated ferrous sulfate
English: green vitriol
Properties: sour, astringent, cool
Channels entered: Lung, Large Intestine, Spleen, Liver

ACTIONS & INDICATIONS:

♦ Dries dampness and transforms phlegm: for abdominal fullness due to jaundice.

♦ Eliminates accumulation and kills parasites: for childhood nutritional impairment due to dysenteric disorder.

♦ Arrests bleeding and tonifies the blood: for bloody stools due to Intestinal wind or pallor due to deficiency of blood.

♦ Relieves toxicity and closes sores: for toxic sores.

CAUTIONS & CONTRAINDICATIONS: Use with caution in cases of weak Stomach. Over-administration can result in vomiting. Incompatible with vinegar.

DOSAGE: 1.5-4.5g. Almost always used in the calcined form.

木芙蓉叶
mù fú róng yè

Pharmaceutical name: Folium Hibisci Mutabilis
Botanical name: *Hibiscus mutabilis* L.
Family: malvaceae

English: hibiscus leaf
Properties: acrid, neutral
Channels entered: Lung, Liver

ACTIONS & INDICATIONS:

♦ Cools the blood and relieves toxicity: for herpes infections and swelling and severe inflammation of abscesses and carbuncles.

♦ Reduces swelling and stops pain: for trauma and contusions, and redness, swelling, and eye pain.

DOSAGE: Sources do not indicate specific dosage as this herb is primarily for external use.

槿皮
jǐn pí

Pharmaceutical name: Cortex Hibisci Syriaci Radicis
Botanical name: *Hibiscus syriacus* L.
Family: malvaceae
English: bark and root bark of the rose of Sharon
Properties: sweet, bitter, cool
Channels entered: Large Intestine, Liver, Spleen

ACTIONS & INDICATIONS:

♦ Clears heat and drains dampness: for bloody stools due to intestinal wind, dysenteric disorders; also for hemorrhoids, rectal prolapse, and vaginal discharge.

♦ Relieves toxicity and arrests itching: for tinea and scabies.

DOSAGE: 3-9g. Usually used externally in a tincture or fumigation.

闹羊花
nào yáng huā

Pharmaceutical name: Inflorescentia Rhododendri Mollis
Botanical name: *Rhododendrum molle* (Bl.) G.Don
Family: ericaceae
English: azalea, yellow azalea
Literal English name: "agitate goat (sheep) flower"
Properties: acrid, warm, extremely toxic
Channel entered: Liver

ACTIONS & INDICATIONS:

♦ Dispels wind and eliminates dampness: for stubborn painful obstruction due to wind-dampness.

♦ Scatters stasis and eliminates swelling: for trauma and injury.

♦ Arrests pain and kills parasites: for tinea.

CAUTIONS & CONTRAINDICATIONS: Contraindicated during pregnancy and in cases of deficiency. See **Toxicity** below.

DOSAGE: 0.3-0.6g

TOXICITY: This substance contains andromedotoxin and rhodotoxin, both of which inhibit cardiopulmonary functions. Symptoms of toxicity include nausea, vomiting, abdominal pain, diarrhea, bradycardia, low blood pressure, difficulty in breathing, and loss of motor function.

蔷薇花
qiáng wēi huā

Pharmaceutical name: Flos Rosae Multiflorae
Botanical name: *Rosa multiflora* Thunb.
Family: rosaceae
English: tea rose, multiflora rose, seven sisters rose
Properties: sweet, cool
Channels entered: none noted

ACTIONS & INDICATIONS:

♦ Clears summerheat. regulates the Stomach, arrests bleeding: for vomiting of blood due to summerheat; also for thirst, dysenteric disorders, malarial disorders, and bleeding from wounds.

CAUTIONS & CONTRAINDICATIONS: Contraindicated in cases of deficiency of source qi.

DOSAGE: 3-6g

茄子秸
qié zǐ jiē

Pharmaceutical name: Caulis Solani Melongenae cum Radicis
Botanical name: *Solanum melongena* L.
Family: solanaceae
English: eggplant vine
Properties: sweet, acrid, cold
Channels entered: none noted

ACTIONS & INDICATIONS:

♦ Relieves toxicity: for dysenteric disorders accompanied by bloody stools, toothache, swelling due to carbuncles, and chilblain sores.

DOSAGE: 9-18g

青粱米
qīng liáng mǐ

Pharmaceutical name: Semen Sentaniae Italicae

Botanical name: *Setaria italica* (L.) Beauv.
Family: poaceae
English: green grain of the foxtail millet
Properties: sweet, slightly cold
Channels entered: none noted

ACTIONS & INDICATIONS:

♦ Tonifies the middle and benefits the qi: for restlessness due to heat patterns, wasting and thirsting syndrome, and dysenteric disorders.

DOSAGE: 15-30g

拳参
quán shēn

Pharmaceutical name: Radix Polygoni Bistortae
Botanical name: *Polygonum bistorta* L.
Family: polygonaceae
English: snakeweed, bistort
Properties: bitter, cool
Channels entered: none noted

ACTIONS & INDICATIONS:

♦ Clears heat and suppresses spasms and convulsions: for spasms and convulsions due to heat; also for tetanus and dysenteric disorders.
♦ Resolves dampness and swelling: for scrofula.

CAUTIONS & CONTRAINDICATIONS: Contradindicated in cases of yin-type sores.

DOSAGE: 3-9g

蛇含石
shé hán shí

Pharmaceutical name: Pyritum Rotundum
English: ferric oxide
Literal English translation: "snake-bearing rock"
Properties: sweet, cold
Channels entered: Pericardium, Liver

ACTIONS & INDICATIONS:

♦ Calms the spirit and settles convulsions: for palpitations and convulsions.
♦ Arrests bleeding and stops pain: for bloody dysenteric disorders, pain of the Heart, and soreness and pain of the joints.

DOSAGE: 6-9g

伸筋草
shēn jīn cǎo

Pharmaceutical name: Herba cum Radice Lycopodii Clavati
Botanical name: *Lycopodium clavatum* L.
Family: lycopodiaceae
English: running pine, staghorn clubmoss
Literal English translation: "extend sinew grass"
Properties: bitter, acrid, warm
Channels entered: Liver, Spleen, Kidney

ACTIONS & INDICATIONS:

♦ Dispels wind and scatters cold, eliminates dampness and swelling, and relaxes the sinews and activates the collaterals: for painful obstruction due to wind, cold, and dampness, especially of the joints; numbness of the skin; weakness of the extremities; trauma and contusions.

CAUTIONS & CONTRAINDICATIONS: Contraindicated during pregnancy and in cases of hemorrhage.

DOSAGE: 9-15g

石灰
shí huī

Pharmaceutical name: Calcite
Chemical name: calcium carbonate
English: limestone, calx
Properties: acrid, warm, toxic
Channels entered: Liver, Spleen

ACTIONS & INDICATIONS:

♦ Dries dampness and kills parasites: for scabies, tinea, and sores due to dampness.

♦ Arrests bleeding and stops pain: for bleeding due to trauma and injury; also for hemorrhoids and rectal prolapse.

♦ Removes tissue decay: for warts.

♦ When administered orally, stops dysenteric diarrhea and uterine hemorrhage.

DOSAGE: Prepared calcite (calcination followed by exposure to water) may be administered orally at a dosage of 3-6g. Raw calcite (calcined only) is for external use only.

松针
sōng zhēn

Pharmaceutical name: Folium Pini
Botanical name: *Pinus tabulaeformis* Carr., *P. massoniana* Lamb., or *P. yunnanensis* Franch.

Family: pinaceae
English: pine needle
Properties: bitter, warm
Channels entered: Heart, Spleen

ACTIONS & INDICATIONS:
♦ Dispels wind and dries dampness: for flaccid obstruction of the wind-damp type; also for trauma and contusions, insomnia, edema, and sores of the damp type.
♦ Kills parasites and stops itching: for scabies and tinea.

DOSAGE: 9-15g; if fresh, 3-6g

松香
sōng xiāng

Pharmaceutical name: Resina Pini
Botanical name: *Pinus massoniana* Lamb.
Family: pinaceae
English: pine resin
Literal English translation: "pine fragrance"
Properties: bitter, sweet, warm, acrid, slightly toxic
Channels entered: Liver, Spleen

ACTIONS & INDICATIONS:
♦ Dispels wind and dries dampness: for wind-damp painful obstruction; also treats leprosy, patchy loss of hair in children, and tinea of the head.
♦ Expels pus and toxin and generates flesh: for abscesses and furuncles/carbuncles.
♦ Stops pain: for sprains.

CAUTIONS & CONTRAINDICATIONS: If administered by itself, pine resin can cause blockage of the Stomach and Intestines; it should therefore always be combined with other ingredients. See **Toxicity** below.

DOSAGE: 0.3-1.5g

TOXICITY: Turpentine is the toxic chemical constituent in pine resin. Preparation of pine resin for medicinal use is by heating in a double boiler in order to volatilize the turpentine content. Symptoms of toxicity include nausea, stomach discomfort, loss of appetite, watery stools, headache, dizziness, weakness, and skin rash.

铜绿
tóng lù

Pharmaceutical name: Robigo Aeris
English: verdigris (the green or bluish deposit of copper carbonates formed on copper, brass, or bronze surfaces)

Literal English translation: "copper green"
Properties: sour, neutral, toxic
Channels entered: Liver, Gallbladder

ACTIONS & INDICATIONS:
- Resolves opacity: for opacity of the eye.
- Removes necrosis and closes lesions: for leg ulcers, carbuncles, hermorrhoids.
- Kills parasites: for tinea.

CAUTIONS & CONTRAINDICATIONS: Contraindicated in cases of weakness and deficiency of blood. See **Toxicity** below.

DOSAGE: 0.9-1.5g

TOXICITY: This substance is toxic in large doses. Symptoms of toxicity include nausea and vomiting, salivation, abdominal pain and diarrhea, and bloody stools.

透骨草
tòu gǔ cǎo

Pharmaceutical name: Herba Speranskiae seu Impatientis
Botanical name: *Speranskia tuberculata* (Bge.) Baill. or *Impatiens balsamina* L.
Family: euphorbiaceae
Literal English translation: "penetrate bone grass"
Properties: acrid, warm
Channels entered: none noted

ACTIONS & INDICATIONS:
- Dispels wind and eliminates dampness: for painful obstruction due to wind-dampness, leg-qi due to cold-dampness; also for the inward sinking of toxin from sores and tinea.
- Relaxes the sinews and invigorates the blood: for muscular tetany.

CAUTIONS & CONTRAINDICATIONS: Contraindicated during pregnancy.

DOSAGE: 9-15g

土大黄
tǔ dà huáng

Pharmaceutical name: Radix Rumicis Madaio
Botanical name: *Rumex madaio* Mak.
Family: polygonaceae
English: dock root
Literal English translation: "local rhubarb"
Properties: acrid, bitter, cold
Channels entered: none noted
Properties and indications:
- Clears heat: for coughing up of blood or Lung abscess with dry stools.
- Moves blood stasis: for trauma and contusions.

- ♦ Kills parasites: for tinea.
- ♦ Clears toxicity: for swelling of abscesses.

DOSAGE: 9-15g

土荆皮
tǔ jīng pí

Pharmaceutical name: Cortex Pseudolaricis Kaempferi Radicis
Botanical name: *Pseudolarix kaempferi* Gord.
Family: pinaceae
English: golden larch rootbark
Properties: acrid, warm, toxic
Channels entered: Lung, Spleen

ACTIONS & INDICATIONS:
- ♦ Kills parasites and arrests itching: for tinea, dermatitis, lichen simplex chronicus.

CAUTIONS & CONTRAINDICATIONS: Not for oral administration. See **Toxicity** below.

DOSAGE: Sources do not indicate specific dosage as this herb is for external use only.

TOXICITY: In mice the LD50 for intravenous injection of pseudolaric acid A and B were 486mg/kg and 423mg/kg respectively. Toxic effects included tremors and stiffening of the head and neck, which resolved after five minutes, and was followed by weakness and labored breathing through the mouth. Toxic effects in rats and dogs included aversion to food, vomiting, watery stools, and bloody stools.

万年青叶
wàn nián qīng yè

Pharmaceutical name: Folium Rohdeae Japonicae
Botanical name: *Rohdea japonica* Roth
Family: liliaceae
English: lily of China leaf
Literal English translation: "thousand year green leaf"
Properties: bitter, astringent, slightly cold
Channels entered: Kidney, Liver

ACTIONS & INDICATIONS:
- ♦ Clears heat and relieves toxicity: for swelling and pain of the pharynx, insect bites and stings, and snakebite.
- ♦ Arrests bleeding: for coughing up of blood and vomiting of blood.
- ♦ Strengthens the Heart and promotes urination: for heart failure.

DOSAGE: 9-15g

芜菁子
wú jīng zǐ

Pharmaceutical name: Semen Brassicae Rapae
Botanical name: *Brassica rapa* L.
Family: brassicaceae
English: seed of the field mustard, rapeseed, canola seed
Properties: acrid, neutral
Channels entered: Liver, Spleen, Lung

ACTIONS & INDICATIONS:

♦ Brightens the eyes: for opacity of the eyes.

♦ Clears heat and drains dampness: for jaundice, dysenteric disorders, and difficult urination.

CAUTIONS & CONTRAINDICATIONS: Contraindicated in cases of deficiency cold.

DOSAGE: 3-9g

虾蟆
xiā má

Pharmaceutical name: Rana Limnocharis
Zoological name: *Rana limnocharis* Boie
Family: ranidae
English: frog
Properties: sweet, cold
Channels entered: Spleen

ACTIONS & INDICATIONS:

♦ Clears heat and relieves toxicity: for swelling due to abscesses, furuncles of the heat type, ulcers of the mouth, and scrofula.

♦ Strengthens the Spleen and reduces accumulation: for childhood nutritional impairment.

DOSAGE: Sources do not indicate specific dosage.

线叶金鸡菊
xiàn yè jīn jī jú

Pharmaceutical name: Folium Coreopsidis Lanceolatae
Botanical name: *Coreopsis lanceolata* L.
Family: compositae
English: coreopsis
Literal English translation: "thready leaf golden chicken chrysanthemum"
Properties: acrid, neutral
Channels entered: none noted

ACTIONS & INDICATIONS:

♦ Dispels blood stasis and eliminates swelling, and clears heat and relieves toxicity: for all types of skin lesions and cuts.

DOSAGE: No dosage indicated as this herb is for external use only.

亚麻子
yà má zǐ

Pharmaceutical name: Semen Lini Usitatissimi
Botanical name: *Linum usitatissimum* L.
Family: linaceae
English: flax seed or linseed
Properties: sweet, neutral
Channel entered: Liver

ACTIONS & INDICATIONS:
♦ For leprosy, hives, loss of hair, and dry stools.

CAUTIONS & CONTRAINDICATIONS: Contraindicated during pregnancy and in cases of weak stomach and loose stools.

DOSAGE: 9-15g

银朱
yín zhū

Pharmaceutical name: Vermilion
Chemical name: mercuric sulfide
English: vermilion
Literal English translation: "silver vermilion"
Properties: acrid, warm, toxic
Channels entered: Heart, Lung, Stomach

ACTIONS & INDICATIONS:
♦ Attacks toxin, kills parasites: for toxic sores, tinea, and scabies.
♦ Dries dampness and dispels phlegm: for chest and abdominal pain due to congested fluids.

CAUTIONS & CONTRAINDICATIONS: Use internally with caution. Incompatible with Magnetitum *(ci shi)* and salty water. See **Toxicity** below.

DOSAGE: 0.2-0.5g powdered when administered orally

TOXICITY: In mice the intravenous LD50 dose is 10g/kg.

樱桃
yīng táo

Pharmaceutical name: Fructus Pruni Pseudocerasi
Botanical name: *Prunus pseudocerasus* Lindl.

Family: rosaceae
English: cherry
Properties: sweet, warm
Channels entered: none noted

ACTIONS & INDICATIONS:
- Benefits qi: for paralysis and the sores of chilblains.
- Dispels wind-dampness: for low back and leg pain due to wind-dampness.

CAUTIONS & CONTRAINDICATIONS: According to many sources, overeating of cherries can result in vomiting, weakness and burning of the ears, or lead to a deficiency-heat type of cough.

DOSAGE: 240-480g when used in decoctions

藏青果
zàng qīng guǒ

Pharmaceutical name: Fructus Terminaliae Chebulae Immaturus
Botanical name: *Terminalia chebula* Retz.
Family: combretaceae
English: immature fruit of myrobalan
Literal English translation: "dark blue fruit"
Properties: sour, bitter, astringent, slightly cold
Channels entered: Lung, Stomach

ACTIONS & INDICATIONS:
- Clears heat and generates fluids, and relieves toxicity, binds up the Intestines, and kills parasites: for diptherial disorders, dysenteric disorders, and similar disorders.

CAUTIONS & CONTRAINDICATIONS: Contraindicated in cases of throat pain due to wind-fire toxin, and in cases of attack by cold.

DOSAGE: 1.5-4.5g

蚤休
zǎo xiū

Pharmaceutical name: Rhizoma Paris Polyphyllae
Botanical name: *Paris polyphylla* Smith
Family: liliaceae
English: Himalayan paris
Literal English translation: "flea rest"
Properties: bitter, acrid, cold, toxic
Channels entered: Heart, Liver

ACTIONS & INDICATIONS:
- Clears heat and relieves toxicity: for deep-seated furuncles and swelling due to abscesses; also for bites and stings of snakes and insects.
- Stops wheezing and cough: for chronic coughing and wheezing.
- Extinguishes wind and arrests tremors: for childhood tremors and muscle twitches.

CAUTIONS & CONTRAINDICATIONS: Contraindicated in cases of constitutional weakness, and fire or heat toxin not due to excess, and yin-type external sores; also contraindicated during pregnancy. See **Toxicity** below.

DOSAGE: 3-9g

TOXICITY: The underground stem is toxic. If overdose occurs, symptoms can include nausea, vomiting, headache, and, in severe cases, tremors.

猪胆
zhū dǎn

Pharmaceutical name: Vesica Fellea Suis
Zoological name: *Sus scrofu domestica* Brisson
English: pig gallbladder
Properties: bitter, cold
Channels entered: Liver, Gallbladder, Lung, Large Intestine

ACTIONS & INDICATIONS:

♦ Clears heat and moistens dryness: for heat patterns causing thirst and dryness; also for dry stools, redness of the eye, discharge of pus from the ear.

♦ Relieves toxicity: for swelling of abscesses and carbuncles; also for dysenteric disorders.

DOSAGE: 3-6g

紫贝
zǐ bèi

Pharmaceutical name: Concha Zibei
Zoological names: *Erosoria caputserpentis* (L.), *Cypraea lynx* (L.), or *Mauritia arabica* (L.)
Family: cypraeidae
English: cowrie
Literal English translation: "purple cowrie"
Properties: salty, neutral
Channels entered: Spleen, Liver

ACTIONS & INDICATIONS:

♦ Clears heat, calms the Liver, calms the spirit, and brightens the eye: for opacity of the eye due to heat toxin, for skin lesion heat toxin that spreads to the eyes in children, and startling causing disturbance of sleep.

DOSAGE: 6-15g

紫荆皮
zǐ jīng pí

Pharmaceutical name: Cortex Cercis Chinensis

Botanical name: *Cercis chinensis* Bge.
Family: caesalpiniaceae
English: bark of the Chinese redbud
Properties: bitter, neutral
Channels entered: Liver, Spleen

ACTIONS & INDICATIONS:

♦ Invigorates the blood and unblocks the channels: for painful obstruction due to wind, cold, dampness; painful obstruction of the throat, amenorrhea; trauma and contusions.

♦ Eliminates swelling and relieves toxicity: for swelling due to abscesses; also for tinea, insect bites and stings, snakebites.

CAUTIONS & CONTRAINDICATIONS: Contraindicated during pregnancy.

DOSAGE: 6-12g

紫苏梗
zǐ sū gěng

Pharmaceutical name: Caulis Perillae Frutescens
Botanical name: *Perilla frutescens* (L.) Britt. var. *crispa* (Thunb.) Hand. -Mazz, or *P. frutescens* (L.) Britt. var *acuta* (Thunb.) Kudo
Family: lamiaceae
English: perilla stem
Properties: acrid, sweet, slightly warm
Channels entered: Spleen, Stomach, Lung

ACTIONS & INDICATIONS:

♦ Regulates qi and disperses constraint: for constrained qi, food accumulation, and a stifling sensation in the chest and diaphragm.

♦ Calms the fetus: for restless fetus.

DOSAGE: 4.5-9g

紫玉簪叶
zǐ yù zān yè

Pharmaceutical name: Folium Hostae Ventricosae
Botanical name: *Hosta ventricosa* (Salisb.) Stearn
Family: liliaceae
English: hosta
Properties: none noted
Channels entered: none noted

ACTIONS & INDICATIONS:

♦ For uterine bleeding and discharge.
♦ For chronic sores.

DOSAGE: Sources do not indicate specific dosage as this herb is primarily for external use.

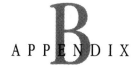

APPENDIX B

General References

Bensky, Dan, and Randall Barolet. *Chinese Herbal Medicine: Formulas & Strategies*. Seattle: Eastland Press, 1990.

Bensky, Dan, and Andrew Gamble. *Chinese Herbal Medicine: Materia Medica*. Rev. ed. Seattle: Eastland Press, 1993.

Berkow, Robert, ed. *The Merck Manual of Diagnosis and Therapy*. 15th ed. Rahway, NJ: Merck Sharp & Dohme Research Laboratories, 1987.

Braun-Falco, O., G. Plewig, H. H. Wolff, and R. K. Winkelman. *Dermatology*. Berlin: Springer-Verlag, 1991.

Dai, Yin-Fang, and Cheng-Jun Liu. *Medicinal Uses of Fruits (Yao yong guo pin)* 药用果品. Nanning: Guangxi People's Publishing House, 1982.

Dou, Guo-Xiang, *Guide to Food Therapy (Yin shi zhi liao zhi nan)* 饮食治疗指南. Jiangsu: Jiangsu Science and Technology Press, 1981.

duVivier, A. *Atlas of Clinical Dermatology*. New York: Saunders, 1986.

Fitzpatrick, Thomas B., et al, eds. *Dermatology in General Medicine: Textbook and Atlas*. New York: McGraw-Hill, 1987.

Gu, Bo-Hua, ed. *Practical Textbook of Traditional Chinese External Diseases (Shi yong zhong yi wai ke xue)* 实用中医外科学. Shanghai: Shanghai Science & Technology Press, 1985.

Jiangsu College of New Medicine. *Encyclopedia of Traditional Chinese Materia Medica (Zhong yao da ci dian)* 中药大辞典. Shanghai: People's Press, 1977.

Marks, R. *Roxburgh's Common Skin Diseases*. 16th ed. London: Chapman & Hall Medical, 1993.

Moschella, Samuel L., and Harry J. Hurley. *Dermatology*. 3rd ed. Philadelphia: W.B. Saunders, 1992.

Orkin, Milton, Howard I. Maibach, Mark V. Dahl. *Dermatology*. East Norwalk, CT: Appleton-Lange, 1991.

Peng, Huai-Ren, ed. *Great Compendium of Famous Chinese Medical Formulas (Zhong hua ming yi fang ji da quan)* 中华名医方剂大全. Beijing: Gold Shield Press, 1990.

Shanghai First Medical College, Huashan Hospital Department of Dermatology. *Manual of Dermatology (Pi fu ke shou ce)*. Rev. ed. 皮肤科手册. Shanghai: Shanghai Science & Technology Press, 1979.

Steigleder, Gerd Klaus, and Howard I. Maibach. *Pocket Atlas of Dermatology*. New York: Thieme-Stratton, 1984.

Xu, Yi-Hou. *Traditional Chinese Dermatology Diagnosis and Treatment (Zhong yi pi fu ke zhen liao xue)* 中医皮肤科诊疗学. Wuhan: Hubei Science & Technology Press, 1986.

Ye, Ju-Quan. *Traditional Chinese Food Medicinals and Folk Prescriptions (Shi wu zhong yao yu pian fang)* 食物中药与便方. Jiangsu: Jiangsu Science and Technology Press, 1980.

Zhang, Jin-Zhang, ed. *Integrated Traditional and Western Treatment of Skin Diseases (Zhong xi yi jie he pi fu xing bing zhi liao xue)* 中西医结合皮肤性病治疗学. Wuhan: Wuhan Press, 1992.

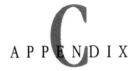

APPENDIX C

Historical References

A Hundred Questions About Infants and Children (Ying tong bai wen) 婴童百问. Lu Bo-Si, 1506.

Collection of Cases on External Diseases (Wai ke yi an hui bian) 外科医案汇编. Yu Jing-He, 1891.

Collection of Records of Redressing Wrongs (Xi yuan ji lu) 洗冤集录. Song Ci-Zhuan, 1247.

Collection of Treatments for Sores (Yang yi da quan) 疡医大全. Gu Shi-Deng, 1760.

Compendium of External Medicine (Wai ke da cheng) 外科大成. Qi Kun, 1665.

Complete Book of Experiences with Sores and Ulcers (Chuang yang jing yan quan shu) 疮疡经验全书. Dou Han-Qing (Song); book was actually published in 1695.

Comprehensive Recording of Sage-like Benefit from the Zheng He Era (Zheng he sheng ji zong lu) 政和圣济总录. Shen Fu, et al., 1122.

Discussion of Cold-induced Disorders (Shang han lun) 伤寒论. Zhang Zhong-Jing, Eastern Han.

Discussion of the Origins of Symptoms of Diseases (Zhu bing yuan hou lun) 诸病源候论. Chao Yuan-Fang, 610.

Discussion of the Origin and Development of Medicine (Yi xue yuan liu lun) 医学源流论. Xu Da-Chun, 1757.

Discussion of Warm Epidemics (Wen yi lun) 温疫论. Wu You-Xing, 1642.

Emergency Formulas to Keep Up One's Sleeve (Zhou hou bei ji fang) 肘后备急方. Ge Hong, 341.

Essence of External Diseases (Wai ke jing yi) 外科精义. Qi De, 1335.

Essentials from the Golden Cabinet (Jin gui yao lue) 金匮要略. Zhang Zhong-Jing, Eastern Han.

Essential Outline of Sores (Yang ke gang yao) 疡科纲要. Zhang Shan-Lei, 1917.

Formulas to Guard Life from Lingnan (Ling nan wei sheng fang) 岭南卫生方. Shi Ji-Hong, Song/Yuan dynasties.

Fundamental Gatherings of Disclosure of Diseases (Jie wei yuan sou) 解围元薮. Shen Zhi-Wen, 1550.

Golden Mirror of the Medical Tradition (Yi zong jin jian) 医宗金鉴. Wu Qian, 1742.

Grand Materia Medica (Ben cao gang mu) 本草纲目. Li Shi-Zhen, 1578.

Health Benefit Treasures (Wei ji bao shu) 卫济宝书. Dong-Xuan Ju-Shi (probable author), c. 1170.

Introduction to Medicine (Yi xue ru men) 医学入门. Li Chan, 1575.

Liu Juan-Zi's Formulas Passed Down from a Spirit (Liu Juan-Zi gui yi fang) 刘涓子鬼遗方. Liu Juan-Zi, Jin dynasty.

Mechanisms and Essentials of Pestilent Sores (Li yang ji yao) 疠疡机要. Xue Ji, 1554.

Omissions from the Grand Materia Medica (Ben cao gang mu shi yi) 本草纲目拾遗. Zhao Xue-Min, 1765.

Principles and Experiences of External Diseases (Wai ke li li) 外科理例. Wang Ji, 1531.

Profound Insights on External Diseases (Wai ke qi xuan) 外科启玄. Shen Dou-Yuan, 1604.

Profound Purpose from the Heavenly Abode (Dong tian ao zhi) 洞天奥旨. Chen Shi-Duo, 1694.

Secret Records on Bayberry Flower Sores (Mei chuang mi lu) 霉疮秘录. Chen Si-Cheng, 1632.

Sores and Ulcers (Chuang yang) 疮疡. Zou Han-Huang, 1840.

Standards of Patterns and Treatments (Zheng zhi zhun sheng) 证治准绳. Wang Ken-Tang, 1602.

Stone Chamber Secret Records (Shi shi mi lu) 石室秘录. Chen Shi-Duo, 1687.

Thousand Ducat Formulas (Qian jin yao fang) 千金要方. Sun Si-Miao, 652.

HISTORICAL REFERENCES

True Lineage of External Medicine (Wai ke zheng zong) 外科正宗.
Chen Shi-Gong, 1617.

Yellow Emperor's Inner Classic (Huang di nei jing) 黄帝内经.
Authors unknown, c. 100 B.C.

Zhou Annals (Zhou li) 周礼. Zhou Gong (putative author), published during Warring States period.

APPENDIX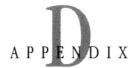

Pinyin-English Cross Reference of Formula Names

A

ān gōng niú huáng wán — Calm the Palace Pill with Cattle Gallstone, 77

B

bā èr dān — Eight-Two Special Powder, 70
bā zhēn tāng jiā jiǎn — Modified Eight-Treasure Decoction, 266
bā zhēn tāng — Eight-Treasure Decoction, 68
bái bān wū hēi tāng — White Spots Pitch-Black Decoction, 293
bái bǐ tāng — White Dagger Sore Decoction, 219
bái diàn fēng wán — White Blotch Wind Pill, 293
bái hǔ tāng — White Tiger Decoction 157
bái huā shé shé cǎo xǐ jì — Oldenlandia Wash, 115
bái xiè fēng dīng — Psoriasis Tincture, 183
bǎi bù dīng — Stemona Tincture, 146
bǎi zhī yóu — Biota Ointment, 268
bài dú yǐn — Defeat Toxin Decoction, 196
bān máo dīng — Mylabris Tincture, 176
bǎo fà tāng — Protect the Hair Decoction, 270
bèi xiè shèn shī tāng — Dioscorea Decoction to Leach Out Dampness [B], 281
bèi xiè shèn shī tāng jiā jiǎn — Modified Dioscorea Decoction to Leach Out Dampness [A], 220
bīng shí sǎn — Borneol and Gypsum Powder, 104
bǔ gǔ zhī dīng zhù shè yè — Psoralea Tincture Injection, 113
bǔ pí wèi xiè yīn huǒ shēng yáng tāng jiā jiǎn — Modified Tonify the Spleen Stomach, Drain Yin Fire, and Raise the Yang Decoction, 232

333

bǔ zhōng yì qì tāng jiā jiǎn — Modified Tonify the Middle and Augment the Qi Decoction, 55
bù mián cā jì — Cotton Cloth Rub, 170

C

cāng bó niú xī fāng — Atractylodes, Phellodendron, and Achyranthes Formula, 187
cāng fū shuǐ xǐ jì — Xanthium and Kochia Wash, 59
chái hú qīng gān tāng — Bupleurum Decoction to Clear the Liver, 74
chōng hé gāo — Flush and Harmonize Plaster, 78
chú chóng jú dīng — Coreopsis Tincture to Eliminate Bugs, 146
chú shī jiě dú tāng — Eliminate Dampness and Relieve Toxicity Decoction, 257
chú shī wèi líng tāng jiā jiǎn — Modified Eliminate Dampness Decoction by Combining Calm the Stomach and Five Ingredient Powder with Poria, 166
chú shī wèi líng tāng — Eliminate Dampness Decoction by Combining Calm the Stomach and Five-Ingredient Powder with Poria, 101
chuān ài tāng — Zanthoxylum and Artemisia Decoction, 144
chuān jiāo dà suàn ní — Zanthoxylum and Allium Paste, 132
cuó chuāng jiān jì — Acne Decoction, 257

D

dà huáng bīng piàn fāng — Rheum and Borneol Formula, 184
dà huáng sǎn — Rheum Powder, 78
dà qīng lián qiáo tāng jiā jiǎn — Modified Daqingye and Forsythia Decoction, 100
dān dú gāo — Erysipelas Plaster, 79
dāng guī sì nì tāng jiā jiǎn — Modified Tangkuei Decoction for Frigid Extremities [A], 152
dāng guī sì nì tāng jiā jiǎn — Modified Tangkuei Decoction for Frigid Extremities [B], 200
dāng guī sì nì tāng — Tangkuei Decoction for Frigid Extremities, 279
dāng shú yǎng xuè tāng — Tangkuei and Cooked Rehmannia Decoction to Nourish the Blood, 45
dǎng shēn jì shēng bǔ yì fāng — Codonopsis and Sangjisheng Tonifying and Augmenting Formula, 242
dì huáng yǐn zǐ jiā jiǎn — Modified Rehmannia Decoction, 138
dì shí zhī fāng — Rehmannia, Gypsum, and Anemarrhena Formula, 227
dì yú èr cāng hú gāo — Sanguisorba, Xanthium, and Atractylodes Paste, 169
diān dǎo sǎn — Upside Down Powder, 258
dīng xiāng bīng piàn sǎn — Clove and Borneol Powder, 250
dōng chóng xià cǎo dīng — Cordyceps Tincture, 269
dòng chuāng gāo — Freeze Sore Plaster, 155
dòng chuāng yóu — Freeze Sore Ointment, 154
dú huó jì shēng tāng jiā jiǎn — Modified Angelica Pubescens and Sangjisheng Decoction, 235

dú wèi huáng qí fāng — Single-Ingredient Astragalus Formula, 232

E

é huáng sǎn — Light-Yellow Powder, 139
èr xiān tāng jiā jiǎn — Modified Two-Immortal Decoction [A], 211
èr xiān tāng jiā jiǎn — Modified Two-Immortal Decoction [B], 223
èr zhì wán jiā jiǎn — Modified Two-Ultimate Pill, 290

F

fáng fēng tōng shèng sǎn — Ledebouriella Powder that Sagely Unblocks, 96
fēng fáng sǎn — Hornet Nest Powder, 57
fēng yóu gāo — Nervous Wind Ointment, 176
fèi zǐ fěn — Miliaria Powder, 247
fèng huáng yī fāng — Phoenix Mantle Formula, 285
fù zǐ lǐ zhōng tāng jiā guì zhī tāng jiā jiǎn — Modified Prepared Aconite Decoction to Regulate the Middle Plus Modified Cinnamon Twig Decoction, 209
fù zǐ lǐ zhōng wán — Prepared Aconite Pill to Regulate the Middle, 278

G

gān lù xiāo dú dān — Sweet Dew Special Pill to Eliminate Toxin, 248
gé gēn qín lián tāng — Pueraria, Scutellaria, and Coptis Decoction, 186
gǒu jǐ shuǐ xǐ jì — Cibotium Wash, 302
guī pí tāng — Restore the Spleen Decoction, 277
guī sháo dì huáng tāng jiā jiǎn — Modified Tangkuei, Peony, and Rehmannia Decoction, 108
guī xiōng fāng — Angelica and Ligusticum Formula, 236
guǐ dān jiāng cán tāng — Buchnera, Moutan, and Batryticatus Decoction, 201
guì zhī jiā dāng guī tāng jiā jiǎn — Modified Cinnamon Twig Decoction Plus Tangkuei, 153
guì zhī má huáng gè bàn tāng — Combined Cinnamon Twig and Ephedra Decoction, 47
guì zhī tāng jiā jiǎn — Modified Cinnamon Twig Decoction [A], 207
guì zhī tāng jiā jiǎn — Modified Cinnamon Twig Decoction [B], 217

H

hǎi ài tāng — Artemisia Argyi Decoction, 268
hé shǒu wū jiǔ — Polygonum Wine, 88
hēi yóu gāo — Black Ointment, 168
hóng bù gāo — Red Cloth Plaster, 63
hóng líng jiǔ — Effective Scarlet Wine, 154
hóng yóu gāo — Red Ointment, 83
hú chòu fěn — Fox Stench Powder, 250
10% hú jiāo jiǔ jīng jìn yè — Ten Percent Ground Pepper Alcohol, 153
hú má wán jiā jiǎn — Modified Linum Pill, 291

hŭ pò èr wū hú gāo — Succinum and Two-Aconite Paste, 169
hŭ pò là fán wán — Succinum, Beeswax, and Alum Pill, 68
huá dài fěn — Talcum and Indigo Powder, 188
huáng lián gāo — Coptis Ointment, 64, 103, 104, 188, 197, 233
huáng lián jiě dú tāng hé sān miào wán — Combined Coptis Decoction to Relieve Toxicity and Three-Marvel Pill, 75
huáng lián jiě dú tāng — Coptis Decoction to Relieve Toxicity, 105
huáng lián jiě dú tāng, wŭ wèi xiāo dú yǐn huà cái — Combined Coptis Decoction to Relieve Toxin and Five-Ingredient Decoction to Eliminate Toxin, 221
huáng qí zǎo xiū yǐn — Astragalus and Paris Decoction, 58
huàn jī sǎn — Change Flesh Powder, 87
huí yáng yù lóng gāo — Jade Dragon Plaster to Restore Yang, 236
huó xuè rùn zào shēng jīn tāng jiā jiǎn — Modified Invigorate the Blood, Moisten Dryness, and Generate Fluids Decoction, 227
huó xuè sàn yū tāng — Invigorate the Blood and Scatter Stasis Decoction, 219

J

jiā wèi cāng zhú gāo — Augmented Atractylodes Gelatin, 301
jiā zhǐ gāo — Paper Sandwich Plaster, 284
jiǎn cǎo sǎn — Clinopodium Powder, 130
jiě dú zǐ jīn gāo — Purple and Gold Plaster to Relieve Toxin, 286
jīn guì shèn qì wán jiā jiǎn — Modified Kidney Qi Pill from the Golden Cabinet, 241
jīn huáng sǎn — Golden-Yellow Powder, 62, 70, 78
jīn líng zǐ sǎn jiā jiǎn — Modified Melia Powder, 102
jīn sù gaō — Golden Plain Plaster, 83
jīng fáng bài dú sǎn jiā jiǎn — Modified Schizonepeta and Ledebouriella Powder to Overcome Toxin, 206
jiǔ yī dān — Nine-One Special Powder, 104
jiǔ zhā bí gāo — Rosacea Paste, 261

K

kè yín fāng — Overcome Psoriasis Formula, 219
kǔ jiāo tāng — Sophora and Zanthoxylum Decoction, 144
kǔ shēn tāng — Sophora Decoction, 89
kǔ suàn cù jìn pào — Sophora and Allium Vinegar Soak, 132

L

lí lú sǎn — Veratrum Powder, 146
lián chuāng gāo — Shin Sore Plaster, 286
liàn jiāo yào yùn — Melia and Zanthoxylum Dry Compress, 237
liáng xuě rùn zào yǐn — Cool the Blood and Moisten Dryness Decoction, 300

liáng xuè huó xuè fāng — Cool and Invigorate the Blood Formula, 275
liáng xuè qīng fèi yǐn — Cool the Blood and Clear the Lung Decoction, 255
liáng xuè wǔ gēn tāng — Cool the Blood Decoction with Five Roots, 275
liáng xuè wǔ huā tāng — Cool the Blood Decoction with Five Flowers, 256
liáng xuè xiāo fēng sǎn jiā jiǎn — Modified Cool the Blood and Eliminate Wind Powder, 226
liáng xuè xiāo fēng sǎn — Cool the Blood and Eliminate Wind Powder, 46
liù shén wán — Six-Miracle Pill, 192, 193
liù wèi dì huáng wán — Six-Ingredient Pill with Rehmannia 283
liù yī sǎn — Six-One Powder, 62
lóng dǎn xiè gān tāng jiā jiǎn — Modified Gentiana Longdancao Decoction to Drain the Liver, 222
lóng dǎn xiè gān tāng — Gentiana Longdancao Decoction to Drain the Liver, 95
lóng kuí shī fū jì — Black Solanum Compress, 54
lú huì bīng zhū wài fū jì — Aloe, Borneol, and Magarita Paste, 103
lù lù tōng shuǐ xǐ jì — Liquidambar Wash, 224
lǜ páo sǎn — Green Robe Powder, 120
lù shì bān tū tāng — Lu Family Decoction for Patchy Baldness, 265

M-N

mǎ chǐ xiàn shuǐ xǐ jì — Portulaca Wash, 97
mǎ qīng shuǐ xǐ jì — Portulaca and Daqingye Wash, 113
mǎ zhú fēng fáng shuǐ xǐ jì — Portulaca, Atractylodes, and Wasp-nest Wash, 110
mài wèi dì huáng tāng — Ophiopogon, Schisandra, and Rehmannia Decoction, 222
máng xiāo xǐ jì — Mirabilitum Wash, 172
mì tuó sēng sǎn — Lithyargyrum Powder, 293
mó fēng gāo — Rub the Wind Ointment, 183-184
mò yín jiān yè — Myrrha and Lonicera Decoction, 164
mù guā bīng láng sǎn — Chaenomeles and Areca Powder, 282
niú gōng liáng xuè fāng — Arctium and Taraxacum Formula to Cool the Blood, 74

P

pí pá qīng fèi yǐn — Eriobotrya Decoction to Clear the Lung, 255
píng wèi sǎn jiā jiǎn — Modified Calm the Stomach Powder, 208
pú dì rěn tāng — Taraxacum, Viola, and Lonicera Decoction, 246
pǔ jì xiāo dú yǐn jiā jiǎn — Modified Universal Benefit Decoction to Eliminate Toxin, 202
pǔ jì xiāo dú yǐn — Universal Benefit Decoction to Eliminate Toxin, 73
pǔ lián gāo — Universally Linked Ointment, 223

Q

qī bǎo měi rán dān — Seven-Treasure Special Pill for Beautiful Whiskers, 266
qī sān dān — Seven-Three Special Powder, 70
qí bái táng — Astragalus and Atractylodes Decoction, 182
qiān jīn sǎn — Thousand Ducat Powder, 109
qián yáng xī fēng tāng — Anchor Yang and Extinguish Wind Decoction, 175
qié zǐ jiē jiān shuǐ — Eggplant Vine Wash, 154
qīng dài gāo — Indigo Ointment, 130
qīng dài kǔ jiāo sǎn — Indigo, Alumen, and Zanthoxylum Powder, 171
qīng dài sǎn — Indigo Powder, 54
qīng guǒ shuǐ xǐ jì — Terminalia Wash, 203
qīng hāo gāo — Artemisia Annua Ointment, 233
qīng hāo yǐn — Artemisia Annua Decoction, 158
qīng jī shèn shī tāng — Clear the Flesh and Leach Out Dampness Decoction, 201
qīng jiě piàn — Clear and Relieve Tablet, 163
qīng liáng fěn — Clearing and Cooling Powder, 158
qīng liáng gāo — Clearing and Cooling Ointment, 53
qīng mù xiāng sǎn — Aristilochia Powder, 249
qīng pí chú shī yǐn — Clear the Spleen and Remove Dampness Decoction, 52
qīng rè jiě dú xǐ jì — Clear Heat and Reduce Toxin Wash, 114
qīng shǔ tāng — Clear Summerheat Decoction, 246
qīng wēn bài dú yǐn jiā jiǎn — Modified Clear Epidemics and Overcome Toxin Decoction, 124
qīng wēn bài dú yǐn — Clear Epidemics and Overcome Toxin Decoction, 76
qīng xuè sōu dú wán — Clear the Blood and Collect the Toxin Pill, 139
qīng yíng tāng jiā jiǎn — Modified Clear the Nutritive Level Decoction, 123
qīng yíng tāng — Clear the Nutritive Level Decoction, 76
qū fǔ shēng jī fāng — Remove Decay and Generate Flesh Formula, 284
qū shī sǎn — Dispel Dampness Powder, 168
qù bān gāo — Remove Spots Ointment, 258
quán chóng fāng — Scorpion Formula, 47

R

rén shēn gù běn wán jiā jiǎn — Modified Ginseng Pill to Stabilize the Root, 97
rén shēn yǎng yíng tāng — Ginseng Decoction to Nourish the Nutritive Qi, 267
ròu cì sǎn — Tissue Thorn Powder, 303
rú yì jīn huáng sǎn jiā jiǎn — Modified Golden-Yellow Powder According to One's Wishes, 64
rú yì jīn huáng sǎn — Golden-Yellow Powder According to One's Wishes, 59
rùn jī gāo — Moisten the Flesh Ointment, 184

S

sān huáng xǐ jì — Three-Yellow Wash, 63

sān shén wán — Three-Miracle Pill, 128

sān xīn dǎo chì sǎn jiā jiǎn — Modified Three-Pith Guide Out the Red Powder, 166

shā shēn mài mén dōng tāng — Glehnia and Ophiopogonis Decoction, 119

shāng lù sǎn — Phytolacca Powder, 294

shé tùi gāo — Exuvia Serpentis Plaster, 82

shé yǎo piàn — Snake Bite Medicine Pills, 149

shēn qí zhī mǔ tāng — Codonopsis, Astragalus, and Anemarrhena Decoction, 53

shén xiào xuǎn yào — Miraculous Tinea Remedy, 131

shén yìng xiāo fēng sǎn jiā jiǎn — Modified Miraculous Extinguish Wind Powder, 292

shēng bàn xià fū tiē — Pinellia Poultice, 109

shēng dì yǎng yīn qīng rè fāng — Rehmannia Formula to Nourish the Yin and Clear Heat, 231

shēng fà bǎo — Generate Hair Treasure, 271

shēng jī sǎn — Generate Flesh Powder, 71

shēng má hé jì — Cimicifuga Combined Formula, 117

shēng xuán yǐn — Rehmannia and Scrophularia Decoction, 221

shī zhěn sǎn — Eczema Powder, 168

shí chāng pǔ bǎi bù tāng — *Acorus and Stemona Wash*, 147

shí cù hú jì — Table Vinegar Paste, 178

shí sì wèi jiàn zhōng tāng — Fourteen-Ingredient Decoction to Strengthen the Middle, 277

shū fēng qīng rè yǐn — Disperse Wind and Clear Heat Decoction, 129

sì jūn zǐ tāng hé èr miào sǎn — Four-Gentleman Decoction Combined with Two-Marvel Powder, 282

sì wù rùn fū tāng jiā jiǎn — Modified Moisten the Skin Decoction with the Four Substances, 175

sì wù tāng jiā wèi — Augmented Four-Substance Decoction, 211

sì wù tāng — Four-Substance Decoction, 105

sì wù tāng,, liù wèi dì huáng tāng hé cái — Combined Four-Substance Decoction and Six-Ingredient Decoction with Rehmannia, 265

T

táo hóng sì wù tāng — Four-Substance Decoction with Safflower and Peach Pit, 256

táo yì shēn hóng tāng — Persica, Leonuris, Salvia, and Carthamus Decoction, 235

tiān wáng bǔ xīn dān — Emperor of Heaven's Special Pill to Tonify the Heart, 193

tiáo wèi chéng qì tāng — Regulate the Stomach and Order the Qi Decoction, 255

tōng luò huó xuè fāng — Unblock the Collaterals and Invigorate the Blood Formula, 276

tōng qiào huó xuè tāng — Unblock the Orifices and Invigorate the Blood Decoction, 268

tòu guì hóng xǐ jì — Speranskia, Cinnamon, and Carthamus Wash, 243
tòu zhěn tāng — Vent the Rash Decoction, 118
tǔ fú líng hé jì — Smilax Combined Formula, 137
tǔ fú líng dà huáng tāng — Smilax and Rheum Decoction, 105
tuō lǐ xiāo dú sǎn — Support the Interior and Eliminate Toxin Decoction, 69

W

wán xuǎn fú píng wán — Spirodela Pill for Stubborn Tinea, 128
wàn líng dān — Ten Thousand Efficacies Special Pill, 86
wēn qīng yǐn jiā jiǎn — Modified Warming and Clearing Decoction, 105
wū shé qū fēng tāng — Zaocys Dispel Wind Decoction, 46
wú gōng fāng — Scolopendra Formula, 240
wú gōng jiàn — Scolopendra Farewell Dinner, 285
wú jīng zǐ sǎn — Brassica Powder, 269
wú zhū yú gāo — Evodia Ointment, 54
wǔ bǎo sǎn — Five-Treasure Powder, 138
wǔ hǔ tāng jiā wèi — Augmented Five-Tiger Decoction, 119
wǔ wèi xiāo dú yǐn — Five-Ingredient Decoction to Eliminate Toxin, 58
wǔ wǔ dān — Five-Five Special Powder, 139
wǔ xiāng sǎn — Five-Fragrance Powder

X

xī jiǎo dì huáng tāng jiā jiǎn — Modified Rhinoceros Horn and Rehmannia Decoction [A], 195
xī jiǎo dì huáng tāng jiā jiǎn — Modified Rhinoceros Horn and Rehmannia Decoction [B], 218
xīn yí qīng fèi yǐn — Magnolia Flower Decoction to Clear the Lung, 94
xīn zhǐ jīng fáng sǎn — Asarum, Dahurica, Schizonepeta, Ledebouriella Powder, 171
xǐ chuāng fāng — Formula to Wash Sores, 54
xìng rén ruǎn gāo — Prunus Ointment, 301
xiān fāng huó mìng yǐn — Sublime Formula for Sustaining Life, 67
xiāng bèi yǎng yíng tāng — Cyperus and Fritillaria Decoction to Nourish the Nutritive Level, 82
xiāng fù mù zéi shuǐ xǐ jì — Cyperus and Equisetum Wash, 110
xiāng shā liù jūn zǐ tāng jiā jiǎn — Modified Six-Gentleman Decoction with Aucklandia and Amomum, 209
xiāo bān qīng dài yǐn — Eliminate Spots with Indigo Decoction, 275
xiāo fēng huà yū tāng — Eliminate Wind and Transform Stasis Decoction, 177
xiāo fēng sǎn jiā jiǎn — Modified Eliminate Wind Powder [A], 174
xiāo fēng sǎn jiā jiǎn — Modified Eliminate Wind Powder [B], 210
xiāo fēng sǎn — Eliminate Wind Powder, 142
xiāo yáo sǎn jiā jiǎn — Modified Rambling Powder [A], 81
xiāo yáo sǎn jiā jiǎn — Modified Rambling Powder [B], 292
xiāo yáo sǎn — Rambling Powder, 102
xiāo yóu yè — Reduce Wart Liquid, 111
xiǎo mǐ qīng tāng — Millet Soup, 187

Y

yā dǎn zǐ fū tiē — Brucea Poultice, 109
yā dǎn zǐ gāo — Brucea Plaster, 114
yā dǎn zǐ yóu — Brucea Liniment, 113
yáng hé tāng jiā jiǎn — Modified Yang-Heartening Decoction, 240
yǎng xuè rùn fū yǐn jiā jiǎn — Modified Nourish the Blood and Moisten the Skin Decoction, 218
yǎng xuè rùn fū yǐn — Nourish the Blood and Moisten the Skin Decoction, 181 299
yǎng xuè rùn fū yǐn — Nourish the Blood and Moisten the Skin Decoction, 44
yǎng xuè xiāo fēng zào shī fāng — Enrich the Blood, Dispel Wind, and Dry Dampness Formula, 241
yǎng yīn shēng jī sǎn — Enrich the Yin and Generate the Flesh Powder, 203
yě jú bài dú tāng — Chrysanthemum Decoction to Defeat Toxin, 61
yě jú niú zǐ tāng — Chrysanthemum and Arctium Decoction, 182
yī hào sǎo fēng wán — Number One Sweep the Wind Pill, 88
yī hào xuǎn yào shuǐ — Number 1 Tinea Liniment, 129
yī sǎo guāng — One Sweep Gone, 143
yì rén chì dòu tāng jiā jiǎn — Modified Coix and Phaseolus Decoction, 101
yín qiáo sǎn jiā jiǎn — Modified Honeysuckle and Forsythia Powder [A], 122-123
yín qiáo sǎn jiā jiǎn — Modified Honeysuckle and Forsythia Powder [B], 207
yín qiáo sǎn — Honeysuckle and Forsythia Powder, 117
yín qiáo sǎn, bái hǔ tāng huà cái — Honeysuckle and Forsythia Powder Combined with White Tiger Decoction, 195
yīng táo jiǔ — Cherry Tincture, 153
yú lín fāng — Fish-Scale Formula, 299
yún nán bái yào — Yunnan White Medicine, 192
yù hóng gāo — Jade Red Ointment, 202
yù lù gāo — Jade Dew Plaster, 98
yù lù sǎn — Jade Dew Powder, 158
yù píng fēng sǎn — Jade Windscreen Powder, 207
yuán huā gān cǎo xǐ jì — Daphne and Licorice Wash, 155
yuán huā shuǐ xǐ jì — Daphne Wash, 59

Z

zēng yè tāng jiā jiǎn — Modified Increase the Fluids Decoction, 197
zhēn zhū sǎn — Magarita Powder, 197
zhī bǎi dìhuáng wán — Anemarrhena, Phellodendron, and Rehmannia Decoction, 96
zhī yì xǐ fāng — Seborrhea Wash, 183
zhǐ zhú sǎn jiā jiǎn — Modified Immature Bitter Orange and Atractylodes Macrocephala Powder, 208
zhì fù tāng — Prepared Aconite Decoction, 200
zhū dǎn zhī wài xǐ fāng — Pig Bile Wash, 185

zhú yè huáng qí tāng — Lophatherus and Astragalus Decoction, 69
zhú yè shí gāo tāng — Lophatherus and Gypsum Decoction, 95
zī gān bǔ shèn fāng — Nourish the Liver and Tonify the Kidney Formula, 231
zī yīn chú shī tāng jiā jiǎn — Modified Enrich the Yin and Eliminate Dampness Decoction, 167
zǐ bǎn tāng — Arnebia and Isatis Decoction, 227
zǐ lán fāng — Lithospermum and Isatis Formula, 108
zǐ lián gāo — Arnebia and Coptis Ointment, 188
zǐ xuè dān — Purple Snow Special Pill, 77
zǐ yù zān gāo — Hosta Ointment, 303
zùi xiān sǎn — Drunken Fairy Powder, 87

Formula Index

A

Acne Decoction *(cuó chuāng jiān jì)*, 257
Acorus and Stemona Wash *(shí chāng pǔ bǎi bù tāng)*, 147
Aloe, Borneol, and Magarita Paste *(lú huì bīng zhū wài fū jì)*, 103
Anchor Yang and Extinguish Wind Decoction *(qián yáng xī fēng tāng)*, 175
Anemarrhena, Phellodendron, and Rehmannia Decoction *(zhī bǎi dìhuáng wán)*, 96
Angelica and Ligusticum Formula *(guī xiōng fāng)*, 236
Arctium and Taraxacum Formula to Cool the Blood *(niú gōng liáng xuè fāng)*, 74
Aristilochia Powder *(qīng mù xiāng sǎn)*, 249
Arnebia and Coptis Ointment *(zǐ lián gāo)*, 188, 223
Arnebia and Isatis Decoction *(zǐ bǎn tāng)*, 227
Artemisia Annua Decoction *(qīng hāo yǐn)*, 158
Artemisia Annua Ointment *(qīng hāo gāo)*, 233
Artemisia Argyi Decoction *(hǎi ài tāng)*, 268
Asarum, Dahurica, Schizonepeta, Ledebouriella Powder *(xīn zhǐ jīng fáng sǎn)*, 171
Astragalus and Atractylodes Decoction *(qí bái tāng)*, 182
Astragalus and Paris Decoction *(huáng qí zǎo xiū yǐn)*, 58
Atractylodes, Phellodendron, and Achyranthes Formula *(cāng bó niú xī fāng)*, 187
Augmented Atractylodes Gelatin *(jiā wèi cāng zhú gāo)*, 301
Augmented Five-Tiger Decoction *(wǔ hǔ tāng jiā wèi)*, 119
Augmented Four-Substance Decoction *(sì wù tāng jiā wèi)*, 211

B

Biota Ointment *(bǎi zhī yóu)*, 268
Black Ointment *(hēi yóu gāo)*, 168, 176, 197
Black Solanum Compress *(lóng kuí shī fū jì)*, 54
Borneol and Gypsum Powder *(bīng shí sǎn)*, 64, 104
Brassica Powder *(wú jīng zǐ sǎn)*, 269
Brucea Liniment *(yā dǎn zǐ yóu)*, 113
Brucea Plaster *(yā dǎn zǐ gāo)*, 114
Brucea Poultice *(yā dǎn zǐ fū tiē)*, 109
Buchnera, Moutan, and Batryticatus Decoction *(guǐ dān jiāng cán tāng)*, 201
Bupleurum Decoction to Clear the Liver *(chái hú qīng gān tāng)*, 74

C

Calm the Palace Pill with Cattle Gallstone *(ān gōng niú huáng wán)*, 77, 197
Chaenomeles and Areca Powder *(mù guā bīng láng sǎn)*, 282
Change Flesh Powder *(huàn jī sǎn)*, 87
Cherry Tincture *(yīng táo jiǔ)*, 153
Chrysanthemum and Arctium Decoction *(yě jú niú zǐ tāng)*, 182
Chrysanthemum Decoction to Defeat Toxin *(yě jú bài dú tāng)*, 61
Cibotium Wash *(gǒu jǐ shuǐ xǐ jì)*, 302
Cimicifuga Combined Formula *(shēng má hé jì)*, 117
Clear and Relieve Tablet *(qīng jiě piàn)*, 163, 166
Clear Epidemics and Overcome Toxin Decoction *(qīng wēn bài dú yǐn)*, 76, 240
Clear Heat and Reduce Toxin Wash *(qīng rè jiě dú xǐ jì)*, 114
Clear Summerheat Decoction *(qīng shǔ tāng)*, 246
Clear the Blood and Collect the Toxin Pill *(qīng xuè sōu dú wán)*, 139
Clear the Flesh and Leach Out Dampness Decoction *(qīng jī shèn shī tāng)*, 201
Clear the Nutritive Level Decoction *(qīng yíng tāng)*, 76
Clear the Spleen and Remove Dampness Decoction *(qīng pí chú shī yǐn)*, 52
Clearing and Cooling Ointment *(qīng liáng gāo)*, 53, 188, 233
Clearing and Cooling Powder *(qīng liáng fěn)*, 48, 158, 188, 228, 247
Clinopodium Powder *(jiǎn cǎo sǎn)*, 130
Clove and Borneol Powder *(dīng xiāng bīng piàn sǎn)*, 250
Codonopsis and Sangjisheng Tonifying and Augmenting Formula *(dǎng shēn jì shēng bǔ yì fāng)*, 242
Codonopsis, Astragalus, and Anemarrhena Decoction *(shēn qí zhī mǔ tāng)*, 53
Combined Cinnamon Twig and Ephedra Decoction *(guì zhī má huáng gè bàn tāng)*, 47
Combined Coptis Decoction to Relieve Toxicity and Three-Marvel Pill *(huáng lián jiě dú tāng hé sān miào wán)*, 75
Combined Coptis Decoction to Relieve Toxin and Five-Ingredient Decoction to Eliminate Toxin *(huáng lián jiě dú tāng, wǔ wèi xiāo dú yǐn huà cái)*, 221
Combined Four-Substance Decoction and Six-Ingredient Decoction with Rehmannia *(sì wù tāng, liù wèi dì huáng tāng huà cái)*, 265

Cool and Invigorate the Blood Formula *(liáng xuè huó xuè fāng)*, 275
Cool the Blood and Clear the Lung Decoction *(liáng xuè qīng fèi yǐn)*, 255
Cool the Blood and Eliminate Wind Powder *(liáng xuè xiāo fēng sǎn)*, 46, 181, 217
Cool the Blood and Moisten Dryness Decoction *(liáng xuě rùn zào yǐn)*, 300
Cool the Blood Decoction with Five Flowers *(liáng xuè wǔ huā tāng)*, 256, 261
Cool the Blood Decoction with Five Roots *(liáng xuè wǔ gēn tāng)*, 275
Coptis Decoction to Relieve Toxicity *(huáng lián jiě dú tāng)*, 105
Coptis Ointment *(huáng lián gāo)*, 64, 103, 104, 188, 197, 233
Cordyceps Tincture *(dōng chóng xià cǎo dīng)*, 269
Coreopsis Tincture to Eliminate Bugs *(chú chóng jú dīng)*, 146
Cotton Cloth Rub *(bù mián cā jì)*, 170, 177
Cyperus and Equisetum Wash *(xiāng fù mù zéi shuǐ xǐ jì)*, 110
Cyperus and Fritillaria Decoction to Nourish the Nutritive Level *(xiāng bèi yǎng yíng tāng)*, 82

D

Daphne and Licorice Wash *(yuán huā gān cǎo xǐ jì)*, 155
Daphne Wash *(yuán huā shuǐ xǐ jì)*, 59
Defeat Toxin Decoction *(bài dú yǐn)*, 196
Dioscorea Decoction to Leach Out Dampness [B] *(bèi xiè shèn shī tāng)*, 281
Dispel Dampness Powder *(qū shī sǎn)*, 168
Disperse Wind and Clear Heat Decoction *(shū fēng qīng rè yǐn)*, 129
Drunken Fairy Powder *(zùi xiān sǎn)*, 87

E

Eczema Powder *(shī zhěn sǎn)*, 168
Effective Scarlet Wine *(hóng líng jiǔ)*, 154, 237
Eggplant Vine Wash *(qié zǐ jiē jiān shuǐ)*, 154
Eight-Treasure Decoction *(bā zhēn tāng)*, 68
Eight-Two Special Powder *(bā èr dān)*, 70, 283
Eliminate Dampness and Relieve Toxicity Decoction *(chú shī jiě dú tāng)*, 257
Eliminate Dampness Decoction by Combining Calm the Stomach and Five-Ingredient Powder with Poria *(chú shī wèi líng tāng)*, 101, 300
Eliminate Spots with Indigo Decoction *(xiāo bān qīng dài yǐn)*, 275
Eliminate Wind and Transform Stasis Decoction *(xiāo fēng huà yū tāng)*, 177
Eliminate Wind Powder *(xiāo fēng sǎn)*, 142
Emperor of Heaven's Special Pill to Tonify the Heart *(tiān wáng bǔ xīn dān)*, 193
Enrich the Blood, Dispel Wind, and Dry Dampness Formula *(yǎng xuè xiāo fēng zào shī fāng)*, 241
Enrich the Yin and Generate the Flesh Powder *(yǎng yīn shēng jī sǎn)*, 203
Eriobotrya Decoction to Clear the Lung *(pí pá qīng fèi yǐn)*, 255, 261
Erysipelas Plaster *(dān dú gāo)*, 79
Evodia Ointment *(wú zhū yúgāo)*, 54
Exuvia Serpentis Plaster *(shé tùi gāo)*, 82

F

Fish-Scale Formula *(yú lín fāng)*, 299
Five-Five Special Powder *(wǔ wǔ dān)*, 139, 283
Five-Fragrance Powder *(wǔ xiāng sǎn)*
Five-Ingredient Decoction to Eliminate Toxin *(wǔ wèi xiāo dú yǐn)*, 58, 148, 162, 249, 256, 261
Five-Treasure Powder *(wǔ bǎo sǎn)*, 138, 166
Flush and Harmonize Plaster *(chōng hé gāo)*, 78, 139
Formula to Wash Sores *(xǐ chuāng fāng)*, 54
Four-Gentleman Decoction Combined with Two-Marvel Powder *(sì jūn zǐ tāng hé èr miào sǎn)*, 282
Four-Substance Decoction *(sì wù tāng)*, 105
Four-Substance Decoction with Safflower and Peach Pit *(táo hóng sì wù tāng)*, 256, 261
Fourteen-Ingredient Decoction to Strengthen the Middle *(shí sì wèi jiàn zhōng tāng)*, 277
Fox Stench Powder *(hú chòu fěn)*, 250
Freeze Sore Ointment *(dòng chuāng yóu)*, 154
Freeze Sore Plaster *(dòng chuāng gāo)*, 155

G

Generate Flesh Powder *(shēng jī sǎn)*, 71, 90, 139, 155, 284, 285
Generate Hair Treasure *(shēng fà bǎo)*, 271
Gentiana Longdancao Decoction to Drain the Liver *(lóng dǎn xiè gān tāng)*, 95, 100
Ginseng Decoction to Nourish the Nutritive Qi *(rén shēn yǎng yíng tāng)*, 267
Glehnia and Ophiopogonis Decoction *(shā shēn mài mén dōng tāng)*, 119, 120
Golden Plain Plaster *(jīn sù gāo)*, 83
Golden-Yellow Powder *(jīn huáng sǎn)*, 62, 70, 78
Golden-Yellow Powder According to One's Wishes *(rú yì jīn huáng sǎn)*, 59, 283
Green Robe Powder *(lǜ páo sǎn)*, 120

H

Honeysuckle and Forsythia Powder *(yín qiáo sǎn)*, 117
Honeysuckle and Forsythia Powder Combined with White Tiger Decoction *(yín qiáo sǎn, bái hǔ tāng huà cái)*, 195
Hornet Nest Powder *(fēng fáng sǎn)*, 57
Hosta Ointment *(zǐ yù zān gāo)*, 303

I

Indigo Ointment *(qīng dài gāo)*, 130, 184, 197, 203, 283
Indigo Powder *(qīng dài sǎn)*, 54, 124, 163, 167, 283
Indigo, Alumen, and Zanthoxylum Powder *(qīng dài kǔ jiāo sǎn)*, 171
Invigorate the Blood and Scatter Stasis Decoction *(huó xuè sàn yū tāng)*, 219

J

Jade Dew Plaster *(yù lù gāo)*, 70, 78, 98, 103
Jade Dew Powder *(yù lù sǎn)*, 58, 62, 63, 158, 163, 247
Jade Dragon Plaster to Restore Yang *(huí yáng yù lóng gāo)*, 236
Jade Red Ointment *(yù hóng gāo)*, 202, 283
Jade Windscreen Powder *(yù píng fēng sǎn)*, 207

L

Ledebouriella Powder that Sagely Unblocks *(fáng fēng tōng shèng sǎn)*, 96
Light-Yellow Powder *(é huáng sǎn)*, 139, 169, 247
Liquidambar Wash *(lù lù tōng shuǐ xǐ jì)*, 224
Lithospermum and Isatis Formula *(zǐ lán fāng)*, 108
Lithyargyrum Powder *(mì tuó sēng sǎn)*, 293
Lophatherus and Astragalus Decoction *(zhú yè huáng qí tāng)*, 69
Lophatherus and Gypsum Decoction *(zhú yè shí gāo tāng)*, 95
Lu Family Decoction for Patchy Baldness *(lù shì bān tū tāng)*, 265

M

Magarita Powder *(zhēn zhū sǎn)*, 197
Magnolia Flower Decoction to Clear the Lung *(xīn yí qīng fèi yǐn)*, 94
Melia and Zanthoxylum Dry Compress *(liàn jiāo yào yùn)*, 237
Miliaria Powder *(fèi zǐ fěn)*, 247
Millet Soup *(xiǎo mǐ qīng tāng)*, 187
Mirabilitum Wash *(máng xiāo xǐ jì)*, 172
Miraculous Tinea Remedy *(shén xiào xuǎn yào)*, 131
Modified Angelica Pubescens and Sangjisheng Decoction *(dú huó jì shēng tāng jiā jiǎn)*, 235
Modified Calm the Stomach Powder *(píng wèi sǎn jiā jiǎn)*, 208
Modified Cinnamon Twig Decoction Plus Tangkuei *(guì zhī jiā dāng guī tāng jiā jiǎn)*, 153
Modified Cinnamon Twig Decoction [A] *(guì zhī tāng jiā jiǎn)*, 207
Modified Cinnamon Twig Decoction [B] *(guì zhī tāng jiā jiǎn)*, 217
Modified Clear Epidemics and Overcome Toxin Decoction *(qīng wēn bài dú yǐn jiā jiǎn)*, 124
Modified Clear the Nutritive Level Decoction *(qīng yíng tāng jiā jiǎn)*, 123
Modified Coix and Phaseolus Decoction *(yì rén chì dòu tāng jiā jiǎn)*, 101
Modified Cool the Blood and Eliminate Wind Powder *(liáng xuè xiāo fēng sǎn jiā jiǎn)*, 226
Modified Daqingye and Forsythia Decoction *(dà qīng lián qiáo tāng jiā jiǎn)*, 100
Modified Dioscorea Decoction to Leach Out Dampness [A] *(bèi xiè shèn shī tāng jiā jiǎn)*, 220
Modified Eight-Treasure Decoction *(bā zhēn tāng jiā jiǎn)*, 266
Modified Eliminate Dampness Decoction by Combining Calm the Stomach and Five Ingredient Powder with Poria *(chú shī wèi líng tāng jiā jiǎn)*, 166

Modified Eliminate Wind Powder [A] *(xiāo fēng sǎn jiā jiǎn)*, 174
Modified Eliminate Wind Powder [B] *(xiāo fēng sǎn jiā jiǎn)*, 210
Modified Enrich the Yin and Eliminate Dampness Decoction *(zī yīn chú shī tāng jiā jiǎn)*, 167
Modified Gentiana Longdancao Decoction to Drain the Liver *(lóng dǎn xiè gān tāng jiā jiǎn)*, 222
Modified Ginseng Pill to Stabilize the Root *(rén shēn gù běn wán jiā jiǎn)*, 97
Modified Golden-Yellow Powder According to One's Wishes *(rú yì jīn huáng sǎn jiā jiǎn)*, 64
Modified Honeysuckle and Forsythia Powder [A] *(yín qiáo sǎn jiā jiǎn)*, 122-123
Modified Honeysuckle and Forsythia Powder [B] *(yín qiáo sǎn jiā jiǎn)*, 207
Modified Immature Bitter Orange and Atractylodes Macrocephala Powder *(zhǐ zhú sǎn jiā jiǎn)*, 208
Modified Increase the Fluids Decoction *(zēng yè tāng jiā jiǎn)*, 197
Modified Invigorate the Blood, Moisten Dryness, and Generate Fluids Decoction *(huó xuè rùn zào shēng jīn tāng jiā jiǎn)*, 227
Modified Kidney Qi Pill from the Golden Cabinet *(jīn guì shèn qì wán jiā jiǎn)*, 241
Modified Linum Pill *(hú má wán jiā jiǎn)*, 291
Modified Melia Powder *(jīn líng zǐ sǎn jiā jiǎn)*, 102
Modified Miraculous Extinguish Wind Powder *(shén yìng xiāo fēng sǎn jiā jiǎn)*, 292
Modified Moisten the Skin Decoction with the Four Substances *(sì wù rùn fū tāng jiā jiǎn)*, 175
Modified Nourish the Blood and Moisten the Skin Decoction *(yǎng xuè rùn fū yǐn jiā jiǎn)*, 218
Modified Prepared Aconite Decoction to Regulate the Middle Plus Modified Cinnamon Twig Decoction *(fù zǐ lǐ zhōng tāng jiā guì zhī tāng jiā jiǎn)*, 209
Modified Rambling Powder [A] *(xiāo yáo sǎn jiā jiǎn)*, 81
Modified Rambling Powder [B] *(xiāo yáo sǎn jiā jiǎn)*, 292
Modified Rehmannia Decoction *(dì huáng yǐn zǐ jiā jiǎn)*, 138
Modified Rhinoceros Horn and Rehmannia Decoction [A] *(xī jiǎo dì huáng tāng jiā jiǎn)*, 195
Modified Rhinoceros Horn and Rehmannia Decoction [B] *(xī jiǎo dì huáng tāng jiā jiǎn)*, 218
Modified Schizonepeta and Ledebouriella Powder to Overcome Toxin *(jīng fáng bài dú sǎn jiā jiǎn)*, 206
Modified Six-Gentleman Decoction with Aucklandia and Amomum *(xiāng shā liù jūn zǐ tāng jiā jiǎn)*, 209
Modified Tangkuei Decoction for Frigid Extremities [A] *(dāng guī sì nì tāng jiā jiǎn)*, 152
Modified Tangkuei Decoction for Frigid Extremities [B] *(dāng guī sì nì tāng jiā jiǎn)*, 200
Modified Tangkuei, Peony, and Rehmannia Decoction *(guī sháo dì huáng tāng jiā jiǎn)*, 108

Modified Three-Pith Guide Out the Red Powder *(sān xīn dǎo chì sǎn jiā jiǎn)*, 166
Modified Tonify the Middle and Augment the Qi Decoction *(bǔ zhōng yì qì tāng jiā jiǎn)*, 55
Modified Tonify the Spleen Stomach, Drain Yin Fire, and Raise the Yang Decoction *(bǔ pí wèi xiè yīn huǒ shēng yáng tāng jiā jiǎn)*, 232
Modified Two-Immortal Decoction [A] *(èr xiān tāng jiā jiǎn)*, 211
Modified Two-Immortal Decoction [B] *(èr xiān tāng jiā jiǎn)*, 223
Modified Two-Ultimate Pill *(èr zhì wán jiā jiǎn)*, 290
Modified Universal Benefit Decoction to Eliminate Toxin *(pǔ jì xiāo dú yǐn jiā jiǎn)*, 202
Modified Warming and Clearing Decoction *(wēn qīng yǐn jiā jiǎn)*, 105
Modified Yang-Heartening Decoction *(yáng hé tāng jiā jiǎn)*, 240
Moisten the Flesh Ointment *(rùn jī gāo)*, 184, 301
Mylabris Tincture *(bān máo dīng)*, 176
Myrrha and Lonicera Decoction *(mò yín jiān yè)*, 164

N

Nervous Wind Ointment *(fēng yóu gāo)*, 176
Nine-One Special Powder *(jiǔ yī dān)*, 83, 104, 155
Nourish the Blood and Moisten the Skin Decoction *(yǎng xuè rùn fū yǐn)*, 181 299
Nourish the Blood and Moisten the Skin Decoction *(yǎng xuè rùn fū yǐn)*, 44
Nourish the Liver and Tonify the Kidney Formula *(zī gān bǔ shèn fāng)*, 231
Number 1 Tinea Liniment *(yī hào xuǎn yào shuǐ)*, 129
Number One Sweep the Wind Pill *(yī hào sǎo fēng wán)*, 88

O

Oldenlandia Wash *(bái huā shé shé cǎo xǐ jì)*, 115
One Sweep Gone *(yī sǎo guāng)*, 143
Ophiopogon, Schisandra, and Rehmannia Decoction *(mài wèi dì huáng tāng)*, 222
Overcome Psoriasis Formula *(kè yín fāng)*, 219

P

Paper Sandwich Plaster *(jiā zhǐ gāo)*, 284
Persica, Leonuris, Salvia, and Carthamus Decoction *(táo yì shēn hóng tāng)*, 235
Phoenix Mantle Formula *(fèng huáng yī fāng)*, 285
Phytolacca Powder *(shāng lù sǎn)*, 294
Pig Bile Wash *(zhū dǎn zhī wài xǐ fāng)*, 185
Pinellia Poultice *(shēng bàn xià fū tiē)*, 109
Polygonum Wine *(hé shǒu wū jiǔ)*, 88
Portulaca and Daqingye Wash *(mǎ qīng shuǐ xǐ jì)*, 113
Portulaca Wash *(mǎ chǐ xiàn shuǐ xǐ jì)*, 97 124, 197

Portulaca, Atractylodes, and Wasp-nest Wash *(mǎ zhú fēng fáng shuǐ xǐ jì)*, 110
Prepared Aconite Decoction *(zhì fù tāng)*, 200
Prepared Aconite Pill to Regulate the Middle *(fù zǐ lǐ zhōng wán)*, 278
Protect the Hair Decoction *(bǎo fà tāng)*, 270
Prunus Ointment *(xìng rén ruǎn gāo)*, 301
Psoralea Tincture Injection *(bǔ gǔ zhī dīng zhù shè yè)*, 113
Psoriasis Tincture *(bái xiè fēng dīng)*, 183
Pueraria, Scutellaria, and Coptis Decoction *(gé gēn qín lián tāng)*, 186
Purple and Gold Plaster to Relieve Toxin *(jiě dú zǐ jīn gāo)*, 286
Purple Snow Special Pill *(zǐ xuě dān)*, 77

R

Rambling Powder *(xiāo yáo sǎn)*, 102
Red Cloth Plaster *(hóng bù gāo)*, 63
Red Ointment *(hóng yóu gāo)*, 83, 90, 193, 283
Reduce Wart Liquid *(xiāo yóu yè)*, 111
Regulate the Stomach and Order the Qi Decoction *(tiáo wèi chéng qì tāng)*, 255
Rehmannia and Scrophularia Decoction *(shēng xuán yǐn)*, 221
Rehmannia Formula to Nourish the Yin and Clear Heat *(shēng dì yǎng yīn qīng rè fāng)*, 231
Rehmannia, Gypsum, and Anemarrhena Formula *(dì shí zhī fāng)*, 227
Remove Decay and Generate Flesh Formula *(qū fǔ shēng jī fāng)*, 284
Remove Spots Ointment *(qù bān gāo)*, 258
Restore the Spleen Decoction *(guī pí tāng)*, 277
Rheum and Borneol Formula *(dà huáng bīng piàn fāng)*, 184
Rheum Powder *(dà huáng sǎn)*, 78
Rosacea Paste *(jiǔ zhā bí gāo)*, 261
Rub the Wind Ointment *(mó fēng gāo)*, 183-184

S

Sanguisorba, Xanthium, and Atractylodes Paste *(dì yú èr cāng hú gāo)*, 169
Scolopendra Farewell Dinner *(wú gōng jiàn)*, 285
Scolopendra Formula *(wú gōng fāng)*, 240
Scorpion Formula *(quán chóng fāng)*, 47
Seborrhea Wash *(zhī yì xǐ fāng)*, 183
Seven-Three Special Powder *(qī sān dān)*, 70, 90, 283
Seven-Treasure Special Pill for Beautiful Whiskers *(qī bǎo měi rán dān)*, 266
Shin Sore Plaster *(lián chuāng gāo)*, 286
Single-Ingredient Astragalus Formula *(dú wèi huáng qí fāng)*, 232
Six-Ingredient Pill with Rehmannia *(liù wèi dì huáng wán)*, 62, 283
Six-Miracle Pill *(liù shén wán)*, 192, 193
Six-One Powder *(liù yī sǎn)*, 62, 158
Smilax and Rheum Decoction *(tǔ fú líng dà huáng tāng)*, 105
Smilax Combined Formula *(tǔ fú líng hé jì)*, 137
Snake Bite Medicine Pills *(shé yào piàn)*, 149

Sophora and Allium Vinegar Soak *(kǔ suàn cù jìn pào)*, 132
Sophora and Zanthoxylum Decoction *(kǔ jiāo tāng)*, 144
Sophora Decoction *(kǔ shēn tāng)*, 3, 89, 143
Speranskia, Cinnamon, and Carthamus Wash *(tòu guì hóng xǐ jì)*, 243
Spirodela Pill for Stubborn Tinea *(wán xuǎn fú píng wán)*, 128
Stemona Tincture *(bǎi bù dīng)*, 48, 146
Sublime Formula for Sustaining Life *(xiān fāng huó mìng yǐn)*, 67, 281
Succinum and Two-Aconite Paste *(hǔ pò èr wū hú gāo)*, 169
Succinum, Beeswax, and Alum Pill *(hǔ pò là fán wán)*, 68
Support the Interior and Eliminate Toxin Decoction *(tuō lǐ xiāo dú sǎn)*, 69
Sweet Dew Special Pill to Eliminate Toxin *(gān lù xiāo dú dān)*, 248

T

Table Vinegar Paste *(shí cù hú jì)*, 178
Talcum and Indigo Powder *(huá dài fěn)*, 188
Tangkuei and Cooked Rehmannia Decoction to Nourish the Blood *(dāng shú yǎng xuè tāng)*, 45
Tangkuei Decoction for Frigid Extremities *(dāng guī sì nì tāng)*, 279
Taraxacum, Viola, and Lonicera Decoction *(pú dì rěn tāng)*, 246
Ten Percent Ground Pepper Alcohol *(10% hú jiāo jiǔ jīng jìn yè)*, 153
Ten Thousand Efficacies Special Pill *(wàn líng dān)*, 86
Terminalia Wash *(qīng guǒ shuǐ xǐ jì)*, 203
Thousand Ducat Powder *(qiān jīn sǎn)*, 109
Three-Miracle Pill *(sān shén wán)*, 128
Three-Yellow Wash *(sān huáng xǐ jì)*, 63, 163, 176, 197, 203, 228, 247
Tissue Thorn Powder *(ròu cì sǎn)*, 303

U

Unblock the Collaterals and Invigorate the Blood Formula *(tōng luò huó xuè fāng)*, 276
Unblock the Orifices and Invigorate the Blood Decoction *(tōng qiào huó xuè tāng)*, 268
Universal Benefit Decoction to Eliminate Toxin *(pǔ jì xiāo dú yǐn)*, 73
Universally Linked Ointment *(pǔ lián gāo)*, 223
Upside Down Powder *(diān dǎo sǎn)*, 258, 261

V

Vent the Rash Decoction *(tòu zhěn tāng)*, 118
Veratrum Powder *(lí lú sǎn)*, 146
Vinegar and Rheum Wash, 133

W

White Blotch Wind Pill *(bái diàn fēng wán)*, 293
White Dagger Sore Decoction *(bái bǐ tāng)*, 219

White Spots Pitch-Black Decoction *(bái bān wū hēi tāng)*, 293
White Tiger Decoction *(bái hǔ tāng)*, 157

X

Xanthium and Kochia Wash *(cāng fū shuǐ xǐ jì)*, 59, 224

Y

Yunnan White Medicine *(yún nán bái yào)*, 192

Z

Zanthoxylum and Allium Paste *(chuān jiāo dà suàn ní)*, 132
Zanthoxylum and Artemisia Decoction *(chuān ài tāng)*, 144
Zaocys Dispel Wind Decoction *(wū shé qū fēng tāng)*, 46

Point Index

BODY POINTS

B

BL-1 *(jing ming)*, 104
BL-12 *(feng men)*, 48, 212, 224
BL-13 *(fei shu)*, 48, 60, 212, 224, 259, 270
BL-15 *(xin shu)*, 40, 48, 60, 259
BL-17 *(ge shu)*, 60, 171, 212
BL-18 *(gan shu)*, 40, 48, 60, 212, 224, 259
BL-20 *(pi shu)*, 40, 48, 212, 224, 259
BL-23 *(shen shu)*, 40, 237, 259, 270
BL-40 *(wei zhong)*, 40, 64, 79, 131, 140, 163, 198, 212, 224
BL-58 *(fei yang)*, 279
BL-60 *(kun lun)*, 140, 156

C

CV-6 *(qi hai)*, 40, 140, 279
CV-24 *(cheng jiang)*, 262

G

GB-14 *(yang bai)*, 104
GB-20 *(feng chi)*, 40, 79, 91, 270
GB-21 *(jian jing)*, 140, 228
GB-30 *(huan tiao)*, 140
GB-31 *(feng shi)*, 40, 131, 237
GB-34 *(yang ling quan)*, 91, 104, 140, 270
GB-41 *(zu lin qi)*, 91, 156

Grow Hair point, 269
GV-4 *(ming men)*, 71
GV-9 *(zhi yang)*, 71
GV-10 *(ling tai)*, 64, 233
GV-11 *(shen dao)*, 71
GV-12 *(shen zhu)*, 48, 60, 104, 212, 224
GV-14 *(da zhui)*, 40, 48, 60, 71, 79, 140, 170, 177, 212, 224, 228
GV-14 *(ming men)*, 237
GV-16 *(feng fu)*, 40
GV-20 *(bai hui)*, 269
GV-23 *(shang xing)*, 270
GV-25 *(su liao)*, 262
GV-26 *(shui gou)*, 79

H

HT-7 *(shen men)*, 170
HT-8 *(shao fu)*, 171

J

jia xia, 294
jiu dian feng, 294

K

K-1 *(yong quan)*, 79, 91
KI-2 *(ran gu)*, 91
KI-9 *(zhu bin)*, 279

L

LI-3 *(san jian)*, 91
LI-4 *(he gu)*, 39, 40, 48, 64, 79, 91, 104, 131, 156, 163, 177, 179, 212, 228, 233, 262, 294
LI-11 *(qu chi)*, 39, 40, 48, 64, 79, 91, 104, 140, 156, 163, 170, 177, 198, 212, 228, 233, 243, 262, 279, 294
LI-15 *(jian yu)*, 131, 140, 228, 243
LI-20 *(ying xiang)*, 233, 262
LR-2 *(xing jian)*, 91, 156, 294
LU-5 *(chi ze)*, 163
LU-10 *(yu ji)*, 91

M

M-HN-3 *(yin tang)*, 262
M-HN-6 *(yu yao)*, 270
M-HN-9 *(tai yang)*, 79, 91, 104, 270
M-HN-13 *(yi ming)*, 270
M-LE-8 *(ba feng)*, 91

M-LE-12 *(qi duan)*, 212
M-UE-1 *(shi xuan)*, 212
M-UE-22 *(ba xie)*, 91
M-UE-9 *(ba xie)*, 156

P

PC-3 *(qu ze)*, 131, 163, 233
PC-6 *(nei guan)*, 79, 140, 179, 198, 212, 279
PC-7 *(da ling)*, 79

S

SI-3 *(hou xi)*, 91
SI-18 *(quan liao)*, 262
SP-6 *(san yin jiao)*, 39, 40, 48, 64, 79, 104, 131, 170, 177, 179, 198, 212, 237, 243, 294
SP-9 *(yin ling quan)*, 171, 237, 243
SP-10 *(xue hai)*, 40, 48, 79, 131, 170, 177, 198, 212, 237
ST 2 *(si bai)*, 104, 233
ST-4 *(di cang)*, 104, 262
ST-5 *(da ying)*, 104, 262
ST-6 *(jia che)*, 104
ST-7 *(xia guan)*, 104
ST-8 *(tou wei)*, 104, 269
ST-25 *(tian shu)*, 79, 212, 279
ST-36 *(zu san li)*, 39, 40, 48, 64, 79, 91, 104, 156, 170, 179, 198, 228, 237, 243, 270, 279
ST-44 *(feng long)*, 79

T

TB-4 *(yang chi)*, 156
TB-5 *(wai guan)*, 270
TB-10 *(tian jing)*, 212
TB-23 *(si zhu kong)*, 270

EAR POINTS

A

Adrenal, 48, 185, 233, 237, 247, 262, 294

C

Cheek, 259

E

Ear Apex, 98, 212
Endocrine, 185, 237, 259, 262
External Nose, 262

H

Heart, 233
Hormone, 294

K

Kidney, 185

L

Liver, 185, 233, 237
Lung, 48, 212, 233, 237, 247, 259, 262, 294

O

Occiput, 48, 185, 212, 237, 247, 294

S

Shenmen, 48, 212, 233, 247
Spleen, 185, 212, 237
Stop Wheezing, 212

T

Testicle, 259

Materia Medica Index

A

Acaciae seu Uncariae, Pasta *(er cha)*, 120, 139, 203, 284, 303
Acanthopanacis Gracilistylus Radicis, Cortex *(wu jia pi)*, 89
Achyranthis Bidentatae, Radix *(niu xi)*, 75, 187, 231, 235, 242, 257, 266, 276
Aconiti Carmichaeli Praeparata, Radix *(zhi chuan wu)*, 89, 90, 169
Aconiti Carmichaeli Praeparata, Radix Lateralis *(fu zi)*, 55, 138, 152, 200, 209, 210, 249, 278, 295
Aconiti Kusnezoffii Praeparata, Radix *(zhi cao wu)*, 88, 89, 169, 170
Aconiti Kusnezoffii Praeparata, Radix, dry-fried *(chao zhi cao wu)*, 236
Aconiti Kusnezoffii, Radix *(cao wu)*, 128
Aconiti, Radix *(wu tou)*, 87
Acori Graminei, Rhizoma *(shi chang pu)*, 79, 88, 90, 120, 143, 144, 147, 158, 249, 291, 294
Adenophorae seu Glehniae, Radix *(sha shen)*, 88, 97, 119, 166, 175, 197, 218, 227, 242, 295
Agastaches seu Pogostemi *(huo xiang)*, 62
Agkistrodon seu Bungarus *(bai hua she)*, 87, 89
Akebiae, Fructus *(ba yue zha)*, 292
Alismatis Orientalis, Rhizoma *(ze xie)*, 52, 57, 58, 68, 95, 96, 101, 113, 167, 201, 208, 222, 227, 241, 246, 281, 283
Alli Sativi, Bulbus *(da suan)*, 132
Allii Fistulosi, Bulbus *(cong bai)*, 268
Allii Tuberosi, Folium *(jiu cai)*, 149, 311
Aloes, Herba *(lu hui)*, 103
Alpiniae Oxyphyllae, Fructus *(yi zhi ren)*, 270
Alumen *(ming fan)*, 4, 68, 113, 114, 115, 120, 143, 150, 182, 183, 187, 249, 303

Alumen Praeparatum *(ku fan)*, 83, 129, 143, 150, 168, 170, 171, 224, 250, 284, 294

Amomi Kravanh, Fructus *(bai dou kou)*, 249, 294

Amomi, Fructus *(sha ren)*, 208, 209

Ampelopsis Japonicae, Radix *(bai lian)*, 53, 97, 152, 295, 305

Andrographitis Paniculatae, Herba *(chuan xin lian)*, 192

Anemarrhenae Asphodeloidis, Rhizoma *(zhi mu)*, 46, 53, 76, 90, 94, 96, 124, 142, 157, 181, 187, 210, 227, 231, 255, 276

Anemarrhenae Asphodeloidis, Rhizoma, dry-fried *(chao zhi mu)*, 167, 195, 223, 242

Angelicae Dahuricae, Radix *(bai zhi)*, 46, 55, 59, 62, 67, 70, 79, 87, 89, 90, 110, 143, 149, 170, 171, 201, 202, 224, 236, 250, 286, 292, 295

Angelicae Pubescentis, Radix *(du huo)*, 79, 87, 224, 235, 286, 295

Angelicae Sinensis, Corpus Radicis *(dang gui tou)*, 89

Angelicae Sinensis, Extremitas Radicis *(dang gui wei)*, 89, 294

Angelicae Sinensis, Radix *(dang gui)*, 4, 45, 46, 55, 58, 67, 69, 70, 75, 82, 87, 89, 95, 96, 102, 103, 106, 108, 142, 152, 153, 154, 167, 175, 178, 181, 184, 200, 201, 202, 210, 211, 217, 218, 220, 221, 222, 223, 227, 235, 236, 241, 242, 256, 257, 265, 266, 267, 270, 271, 276, 277, 279, 282, 286, 292, 293, 294, 299, 301

Antelopis, Cornu *(ling yang jiao)*, 77, 242

Aquilariae, Lignum *(chen xiang)*, 77, 249

Arctii Lappae, Fructus *(niu bang zi)*, 74, 75, 117, 118, 119, 142, 182, 202, 210, 227

Arctii Lappae, Fructus, dry-fried *(chao niu bang zi)*, 88, 174, 195, 207

Arecae Catechu, Pericarpium *(da fu pi)*, 81

Arecae Catechu, Semen *(bing lang)*, 131, 168, 170, 282

Arisaematis, Rhizoma *(tian nan xing)*, 59, 62

Arisaematis, Rhizoma, roasted *(wei nan xing)*, 236

Aristolochiae Fangchi, Radix *(fang ji)*, 149, 167, 200, 235

Aristolochiae, Radix *(qing mu xiang)*, 77, 139, 249

Arnebiae seu Lithospermi, Radix *(zi cao)*, 97, 102, 108, 113, 118, 123, 178, 184, 188, 195, 201, 202, 218, 226, 227, 275, 300

Arsenic, calcined *(bai pi shuang)*, 109

Artemisiae Annuae Recens, Herba *(xian qing hao)*, 158

Artemisiae Annuae, Herba *(qing hao)*, 53, 149, 158, 228, 231, 233, 242

Artemisiae Argyi, Folium *(ai ye)*, 59, 144, 224, 268

Artemisiae Yinchenhao, Herba *(yin chen hao)*, 52, 187, 212, 249, 275

Asari, Herba cum Radice *(xi xin)*, 87, 110, 152, 155, 171, 200, 279, 303

Asbestos *(shi hui mu)*, 87

Asparagi Cochinchinensis, Testa *(tian men dong)*, 45, 53, 88, 97, 181, 197, 218, 227

Astragali Membranacei, Radix *(huang qi)*, 45, 52, 53, 55, 62, 69, 70, 97, 152, 166, 181, 182, 192, 197, 207, 211, 222, 232, 233, 240, 242, 267, 271, 277, 299

Astragali Membranacei, Radix, honey-toasted *(zhi huang qi)*, 58, 278

Astragali, Semen *(sha yuan ji li)*, 293
Atractylodis Macrocephalae, Rhizoma *(bai zhu)*, 52, 53, 55, 68, 70, 81, 96, 101, 102, 108, 182, 200, 201, 207, 208, 209, 241, 242, 267, 277, 278, 282, 299
Atractylodis Macrocephalae, Rhizoma, charred *(bai zhu tan)*, 210
Atractylodis Macrocephalae, Rhizoma, dry-fried *(chao bai zhu)*, 82, 209
Atractylodis, Rhizoma *(cang zhu)*, 52, 53, 59, 63, 75, 78, 86, 88, 89, 101, 110, 112, 128, 142, 163, 169, 187, 200, 201, 208, 210, 220, 224, 232, 241, 242, 282, 291, 292, 301
Aucklandiae Lappae, Radix *(mu xiang)*, 139, 149, 209, 219, 224, 249, 277, 282
Averrhoae Carambolae, Fructus *(yang tao)*, 212-3

B

Bambusae in Taeniis, Caulis *(zhu ru)*, 202
Beans, black, 124
Begoniae Fimbristipulatae, Herba *(zi bei tian kui)*, 58, 149, 163
Belamcandae Chinensis, Rhizoma *(she gan)*, 119, 249
Benincasae Hispidae, Epicarpium *(dong gua pi)*, 163, 167
Bidentis Bipinnatae, Herba *(gui zhen cao)*, 149, 309
Biotae Orientalis, Cacumen *(ce bai ye)*, 89, 268
Biotae Orientalis, Semen *(bai zi ren)*, 45, 270
Bletillae Striatae, Rhizoma *(bai ji)*, 130, 131, 184
Bombycis Mori, Excrementum *(can sha)*, 48
Bombyx Batryticatus *(jiang can)*, 57, 74, 128, 182, 201, 241
Borax *(peng sha)*, 120, 203
Borneol *(bing pian)*, 64, 71, 77, 103, 104, 114, 120, 138, 154, 158, 168, 169, 170, 184, 224, 247, 250
Brassicae Rapae, Semen *(wu jing zi)*, 269, 322
Breast milk, 149
Broussonetiae Papyriferae, Folium *(chu ye)*, 149, 307
Brucae Javanicae, Fructus *(ya dan zi)*, 109, 113, 114, 303
Bubali, Cornu *(shui niu jiao)*, 76, 77, 78, 124, 158, 195-196, 203, 218, 242, 276
Buchnerae Cruciatae, Herba *(gui yu jian)*, 201, 219, 222, 240, 308
Bufonis, Secretio *(chan su)*, 150
Bupleuri, Radix *(chai hu)*, 74, 75, 95, 102, 158, 167, 201, 224, 228, 232, 276
Buthus Martensi *(quan xie)*, 47, 87, 129, 240, 292, 294

C

Calcite *(shi hui)*, 249, 318
Calcitum *(han shui shi)*, 77, 168, 169, 218, 232, 250
Calculus Bovis *(niu huang)*, 77
Calomelas *(qing fen)*, 63, 88, 109, 139, 143, 168, 169, 170, 171, 176, 197, 202, 203, 262, 284, 286, 293
Camphora *(zhang nao)*, 129, 143, 154, 155, 170, 258
Campsitis Grandiflora, Flos *(ling xiao hua)*, 228, 242, 256, 313
Cannabis Sativae, Semen *(huo ma ren)*, 45, 181, 219, 220, 228
Carpesii seu Daucusi, Fructus *(he shi)*, 114

Carthami Tinctorii, Flos *(hong hua)*, 45, 108, 114, 123, 153, 155, 163, 181, 218, 219, 228, 232, 235, 236, 242, 243, 256, 268, 276, 291, 292
Caryophylli, Flos *(ding xiang)*, 78, 139, 250
Cassiae, Semen *(jue ming zi)*, 228, 295
Celosiae Argenteae, Semen *(qing xiang zi)*, 97
Celosiae Cristatae, Inflorescentia *(ji guan hua)*, 256, 310
Cercis Chinensis, Cortex, dry-fried *(chao zi jing pi)*, 79, 325
Cervi Degelatinatium, Cornu *(lu jiao shuang)*, 242
Chaenomelis Lagenariae, Fructus *(mu gua)*, 90, 282
Cherry pits, 121
Chili peppers, 64, 154
Chrysanthemi Indici, Flos *(ye ju hua)*, 58, 61, 74, 143, 149, 158, 163, 182, 221, 222, 256, 257
Chrysanthemi Morifolii, Flos *(ju hua)*, 78, 87, 90, 97, 100, 268
Cibotii Barometz, Rhizoma *(gou ji)*, 222, 302
Cicadae, Periostracum *(chan tui)*, 46, 118, 123, 142, 149, 163, 167, 177, 181, 182, 210, 212, 226, 227, 241, 299
Cicadae, Periostracum, dry-fried *(chao chan tui)*, 129
Cilantro, 121
Cimicifugae, Rhizoma *(sheng ma)*, 45, 55, 74, 77, 94, 97, 117, 181, 184, 201, 232
Cinnabaris *(zhu sha)*, 4, 68, 71, 77, 78, 109, 138, 176, 177, 193
Cinnamomi Cassiae, Cortex *(rou gui)*, 6, 55, 90, 101, 138, 152, 155, 200, 236, 240, 267, 271, 278
Cinnamomi Cassiae, Medulla *(gui zhi xin)*, 166
Cinnamomi Cassiae, Ramulus *(gui zhi)*, 47, 89, 152, 153, 200, 206, 210, 217, 242, 243, 279, 299
Cirsii Japonici, Herba seu Radix *(da ji)*, 149
Cistanches Deserticolae, Herba *(rou cong rong)*, 138, 223, 266, 278
Citri Aurantii, Fructus *(zhi ke)*, 62, 106
Citri Aurantii, Fructus, dry-fried *(chao zhi ke)*, 167, 228
Citri Reticulatae Viride, Pericarpium *(qing pi)*, 81, 102, 220, 276
Citri Reticulatae, Pericarpium *(chen pi)*, 59, 62, 67, 74, 82, 101, 110, 166, 201, 202, 208, 209, 219, 250, 267, 282, 302
Citri seu Ponciri Immaturus, Fructus *(zhi shi)*, 67
Citri seu Ponciri Immaturus, Fructus, dry-fried *(chao zhi shi)*, 208
Clematidis, Radix *(wei ling xian)*, 47, 59, 87, 89, 111, 132, 137, 155, 212, 294
Clinopodii, Herba *(jian dao cao)*, 130, 310
Cnidii Monnieri, Fructus *(she chuang zi)*, 90, 110, 114, 129, 143, 183, 293
Coconut, 163, 177
Codonopsitis Pilosulae, Radix *(dang shen)*, 53, 55, 62, 152, 200, 209, 232, 240, 241, 242, 267, 292, 299
Coicis Lachryma-jobi, Semen *(yi yi ren)*, 53, 62, 89, 97, 101, 108, 111, 112, 123, 163, 167, 182, 195, 220, 222, 228, 242, 257, 281
Copper Sulfate, 303
Coptidis, Rhizoma *(huang lian)*, 46, 62, 64, 68, 75, 76, 77, 103, 105, 106, 124, 132, 149, 168, 171, 172, 187, 188, 196, 201, 202, 221, 222, 255, 275

Coptidis, Rhizoma, dry-fried *(chao huang lian)*, 232
Coptidis, Rhizoma, wine-fried *(jiu chao huang lian)*, 74
Cordyceps Sinensis *(dong chong xia cao)*, 269
Coreopsidis Lanceolatae, Folium *(xian ye jin ji ju)*, 146, 322
Coriandrum, Herba *(hu sui)*, 121
Corii Asini, Gelatinum *(e jiao)*, 4
Corni Officinalis, Fructus *(shan zhu yu)*, 96, 138, 167, 222, 231, 241, 265, 283
Cornu Cervi, Gelatinum *(lu jiao jiao)*, 152
Cortex Moutan Radicis, Cortex, dry-fried *(chao mu dan pi)*, 101, 123, 174, 195, 207, 211, 218, 222, 223, 226, 232, 241, 265
Cortex Phellodendri, Cortex, dry-fried *(chao huang bai)*, 139, 166, 169, 223
Corydalis Yanhusuo, Rhizoma *(yan hu suo)*, 102
Crataegi, Fructus *(shan zha)*, 153, 182, 209
Croton Tiglii Praeparata, Semen *(ba dou shuang)*, 139
Croton Tiglii, Semen *(ba dou)*, 79, 130
Cucumber vine, 55
Curculiginis Orchioidis, Rhizoma *(xian mao)*, 211, 223
Curcumae Ezhu, Rhizoma *(e zhu)*, 108, 177, 219, 220
Curcumae Longae, Rhizoma *(jiang huang)*, 62, 103, 152
Curcumae, Tuber *(yu jin)*, 59, 77, 102, 226, 236, 292
Cuscutae Chinensis, Semen *(tu si zi)*, 6, 90, 211, 223, 265, 266, 270
Cyathulae Officinalis, Radix *(chuan niu xi)*, 90, 220
Cynanchi Baiwei, Radix *(bai wei)*, 62, 97
Cyperi Rotundi, Rhizoma *(xiang fu)*, 48, 52, 82, 108, 110, 209, 276, 303

D

Daphnes Genkwa, Flos *(yuan hua)*, 59, 155
Daqingye, Folium *(da qing ye)*, 100, 108, 113, 123, 182, 207, 255, 300
Dendrobii, Herba *(shi hu)*, 87, 197, 227, 270, 300
Dictamni Dasycarpi Radicis, Cortex *(bai xian pi)*, 47, 129, 137, 163, 166, 174, 182, 187, 197, 206, 217, 220, 222, 228, 241, 257, 299, 301
Dioscoreae Bulbiferae, Tuber *(huang yao zi)*, 64
Dioscoreae Hypoglaucae, Rhizoma *(bei xie)*, 67-68, 112, 220, 281
Dioscoreae Oppositae, Radix *(shan yao)*, 53, 58, 82, 96, 97, 166, 175, 195, 197, 240, 241, 283, 299
Dipsaci Asperi, Radix *(xu duan)*, 232, 270
DMSO, 176
Dolichoris Lablab, Semen *(bian dou)*, 119
Draconis, Os *(long gu)*, 108, 175, 211, 286
Draconis, Os, calcined *(duan long gu)*, 168
Draconis, Sanguis *(xue jie)*, 139, 202, 203, 284, 303

E

Ecliptae Prostratae, Herba *(han lian cao)*, 211, 231, 270, 291
Egg, 284, 285

Eggplant vine, Japanese 154
Ephedrae, Herba *(ma huang)*, 4, 47, 87, 96, 117, 119, 184, 206, 217
Ephedrae, Herba, prepared *(zhi ma huang)*, 240
Epimedii, Herba *(yin yang huo)*, 211, 223, 241
Equiseti Hiemalis, Herba *(mu zei)*, 48, 88, 110, 111, 203
Eriobotryae Japonicae, Folium *(pi pa ye)*, 94, 119, 255
Erythrinae, Cortex *(hai tong pi)*, 128
Eucommiae Ulmoidis, Cortex, dry-fried *(chao du zhong)*, 228
Eupatorii Fortunei, Herba *(pei lan)*, 62, 102
Euphoriae Longanae, Arillus *(long yan rou)*, 131, 193, 277
Euphoriae Longanae, Semen *(long yan he)*, 250, 314
Evodiae Rutaecarpae, Fructus *(wu zhu yu)*, 48, 54, 59

F

Fellea Suis, Vesica *(zhu dan)*, 185, 325
Fig, 287
Fig leaf, 295
Forsythiae Suspensae, Fructus *(lian qiao)*, 46, 52, 61, 74, 75, 76, 81, 96, 100, 105, 117, 118, 123, 124, 153, 182, 195, 196, 202, 207, 220, 222, 232, 241, 246, 249, 258
Forsythiae Suspensae, Semen *(lian qiao xin)*, 166
Fritillariae Cirrhosae, Bulbus *(chuan bei mu)*, 193, 221, 249
Fritillariae Thunbergii, Bulbus *(zhe bei mu)*, 58, 62, 67, 81, 119
Fritillariae, Bulbus *(bei mu)*, 82
Fructus Sophorae Japonicae Immaturus, Fructus, dry-fried *(chao huai hua mi)*, 47

G

Gardeniae Jasminoidis, Fructus *(zhi zi)*, 68, 75, 76, 77, 90, 94, 95, 96, 101, 106, 124, 196, 201, 221, 227, 257, 275
Gardeniae Jasminoidis, Fructus, charred *(zhi zi tan)*, 221, 226
Gardeniae Jasminoidis, Fructus, dry-fried *(chao zhi zi)*, 52, 62
Gastrodiae Elatae, Rhizoma *(tian ma)*, 45, 87, 90, 181
Gecko *(ge jie)*, 81
Gentianae Longdancao, Radix, dry-fried *(chao long dan cao)*, 97
Gentianae Qinjiao, Radix *(qin jiao)*, 89, 95, 150, 175, 203, 206, 240
Gigeriae Galli, Endothelium Corneum *(ji nei jin)*, 299
Gingko leaves, 304
Ginseng, Radix *(ren shen)*, 4, 68, 69, 70, 82, 95, 192, 255, 267, 271, 276, 277, 278, 282
Gleditsiae Sinensis, Fructus *(zao jiao)*, 47, 129
Gleditsiae Sinensis, Spina *(zao jiao ci)*, 47, 62, 67, 69, 129
Globefish eye *(he tun mu)*, 303
Glycine Max, Semen *(hei da dou)*, 232, 267, 309
Glycines Germinatum, Semen *(dou juan)*, 257

Glycyrrhizae Uralensis, Radix *(gan cao)*, 3, 45, 46, 59, 62, 63, 67, 69, 74, 75, 76, 79, 82, 87, 88, 94, 95, 96, 97, 101, 102, 106, 117, 118, 119, 120, 123, 124, 137, 142, 149, 155, 158, 167, 177, 181, 182, 187, 195, 196, 201, 202, 206, 207, 208, 209, 210, 211, 217, 221, 222, 226, 240, 241, 242, 246, 256, 258, 275, 276, 282, 286, 291, 299

Glycyrrhizae Uralensis, Radix, honey-toasted *(zhi gan cao)*, 47, 55, 68, 77, 95, 102, 152, 157, 200, 210, 267, 277, 278, 279, 282

Goat's milk, 150

Gold *(huang jin)*, 78

Grapefruit, 213

Guanzhong, Rhizoma *(guan zhong)*, 100

Gummi Olibanum *(ru xiang)*, 67, 109, 153, 303

Gummi Olibanum, dry-fried *(chao ru xiang)*, 55

Gypsum *(shi gao)*, 46, 54, 76, 77, 95, 96, 119, 124, 130, 142, 157, 174, 181, 195, 196, 210, 218, 227, 242, 255, 276

Gypsum, calcined *(duan shi gao)*, 69, 70, 94, 104, 139, 168, 169, 203, 283

H

Haematitum *(dai zhe shi)*, 175, 228, 265

Haliotidis, Concha *(shi jue ming)*, 97, 100

Halloysitum Rubrum *(chi shi zhi)*, 109, 167, 182

Hedyotidis Diffusae, Herba *(bai hua she she cao)*, 114, 115, 231

Hibisci Mutabilis, Folium *(mu fu rong ye)*, 98, 158, 231, 314

Hibisci Syriaci Radicis, Cortex *(jin pi)*, 170, 315

Homalomenae Occultae, Rhizoma *(qian nian jian)*, 90, 222

Honey, 301

Hostae Ventricosae, Folium *(zi yu zan ye)*, 303, 326

Houttuyniae Cordatae, Herba cum Radice *(yu xing cao)*, 55

Hydnocarpi Anthelminticae, Semen *(da feng zi)*, 89, 129, 143, 170, 258

Hydrargyrioxydum rubrum *(hong fen)*, 258, 309

I

Imperatae Cylindricae, Rhizoma *(bai mao gen)*, 97, 275

Indigo Pulverata Levis *(qing dai)*, 54, 120, 124, 130, 171, 188, 197, 203, 275

Isatidis seu Baphicacanthi, Radix *(ban lan gen)*, 74, 97, 108, 111, 115, 124, 192, 202, 207, 221, 227, 275

J

Japanese star fruit, 212

Jixueteng, Radix et Caulis *(ji xue teng)*, 45, 167, 231, 235, 236, 292

Kochiae Scopariae, Fructus *(di fu zi)*, 48, 59, 90, 102, 129, 143, 163, 166, 174, 178, 187, 228, 293, 299

L

Lapis Micae seu Chloriti *(meng shi)* 6, 90

Lard, 301
Lasiosphere seu Calvatiae, Fructificatio *(ma bo)*, 74
Ledebouriellae Divaricatae, Radix *(fang feng)*, 45, 46, 67, 75, 87, 88, 89, 96, 101, 129, 142, 167, 171, 174, 177, 182, 184, 206, 207, 208, 209, 210, 211, 217, 268, 291, 293, 299
Lemnae seu Spirodelae, Herba *(fu ping)*, 48, 128, 206, 212, 291
Lemon, 131
Leonuri Heterophylli, Herba *(yi mu cao)*, 48, 167, 212, 231, 236, 275, 292
Ligustici Chuanxiong, Radix *(chuan xiong)*, 45, 62, 69, 70, 75, 82, 87, 88, 89, 96, 106, 108, 200, 211, 217, 235, 236, 241, 256, 257, 266, 267, 268, 271, 278, 293, 294, 299
Ligustici, Rhizoma et Radix *(gao ben)*, 268
Ligustri Lucidi, Fructus *(nu zhen zi)*, 211, 231, 265, 266, 267, 270, 291, 293
Lilii, Bulbus *(bai he)*, 94
Lime, 53
Linderae Strychnifoliae, Radix *(wu yao)*, 87, 209
Lini Usitatissimi, Semen *(ya ma zi)*, 291, 323
Liquidambaris Taiwanianae, Fructus *(lu lu tong)*, 131, 200, 220, 224, 240, 292
Lithargyrum *(mi tuo seng)*, 250, 262, 293
Lonicerae Japonicae, Flos *(jin yin hua)*, 46, 48, 55, 57, 58, 61, 67, 70, 74, 76, 78, 90, 100, 102, 105, 117, 118, 123, 129, 137, 143, 149, 153, 162, 164, 182, 187, 195, 197, 202, 207, 221, 222, 242, 246, 257
Lonicerae Japonicae, Flos, charred *(jin yin hua tan)*, 195, 218
Lonicerae Japonicae, Ramus *(ren dong teng)*, 220, 246
Lophatheri Gracilis, Herba *(dan zhu ye)*, 62, 69, 76, 95, 117, 123, 170, 196, 246
Luffae, Fasciculus Vascularis *(si gua luo)*, 48, 103, 106, 242
Lumbricus *(di long)*, 87, 207, 231
Lycii Radicis, Cortex *(di gu pi)*, 167, 207, 231, 242
Lycii, Fructus *(gou qi zi)*, 88, 211, 231, 266, 270, 293, 299
Lycopi Lucidi, Herba *(ze lan)*, 220, 236, 276
Lycopodii Clavati, Herba cum Radice *(shen jin cao)*, 222, 235, 318
Lysimachiae Foeni-Graci, Herba cum Radice *(ling ling xiang)*, 249, 312
Lysimachiae, Herba *(jin qian cao)*, 48

M

Mactrae Quadrangularis, Concha Pulvis *(ge li fen)*, 168, 308
Magarita *(zhen zhu)*, 63, 77, 103, 138, 197
Magnetitum *(ci shi)*, 77, 175, 292
Magnoliae Officinalis, Cortex *(hou po)*, 59, 63, 101, 201, 208
Magnoliae, Flos *(xin yi hua)*, 94
Mango skin, 163
Manitis Pentadactylae, Squama *(chuan shan jia)*, 67
Manitis Pentadactylae, Squama, prepared *(chuan shan jia)*, 89
Margaritaferae, Concha *(zhen zhu mu)*, 175, 207

Massa Fermentata *(shen qu)*, 209, 249
Medulla Junci Effusi, Medulla *(deng xin cao)*, 69, 101, 201
Melanteritum, calcined *(duan lu fan)*, 286, 314
Meliae Toosendan, Fructus *(chuan lian zi)*, 102, 237
Melon, bitter, 71
Menispermi Daurici, Rhizoma *(bian fu ge gen)*, 219, 307
Menthae Haplocalycis, Herba *(bo he)*, 74, 96, 117, 120, 182, 203, 212, 249, 268
Menthol, 183
Mercuric Oxide *(sheng yao)*, 139
Mimium *(qian dan)*, 63, 70, 83, 104, 111, 176, 283, 284, 286, 303
Mint, 247
Mirabilitum *(mang xiao)*, 78, 96, 111, 172, 196, 256
Mirabilitum Purum *(xuan ming fen)*, 62
Momordicae Cochinchinensis, Semen *(mu bie zi)*, 87, 143
Mori Albae Radicis, Cortex *(sang bai pi)*, 255
Mori Albae Recens, Folium *(xian sang ye)*, 150
Mori Albae, Ramulus *(sang zhi)*, 235
Mori Albae, Folium *(sang ye)*, 97, 119, 294
Mori Albae, Fructus *(sang shen)*, 265, 266, 270, 291
Morindae Officinalis, Radix *(ba ji tian)*, 138, 152, 223, 241, 266
Moschus, Secretio *(she xiang)*, 77, 102, 203, 249, 268
Moutan Radicis, Cortex *(mu dan pi)*, 74, 76, 96, 100, 112, 124, 149, 163, 182, 196, 201, 227, 231, 255, 257, 281, 283, 300
Moutan Radicis. Cortex, charcoled *(mu dan pi tan)*, 81
Mulberry sap, 131
Mung beans, 247
Mutong, Caulis *(mu tong)*, 95, 101, 142, 166, 201, 249, 258, 279
Mylabris *(ban mao)*, 4, 131, 176, 271
Myrrha *(mo yao)*, 67, 109, 153, 164, 284, 303
Myrrha, dry-fried *(chao mo yao)*, 55

N

Nardostachydis, Rhizoma et Radix *(gan song)*, 269, 307
Nelumbinis Nuciferae, Semen *(lian zi)*, 193
Niter *(xiao shi)*, 78
Nonglutinous rice *(geng mi)*, 95, 157
Notoginseng, Radix *(san qi)*, 192
Notopterygii, Radix et Rhizoma *(qiang huo)*, 46, 57, 58, 167, 182, 184, 200, 217, 232, 266, 286, 293

O

Ophiopogonis Japonici. Tuber *(mai men dong)*, 45, 52, 53, 69, 76, 94, 97, 119, 181, 197, 218, 222, 227, 242, 270, 278, 295, 300
Ostreae, Concha *(mu li)*, 108, 175, 182, 207, 211, 232

P

Paeoniae Lactiflorae, Radix *(bai shao)*, 47, 53, 69, 70, 82, 102, 108, 175, 178, 206, 211, 219, 231, 242, 256, 266, 267, 277, 293

Paeoniae Lactiflorae, Radix, dry-fried *(chao bai shao)*, 81, 96, 97, 102, 152, 167, 175, 210, 219, 227, 267, 292

Paeoniae Rubrae, Radix *(chi shao)*, 53, 57, 67, 74, 75, 76, 79, 87, 100, 101, 102, 106, 108, 124, 153, 195, 196, 200, 201, 202, 217, 218, 219, 220, 221, 222, 226, 231, 232, 235, 236, 241, 246, 255, 265, 266, 268, 275, 276, 282, 293

Paeoniae Rubrae, Radix, dry-fried *(chao chi shao)*, 236

Paeoniae, Radix *(shao yao)*, 279

Panacis Quinquefolii, Radix *(xi yang shen)*, 97

Papaya, unripe 55, 131, 164

Paris Polyphyllae, Rhizoma *(zao xiu)*, 58, 64, 178, 324

Pepper, ground 153

Perillae Frutescentis, Caulis *(zi su geng)*, 242, 326

Perillae Frutescentis, Folium *(zi su ye)*, 149, 282

Perillae Frutescentis, Fructus *(su zi)*, 120

Persicae, Semen *(tao ren)*, 45, 108, 153, 178, 181, 219, 236, 242, 256, 258, 268, 271, 276

Peucedani, Radix *(qian hu)*, 119

Phaseoli Calcarati, Semen *(chi xiao dou)*, 58, 101, 167, 195, 197, 219

Phaseoli Radiati, Semen *(lu dou)*, 232, 247

Phaseoli Radiati, Testa *(lu dou yi)*, 97, 101, 123, 149, 195, 197, 222

Phellodendri, Cortex *(huang bai)*, 47, 54, 59, 62, 63, 75, 78, 90, 96, 103, 105, 112, 120, 124, 130, 143, 149, 163, 168, 169, 171, 172, 187, 203, 220, 221, 223, 232, 241, 255, 281, 282

Phragmitis Communis Recens, Rhizoma *(xian lu gen)*, 117

Phytolaccae, Radix *(shang lu)*, 295

Picrorhizae, Rhizoma *(hu huang lian)*, 170

Pine seeds, 156

Pinelliae Ternatae, Rhizoma *(ban xia)*, 69, 95, 202, 268, 278

Pinelliae Ternatae, Rhizoma, ginger-prepared *(jiang ban xia)*, 209

Pinelliae Ternatae, Rhizoma, untreated *(sheng ban xia)*, 109

Pini, Folium *(song zhen)*, 89, 318

Pini, Gummi *(song xiang)*, 286

Pini, Resina *(song xiang)*, 63, 319

Piperis Nigri, Fructus *(hu jiao)*, 150, 250

Plantaginis, Herba *(che qian cao)*, 97, 102

Plantaginis, Semen *(che qian zi)*, 62, 68, 95, 102, 166, 246

Platycodi Grandiflori, Radix *(jie geng)*, 69, 74, 76, 82, 96, 117, 118, 119, 123, 196, 197, 221, 228, 232, 257

Plum, sour 163

Plumula Nelumbinis Nuciferae, Plumula *(lian xin)*, 166, 231

Polygalae Tenuifoliae, Radix *(yuan zhi)*, 158, 267

Polygalae Tenuifoliae, Radix, prepared *(zhi yuan zhi)*, 277

Polygonati Odorati, Rhizoma *(yu zhu)*, 119, 197
Polygonati, Rhizoma *(huang jing)*, 231
Polygoni Bistortae, Radix *(quan shen)*, 291, 317
Polygoni Cuspidati, Radix et Rhizoma *(hu zhang)*, 231, 295
Polygoni Multiflori, Caulis *(ye jiao teng)*, 178, 270, 292
Polygoni Multiflori, Radix *(he shou wu)*, 45, 87, 88, 90, 108, 167, 175, 211, 218, 223, 227, 231, 241, 266, 267, 270, 292, 293, 299
Polypori Umbellati, Sclerotium *(zhu ling)*, 101, 166, 220
Pomegranate skin, fresh, 55
Poriae Cocos Pararadicis, Sclerotium *(fu shen)*, 265
Poriae Cocos Rubrae, Sclerotium *(chi fu ling)*, 57, 62, 101, 166, 208, 281
Poriae Cocos, Cortex *(fu ling pi)*, 53, 101, 163, 166, 174, 195
Poriae Cocos, Sclerotium *(fu ling)*, 52, 68, 70, 82, 96, 102, 123, 166, 182, 209, 210, 222, 223, 231, 240, 266, 267, 277, 278, 282, 283, 292
Portulacae Oleraceae, Herba *(ma chi xian)*, 97, 101, 102, 108, 110, 113, 114, 158, 295
Prunellae Vulgaris, Spica *(xia ku cao)*, 81, 108
Pruni Armeniacae, Semen *(xing ren)*, 47, 119, 170, 217, 232, 258, 301
Pruni Mume, Fructus *(wu mei)*, 114, 209, 210, 304
Pruni Pseudocerasi, Fructus *(ying tao)*, 153, 323
Pruni, Semen *(yu li ren)*, 45, 181
Pseudolaricis Kaempferi Radicis, Cortex *(tu jing pi)*, 129, 130, 131, 183, 321
Psoraleae Corylifoliae, Fructus *(bu gu zhi)*, 114, 266, 270, 271
Puerariae, Radix *(ge gen)*, 118, 187, 236
Punicae Granati, Pericarpium *(shi liu pi)*, 54, 55 131, 132
Pyritum Rotundum *(she han shi)*, 109, 317
Quisqualis Indicae, Fructus *(shi jun zi)*, 132

R

Rana Limnocharis *(xia ma)*, 89, 322
Raspberries, 164
Realgar *(xiong huang)*, 63, 64, 68, 77, 83, 87, 149, 150, 170, 171, 284, 293, 294
Realgar, calcined *(duan xiong huang)*, 109
Rehmanniae Glutinosae Conquitae, Radix *(shu di huang)*, 45, 53, 69, 82, 89, 96, 108, 138, 167, 175, 181, 211, 218, 222, 227, 231, 236, 240, 241, 242, 256, 266, 267, 278, 283, 299
Rehmanniae Glutinosae, Radix *(sheng di huang)*, 45, 46, 52, 53, 69, 75, 76, 81, 89, 95, 97, 100, 102, 103, 105, 123, 124, 142, 149, 163, 166, 174, 175, 178, 181, 182, 195, 196, 197, 201, 202, 207, 210, 211, 218, 219, 220, 221, 222, 226, 227, 231, 241, 255, 265, 270, 275, 276, 292, 293, 299, 300
Rehmanniae Glutinosae, Radix, charred *(di huang tan)*, 195
Rhei Praeparata, Radix et Rhizoma *(zhi da huang)*, 275
Rhei, Radix et Rhizoma *(da huang)*, 54, 59, 62, 63, 67, 78, 96, 100, 105, 133, 163, 170, 182, 184, 185, 197, 256, 258
Rhei, Radix et Rhizoma, wine-fried *(jiu chao da huang)*, 62, 228
Rhinoceri, Cornu *(xi jiao)*, 76, 77, 78, 195, 203, 218, 276

Rhododendri Mollis, Inflorescentia *(nao yang hua)*, 295, 315
Rhois Chinensis, Fermentatio Galla *(bai yao jian)*, 120, 306
Rhois Chinensis, Galla *(wu bei zi)*, 54, 114, 168, 169, 284, 294, 303
Rhois Chinensis, Galla, dry-fried *(chao wu bei zi)*, 109
Ricini Communis, Semen *(bi ma zi)*, 79, 82, 306
Robigo Aeris *(tong lü)*, 120, 319
Rohdeae Japonicae, Folium *(wan nian qing ye)*, 149, 321
Rosae Multiflorae, Flos *(qiang wei hua)*, 231, 316
Rosae Rugosae, Flos *(mei gui hua)*, 256
Rubi Chingii, Fructus *(fu pen zi)*, 270, 293
Rubiae Cordifoliae, Radix *(qian cao)*, 149, 275, 276, 295, 300
Rumicis Madaio, Radix *(tu da huang)*, 132, 320

S

Salviae Miltiorrhizae, Radix *(dan shen)*, 76, 87, 114, 167, 192, 195, 201, 210, 220, 223, 231, 235, 236, 240, 242, 266, 271, 291, 292, 299
Sambuci Williamsii, Ramulus *(jie gu mu)*, 275, 311
Sangjisheng, Ramulus *(sang ji sheng)*, 228, 235, 242
Sanguisorbae Officinalis, Radix *(di yu)*, 170, 218
Santali Albi, Lignum *(tan xiang)*, 184, 249
Sappan, Lignum *(su mu)*, 212, 219, 236, 242
Schisandrae Chinensis, Fructus *(wu wei zi)*, 45, 82, 167, 178, 192, 222, 231, 242, 267, 270
Schizonepetae Tenuifoliae, Herba seu Flos *(jing jie)*, 45, 46, 67, 87, 89, 96, 117, 120, 123, 129, 142, 171, 174, 177, 181, 182, 206, 207, 209, 211, 226, 266, 269, 293
Scolopendra Subspinipes *(wu gong)*, 82, 240, 286
Scrophulariae Ningpoensis, Radix *(xuan shen)*, 58, 61, 74, 76, 77, 100, 123, 124, 153, 166, 196, 197, 218, 219, 220, 221, 227, 231, 232, 262, 265, 275, 300
Scutellariae Baicalensis, Radix *(huang qin)*, 45, 46, 62, 63, 68, 69, 74, 75, 76, 77, 94, 95, 96, 100, 106, 124, 128, 153, 163, 167, 168, 181, 182, 187, 195, 196, 202, 221, 222, 223, 226, 227, 249, 255, 257, 295, 300
Scutellariae Baicalensis, Radix, dry-fried *(chao huang qin)*, 232
Scutellariae Baicalensis, Radix, wine-fried *(jiu chao huang qin)*, 74
Sentaniae Italicae, Semen *(qing liang mi)*, 187, 316
Serpentis, Exuviae *(she tui)*, 82
Serpentis, Periostracum *(she yi)*, 291
Sesami Indici, Semen *(hei zhi ma)*, 88, 89, 142, 175, 210, 265, 291, 293, 299
Siegesbeckiae, Herba, wine-steamed *(jiu zhi xi xian cao)*, 128
Sinapis Albae, Semen *(bai jie zi)*, 271, 294
Smilacis Glabrae, Rhizoma *(tu fu ling)*, 105, 106, 112, 137, 138, 187, 202, 220, 221, 257
Smithsonitum *(lu gan shi)*, 71
Snail, 150

Sojae Praeparatum, Semen *(dan dou chi)*, 117
Solani Melongenae cum Radicis, Caulis *(qie zi jie)*, 154, 316
Solani Nigri, Herba *(long kui)*, 54, 158, 313
Sophorae Flavescentis, Radix *(ku shen)*, 46, 47, 54, 63, 88, 90, 106, 110, 114, 128, 129, 132, 142, 143, 144, 149, 166, 174, 178, 181, 182, 183, 187, 197, 208, 210, 212, 219, 228, 291, 299
Sophorae Japonicae Immaturus, Fructus *(huai hua mi)*, 182
Sophorae Tonkinensis, Radix *(shan dou gen)*, 82, 202, 207
Soy bean residue, 287
Sparganii Stoloniferi, Rhizoma *(san leng)*, 177, 219
Speranskiae, Herba seu Impatientis *(tou gu cao)*, 243, 294, 320
Spider web, 304
Stalactitum *(e guan shi)*, 71, 138
Stellerae seu Euphorbiae, Radix *(lang du)*, 90, 114, 312
Stemonae, Radix *(bai bu)*, 55, 114, 131, 147, 224
Strychni, Semen, dry-fried *(chao ma qian zi)*, 79
Succinum *(hu po)*, 68, 71, 138, 158, 169
Sugar, powdered white, 287
Sulphur *(liu huang)*, 129, 143, 171, 224, 258, 262, 293
Sunflower seeds, raw, 121

T

Talcum *(hua shi)*, 54, 62, 71, 77, 96, 101, 130, 158, 182, 188, 246, 247, 249, 258, 281
Taraxaci Mongolici, Herba cum Radice *(pu gong ying)*, 55, 57, 58, 61, 74, 149, 162, 195, 220, 221, 222, 246
Taraxaci Mongolici, Herba cum Radice Recens *(xian pu gong ying)*, 149
Tea, green 120
Terminaliae Chebulae Immaturus, Fructus *(zang qing guo)*, 203, 324
Tetrapanacis Papyriferi, Medulla *(tong cao)*, 112, 281
Tribuli Terrestris, Fructus *(bai ji li)*, 46, 88, 89, 181, 193, 211, 241, 291, 293, 300
Tribuli Terrestris, Fructus, dry-fried *(chao bai ji li)*, 128
Trichosanthis Kirilowii, Radix *(tian hua fen)*, 45, 59, 63, 67, 75, 88, 119, 181, 192, 219, 221, 246, 275, 300
Trigonellae Foeni-graeci, Semen *(hu lu ba)*, 242
Trogopterori seu Pteromi, Excrementum *(wu ling zhi)*, 149
Trollii, Flos *(jin lian hua)*, 203, 311
Tung Oil, 286
Tussilagi Farfarae, Flos *(kuan dong hua)*, 167
Typhonii Gigantei, Rhizoma *(bai fu zi)*, 89, 267, 291

U

Uncariae, Ramulus cum Uncis *(gou teng)*, 89, 97, 128, 175, 197, 218, 223, 228

V

Vaccariae Segetalis, Semen *(wang bu liu xing)*, 178, 183, 276
Veratri, Rhizoma et Radix *(li lu)*, 146
Vermilion *(yin zhu)*, 284, 324
Vespae, Nidus *(lu feng fang)*, 57, 82, 110, 111, 149, 178
Vinegar, rice, 55, 79, 131, 133, 164, 171, 177, 178
Violae Yedoensitis, Herba cum Radice *(zi hua di ding)*, 57, 58, 61, 149, 162, 220, 221, 246, 258
Viticis, Fructus *(man jing zi)*, 88, 182, 269

W

Walnut, green outer hull of unripe, 177
Wine, rice 146
Wintermelon skin, 212
Xanthii Sibirici, Fructus *(cang er zi)*, 48, 59, 89, 128, 155, 167, 169, 183, 208, 212, 292
Xanthii Sibirici, Herba *(cang er zi)*, 138, 150

Z

Zanthoxyli Bungeani, Fructus *(chuan jiao)*, 59, 114, 115, 131, 132, 143, 144, 155, 170, 171, 172, 178, 237, 250, 268
Zaocys Dhumnades *(wu shao she)*, 46, 87, 167, 178
Zibei, Concha *(zi bei)*, 175, 325
Zingiberis Officinalis Recens, Rhizoma *(sheng jiang)*, 47, 64, 69, 152, 206, 267, 268, 270, 276
Zingiberis Officinalis, Rhizoma *(gan jiang)*, 69, 82, 150, 153, 155, 200, 209, 278, 295
Zingiberis Officinalis, Rhizoma, roasted *(wei gan jiang)*, 236
Zizyphi Jujubae, Fructus *(da zao)*, 47, 69, 82, 152, 175, 200, 267, 268, 276, 278, 279
Zizyphi Spinosae, Semen *(suan zao ren)*, 45, 277
Zizyphi Spinosae, Semen, dry-fried *(chao suan zao ren)*, 299

General Index

A

A Hundred Questions About Infants and Children, 121
Abscesses, definition of, 65
Acne rosacea, 11, 21
Acne, 8, 21, 253-9
Acupuncture, general treatments for skin disorders, 39-41
Acyclovir, 98
Alcohol, problems with, 49
Alopecia, 231, 263-71
Anger, 8, 178
Antibiotics, 192
Anticoagulants, 193
Atrophy disorder, 238

B

Barbiturates, 192
Basic Questions, 7, 8, 9, 31, 72, 84, 204, 234, 245, 259
Bayberry flower sores, 135
Benzodiazepines, 193
Blood deficiency, 44, 205, 210, 298
   and wind-dryness, 174, 176
   and yin deficiency, 265, 268
   and qi deficiency with toxin, 69
Blood dryness, 167, 180, 195
Blood heat, 44, 205, 210, 217, 256, 261, 299
   giving rise to wind, 265
Blood invigorating, 32

Blood nourishing, 31
Blood stasis, 205, 219, 230, 267, 271, 282
　　and damp toxin, 257
Blood cooling, 31
Blood, reckless movement of, 274
Bloodletting, 4, 98, 156, 212
Boiling rash, 245
Boils, 20
Bromhidrosis, 248-52

C

Cancer, 43
Carbuncles, 20, 57, 61, 65-72
Chao Yuan-Fang, 3, 72, 141, 245
Chen Shi-Duo, 141, 253
Chen Si-Cheng, 5
Chickenpox, 51, 121-5
Chilblain, 151-6
Chlorothiazide, 193
Cold congealing, 278, 291
Cold-dampness, 235, 239, 240
Collagen-vascular diseases, 229
Collection of Records on Redressing Wrongs, 191
Collection of Treatments for Sores, 145
Compendium of External Medicine, 43, 259
Complete Book of External Medicine, 80
Complete Book of Ulcer Experience, 4, 51, 279
Conception and penetrating vessels, disharmony between, 206, 211, 223
Concise Prescriptions from the Golden Casket, 2, 3
Connective tissue diseases, 229
Consciousness, impaired, 77
Constipation, 62, 67
Constitutional insufficiency, 199
Corns, 302-4
Crack, 26
Cradle cap, 180
Crust scab, 26
Cupping, 42, 105, 212, 224
　　blood letting and, 79-80
Cutaneous needling., 270, 294

D

Damp toxin, 94, 257, 258
Damp-heat, 52, 128, 220, 291, 300
　　accumulation of, 57, 122
　　in the Intestines and Stomach, 180

in the lower burner, 95, 281
in the skin of the perineum, 112
in the Spleen channel, 99, 101
sinking, 276
toxin, 52, 61, 67
transforming into fire, 73
wind and, 128
with phlegm, 8
Damp-summerheat, 61
Damp-toxin sores, 161
Dampness dispelling, 31
Decoctions, 33-4
Delirium, 77
Dermatitis, 21, 43, 52, 81, 161-89
   acute, 22
   atopic 165-72
   contact, 3, 43, 99, 161-4
   diaper, 186-9
   exfoliative, 22
   seborrheic, 179-85
Dermatomyositis, 238-43
Diabetics, 67
Diet, improper, 8
Discussion of Cold-induced Disorders, 2
Discussion of the Origins of Symptoms of Diseases, 3, 7, 23, 72, 99, 107, 127, 141, 145, 245, 248, 263, 289, 297
Divine Pivot, 2, 4, 43, 107
Dou Han-Qing, 4, 80
Drug eruptions, 22, 191-8

E

Eczema, 21
Elephantiasis, 72
Elimination strategy, 29
Emergency Formulas to Keep Up One's Sleeves, 93
Epidermophyton, 127
Erosions, 26, 178, 182
Erysipelas, 11, 72-80
   of the leg, 8
   waist-binding, 99
Erysipeloid, 73
Erythema multiforme, 192, 198-204
Erythroderma, exfoliative, 193
Essence of External Diseases, 4
Essence transformation, 137
Excoriation, 26

Expulsion strategy, 30
External invasion., 290
Eyes, 97, 107

F

Fever,
    and chills, 67
    high, 77, 242
    persistent low, 231, 242
Fire,
    blazing in the Liver channel, 99, 100
    exuberant, 174, 230
Fire toxin, 75, 149, 201, 220. *See also* Heat toxin
    covering the head, 72
    insufficient fluids and, 69
    extreme, 66
Fire-phlegm, 81
Fluid pock, 121
Fluids, dysfunctions of, 69, 300
Folliculitis, 56-60, 61
Foods, spicy, 47
Foot, old festering, 280
Fox Stench, 248
Foxglove, 192
Freeze Sores, 151
Fumigation, 37
Furuncles, 20, 57, 60-5

G

Ghost shaven head, 263
Golden Mirror of the Medical Tradition, 86, 88, 100, 179, 198, 215, 302
Governing vessel, 71
Grand Materia Medica, 131, 135

H

Head lesions, 182
Heat clearing 31
Heat,
    accumulated, 61, 95, 261
    affecting the blood level, 123
    deficiency, 96
    fetal, 166
    furuncles, 61
    in the qi level, 122
    incipient, 117
    pent-up, 120

Heat toxin, 75, 118, 220, 239, 258, 256 261
   accumulation of, 62
Herpes simplex, 93-8
Herpes zoster, 72, 94, 98-106
Hives, 21, 22. *See also* Urticaria
Human papilloma virus, 107, 112

I

Ichthyosis, 297-301
Impetigo, 51-6, 94
Infusions, 37-8
Inner Classic, 2, 65
Insect bites, 43, 147-50
Insect toxin, 142
Intestinal parasites, 209
Intestines and Stomach, damp-heat in, 180
Itching and pain, severe, 97
Itching, overview of differential diagnosis, 22-4. *See also* Pruritis

J

Joint pain, 231

K

Kidney and Liver, yin deficiency of, 222, 282
Kidney and Lung, yin deficiency of, 81
Kidney and Spleen yang, deficiency of, 239, 241, 277
Kidney tonifying, 33
Kidney yin deficiency, 290, 292

L

Lacquer sores, 161
Leprosy, 4, 84-91
Leukemia, 43
Lice, 43, 144-7
   snake, 215
Lichen simplex chronicuS, 43, 173-9
Lingnan Hygiene Formulas, 135
Liu Juan-Zi's Formulas Passed Down From A Spirit, 60, 93
Liver and Gallbladder channels, damp toxin in, 94
Liver and Kidney insufficiency, 222, 282
Liver,
   blood, deficiency, 44
   fire, 99, 100, 174
       qi constraint, 290, 292
Liver/Spleen damp-heat, 73, 74

Lower burner, damp-heat in, 95, 281
Lung and Kidney, yin deficiency of, 81
Lung and Stomach channels, heat in, 94 261
Lung heat, 118, 254
Lupus Erythematosus, Systemic, 21, 22, 229-34
Lupus vulgaris, 80-4
Lymphedema, chronic, 72
Lymphoma, 43

M

Macule, 25
Malevolent disease, 84
Measles, 115-21
Medicinal fumigation, 224
Medicinal spills, 38
Medicinal wines, 35
Melasma, 11, 21
Meprobamate, 193
Microporum, 127
Miliaria, 43, 245-8
Moistening dryness, 32
Moles, 107
Morbilliform eruptions, 192
Moxibustion, 41-2, 111, 150, 212, 294
    indirect, 105, 156, 270, 285
Mycobacterium leprae, 84
Mycobacterium tuberculosis, 80
Mycosis, 81

N

Neurodermatitis, 128. *See also* Lichen simplex chronicus
Nodule, 25
Nonsteroidal anti-inflammatory drugs, 193
Numbness, overview of differential diagnosis, 24

O

Ointments, 36
Omissions from the Grand Materia Medica, 90

P

Pain,
    overview of differential diagnosis, 24
    post-herpetic, 102
    severe with itching, 97

Painful Obstruction,
    muscle, 238
    skin, 234
Palpitations, 242
Papule, 25
Pediculosis, 43, 144-7
Pemphigus, 14, 20, 22
Penetrating and conception vessels, disharmony between, 206, 211, 223
Penicillins, 193
Pensiveness, 8
Perineum, damp-heat lodged in, 112
Petechiae, 11
Phenolphthalein, 193
Photosensitivity, 22
Pigmentation, 26
Pills, 34-35
Pityriasis rosea, 128, 225-8
Plaque, 25
Plasters, 37
Plum blossom needling, 177, 224
Polycythemia, 43
Powders, 34, 36
Profound Insights on External Diseases, 107, 157, 186
Profound Purpose from the Heavenly Abode, 151, 253
Pseudomonas, 56
Psoriasis, 81, 128, 180, 215-25
Purpura, 22, 273-9
Purpuric eruptions, 193
Pustule, 25

Q

Qi and blood,
    deficiency of, 57, 62, 68, 266, 269
    deficiency of and toxin, 66, 69
    stagnation of, 100, 102, 232, 261
Qi deficiency, 230
Qi Kun, 259
Qi transformation, 137

R

Rash, damp 161
Raynaud's syndrome, 14
Red traveling rouge, 72
Restlessness, 207
Ringworm, 85
Rosacea, 259-62

Rubella, 116
Rubeola, see Measles, 115

S

Scabies, 3, 25, 43, 141-4
Scales, 25
Scar, 26
Scleroderma, 14, 234-8
Secret Records on Bayberry Flower Sores, 5, 135
Septicemia, 75
Shellfish, problems with, 49
Shen Dou-Yuan, 107, 157
Shingles, 11 20-1, 22
Shortness of breath, 242
Silver Scale Disease, 215
Softening Masses, 33
Sores, 161
    cat eye, 198
    fire band, 99
    ghost face, 229
    goat's beard, 56
    hairline, 56
    heat, 11, 93
    heavenly blister, 51
    mouth, 11
    nape-collar, 173
    neglected tailbone, 186
    open with pus, 10
    pustular, 51
    shin, 279
    snake burrow, 99
    snake cluster, 99
    spider, 99
    sunshine, 157
    swallow's nest, 56
    sugar, 115
    wheat bran, 115
    white dagger, 215
    yellow fluid, 51
Spleen and Kidney yang, deficiency of, 239, 241, 277
Spleen channel, damp-heat in, 99, 101
Spleen deficiency leading to preponderance of dampness, 282
Spleen not governing blood, 277
Spleen/Stomach dysfunction, 205
Spleen/Stomach, accumulated heat in, 95

Spots,
   red, 8
   purple, 273
Staphylococcus aureus, 51, 56, 61, 65
Stomach and Lung channel problems, 94, 261
Stomach heat, 255
Stone Chamber Secret Records, 141
Streptococci, ß-hemolytic, 51, 72
Sulfonamides, 192
Summerheat, 62
Sun Si-Miao, 4, 72
Sunburn, 157-9
Supplement to Thousand Ducat Formulas, 3
Suppuration, slow, 62
Sweat glands, inflammation of, 10
Sweats, night, 231
Swellings, 8
Syphilis, 5, 135-40
   secondary, 112
   tertiary, 81

T

Tetracyclines, 193
Thorns, white, 253
Thousand day sores, 107
Thousand Ducat Formulas, 3, 72
Tinctures, 38
Tinea, 161
   commode, 161
   corporis, 12, 127-33
   cow skin, 173
   cruris, 21
   pine skin, 215
   round, 127
   snake skin, 297
   versicolor, 85
Tonification strategy, 30
Toxic epidermal necrolysis, 193
Toxic heat combined with wind, 194
Toxin arising from the interior, 72
Toxin, qi and blood deficiency with, 69
Toxin, sinking of, 119
Toxin, spotted, 273
Treponema pallidum, 135
Trichophyton, 127
True Lineage of External Medicine, 148, 173
True Lineage of External Medicine, 191

U

Ulcers, 7, 26 152
   leg, 279-87
Urticaria, 9, 43, 199, 204-13

V

Varicella-zoster virus, 99, 122
Vesicle, 25
Vulvitis, 21

W

Wang Bing, 20
Wang Qing-Ren, 271
Warming and clearing, 32
Warts,
   common, 106-11
   venereal, 112-5
Washes, 36
Wheal, 25
Wind, 44
  big, 84
  damp-heat and, 128
  dispelling, 30
  extinguishing, 31
  face traveling, 179
  fish scale, 297
  four bends, 165
  glossy, 263
  malevolent, 84
  numb, 84
  pestilence, 84
  rash, 204
  tinea, 225
  white blotch, 289
  white variegated, 289
Wind-cold, 44, 205, 206, 217
Wind-dampness, 44, 85, 205, 208
Wind-dryness, 174, 290, 298, 299
Wind-heat, 73, 205, 207
  blood dryness and, 180
  dampness and, 174, 176
  seasonal, 116, 122
  toxin from, 67, 94
  upper burner affected by, 94, 117
Wind-toxin, 149
Wine dregs nose, 259

Y

Yang deficiency, 239, 241, 27
Yin and blood, deficiency of, 265, 268
Yin deficiency, 62, 81, 230, 231, 282, 290, 292
    exuberant fire and, 231

Z

Zhao Xue-Min, 90
Zhou Annals, 1, 2